Exercises in Radiological Diagnosis

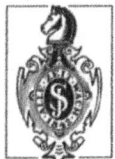

Catherine Roy

Ultrasound
of the Abdomen

114 Radiological Exercises for Students and
Practitioners

With 228 Illustrations

Springer-Verlag
Berlin Heidelberg New York
London Paris Tokyo

Dr. CATHERINE ROY

Hospices Civils de Strasbourg
Centre Hospitalier Régional
Service de Radiologie 1
1, Place de l'Hôpital
F-67091 Strasbourg Cedex

Translated from the French by

MARIE-THÉRÈSE WACKENHEIM

Library of Congress Cataloging-in-Publication Data. Roy, Catherine, 1955- [Echographie abdominale. English] Ultrasound of the abdomen : 114 radiological exercises for students and practitioners / Catherine Roy ; [translated from the French by Marie-Thérèse Wackenheim]. p. cm.–(Exercises in radiological diagnosis) Translation of: Echographie abdominale. Includes index.

ISBN-13: 978-3-540-16546-0   e-ISBN-13: 978-3-642-71199-2
DOI: 10.1007/978-3-642-71199-2

1. Abdomen–Diseases–Diagnosis–Problems, exercises, etc. 2. Abdomen–Imaging–Problems, exercises, etc. 3. Diagnosis, Ultrasonic–Problems, exercises, etc. I. Title. II. Series. [DNLM: 1. Abdomen–pathology–examination questions. 2. Ultrasonic Diagnosis–examination questions. WI 18 R888e] RC944.R6913 1988 617'.5507543–dc19
87-37654

© Springer-Verlag Berlin Heidelberg 1988

The use of registered names, trademarks, etc. in this publication does not imply, even in the absence of a specific statement, that such names are exempt from the relevant protective laws and regulations and therefore free for general use.

Product Liability: The publisher can give no guarantee for information about drug dosage and application thereof contained in this book. In every individual case the respective user must check its accuracy by consulting other pharmaceutical literature.

2127/3130-543210

Foreword

This book, the seventh in the series Exercises in Radiological Diagnosis, deals with sonography, an imaging procedure in which the ability of the radiologist plays an exceptionally important role. The author, Catherine Roy, has very extensive experience in the clinical use of sonography. She has selected the images, which are of excellent quality, with great care to illustrate a wide range of conditions and has supplemented them by commentaries and discussions which are easy to comprehend.

The systematic use of schematic drawings to interpret the images makes it possible for the reader to follow the author's approach without any difficulty. Schematic drawings are particularly important in sonography because the relationship between the details in the images and the anatomy may be very weak.

Images, schematic drawings, and text (both commentaries and interpretations) are three didactic elements which Catherine Roy has skill-fully combined in these exercises into an excellent whole.

A. WACKENHEIM

Contents

Introduction

Ultrasound imaging of the abdomen has now become a routine investigation. It has brought about changes in the procedure of additional investigations and even rendered part of conventional radiology redundant, particularly that concerning the bile ducts.

These exercises are meant for students or physicians who already have basic knowledge of ultrasound diagnosis.

It has not been possible to cover the entire spectrum of abdominal pathology, especially trauma, with 114 cases.

Each of the five chapters relates to an abdominal organ. The book has been organized as follows:

Cases   1– 32: gallbladder and bile ducts
Cases   33– 70: liver
Cases   71– 79: pancreas
Cases   80– 87: suprarenal glands
Cases   88–103: kidneys
Cases 104–114: spleen and miscellaneous structures.

Each exercise comprises one to four sonograms and subsequent comparison with corresponding computed tomography. Besides the annotated description of the scans and of the diagnosis, there is sonological and/or clinical comment. Within each chapter the diagnostic difficulty is progressive. Cases 1, 2, 3, 4, 22, 23, 24, 25, 33, 34 and 71 present normal findings.

I wish to acknowledge and thank Dr. Morel for his participation.

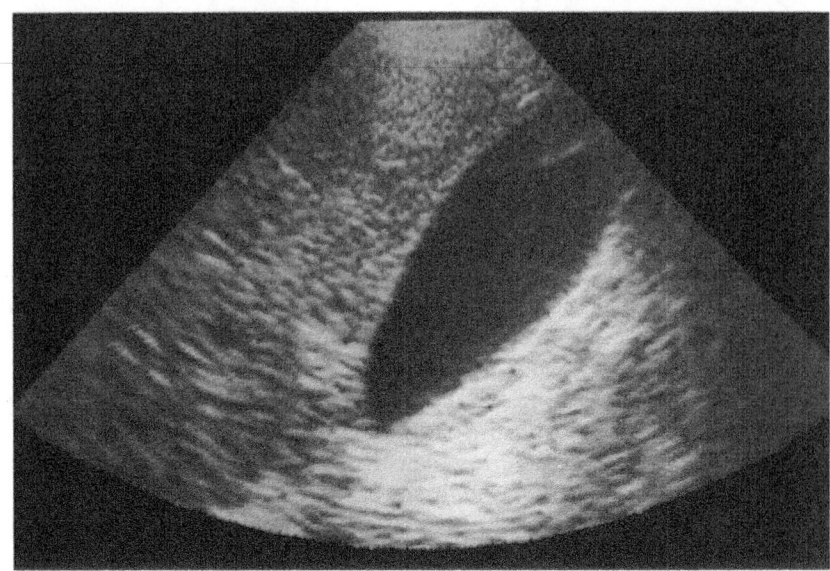

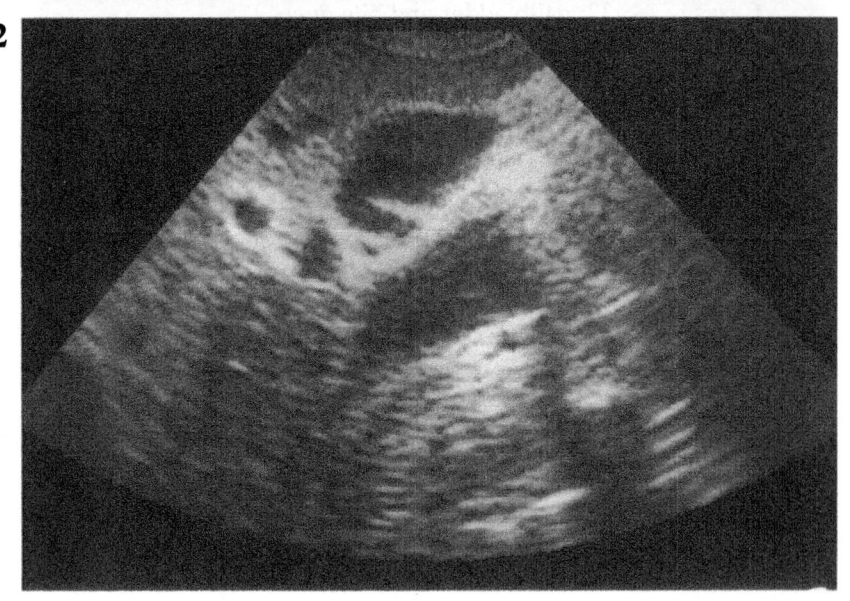

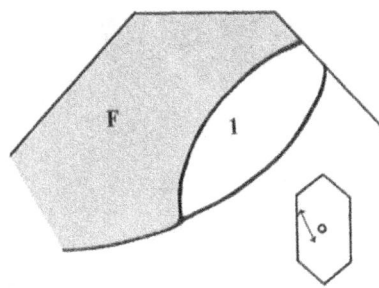

F liver
1 gallbladder
2 inferior vena cava
3 portal vein
4 duodenal gas
5 right renal artery

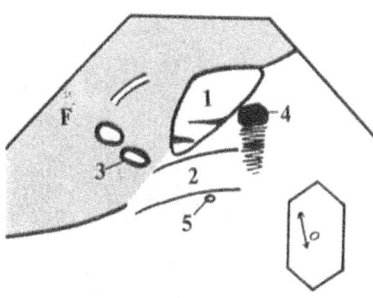

Cases 1 and 2

In analysis of the gallbladder, sonography has triumphed, since it has supplanted and even eliminated oral cholecystography. In adults, abdominal ultrasound imaging is carried out with a 3 or 3.5 MHz transducer. It is a rapid, conclusive and reproducible investigation which does not depend upon hepatic function or require the use of ionizing radiation. The only constraint is that it must be performed in a patient who has been fasting for at least 12 h.

Whatever the patient's symptoms, abdominal ultrasonography should visualize the gallbladder. With real-time instrumentation the gallbladder is visualized in the first seconds of the examination. The orientation of the transducer must be modified so as to obtain the image of the organ's long axis. It should then be rotated perpendicular to that axis to obtain the transverse axis. The entire region must then be scanned with regard to these two axes.

In some cases several expedients may be necessary:
– Breath-holding in deep inspiration lowers the liver.
– The left lateral decubitus position lowers the gallbladder below the costal margin.
– In slender patients the gallbladder is often low, superficial and subcutaneous. Its study requires the interposition of a waterbag between the transducer and the skin, or the utilization of a higher frequency transducer (5 MHz).
– Intercostal scans are indispensable when the gallbladder remains hidden in the subcostal position.

When these manocuvres have failed to visualize the gallbladder, it should be kept in mind that there is considerable variation in the position of this organ, which may be found in the right iliac fossa, the epigastrium or even the left hypochondrium. However, the location of the gallbladder neck is constant. The gallbladder bed (cystic fossa) of the liver is situated in the right anteroposterior groove between the quadrate lobe (segment IV) and segment V. These landmarks are of importance when one searches for a contracted gallbladder.

3

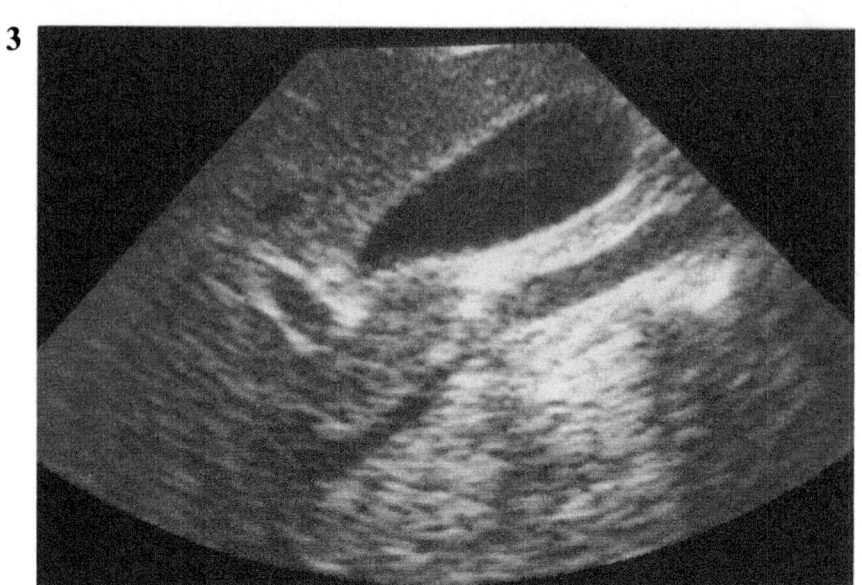

4

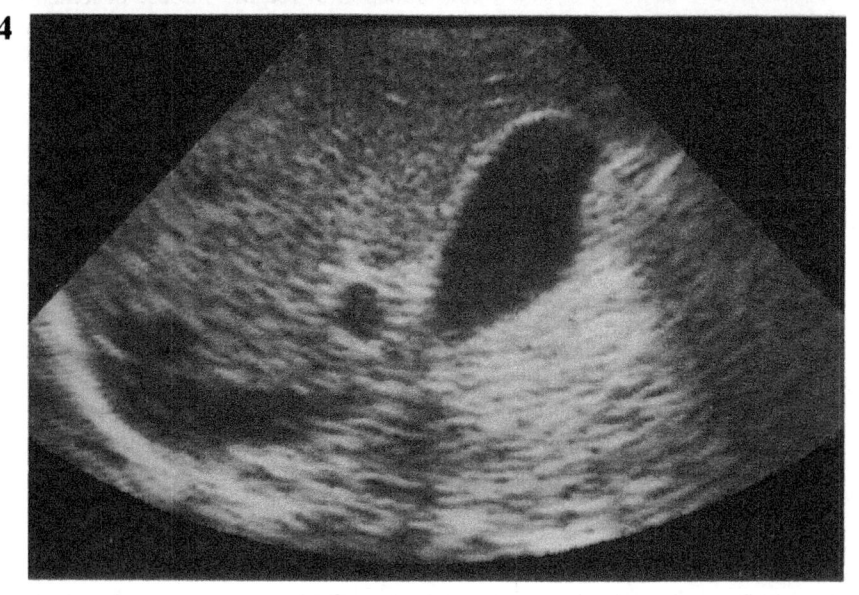

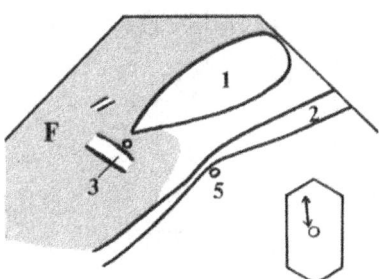

F liver   **3**
1 gallbladder   **4**
2 inferior vena cava
3 portal vein
4 duodenal gas
5 right renal artery
6 middle suprahepatic vein
7 acoustic shadowing of the gallbladder
    wall

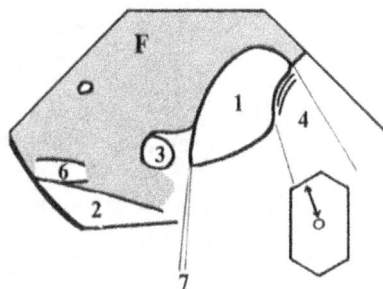

Cases 3 and 4

There is considerable variation in the gallbladder's configuration. Depending on the orientation of the ultrasound beam, the organ appears oval on longitudinal scans and rounded on transverse scans. There are, moreover, multiple morphological variations: bilobate (Case 2), trilobate, or merely bent with visualization of the infundibulum (Case 19). The latter configuration should not be confused with a polypoid formation or with lithiasis.

The gallbladder's size is also variable. A maximal length of 10 cm with a maximal transverse diameter of 4 cm is usually considered normal. Size is, however, closely related to shape. Some gallbladders are elongated (longer than 10 cm) but have a smaller transverse diameter, whereas others are more rounded with a transverse diameter of about 4 cm.

The thickness of the gallbladder wall ranges from 1 to 2 mm. The anterior wall is always well visualized, whereas the posterior wall, in contact with gastrointestinal structures, is less easily displayed (Case 1).

In Case 3, note the relationship of the gallbladder to the inferior vena cava and the right renal artery.

Note also the position of the duodenal gas which makes an imprint on the fundus of the gallbladder in Case 4; this is not present in Case 2.

5

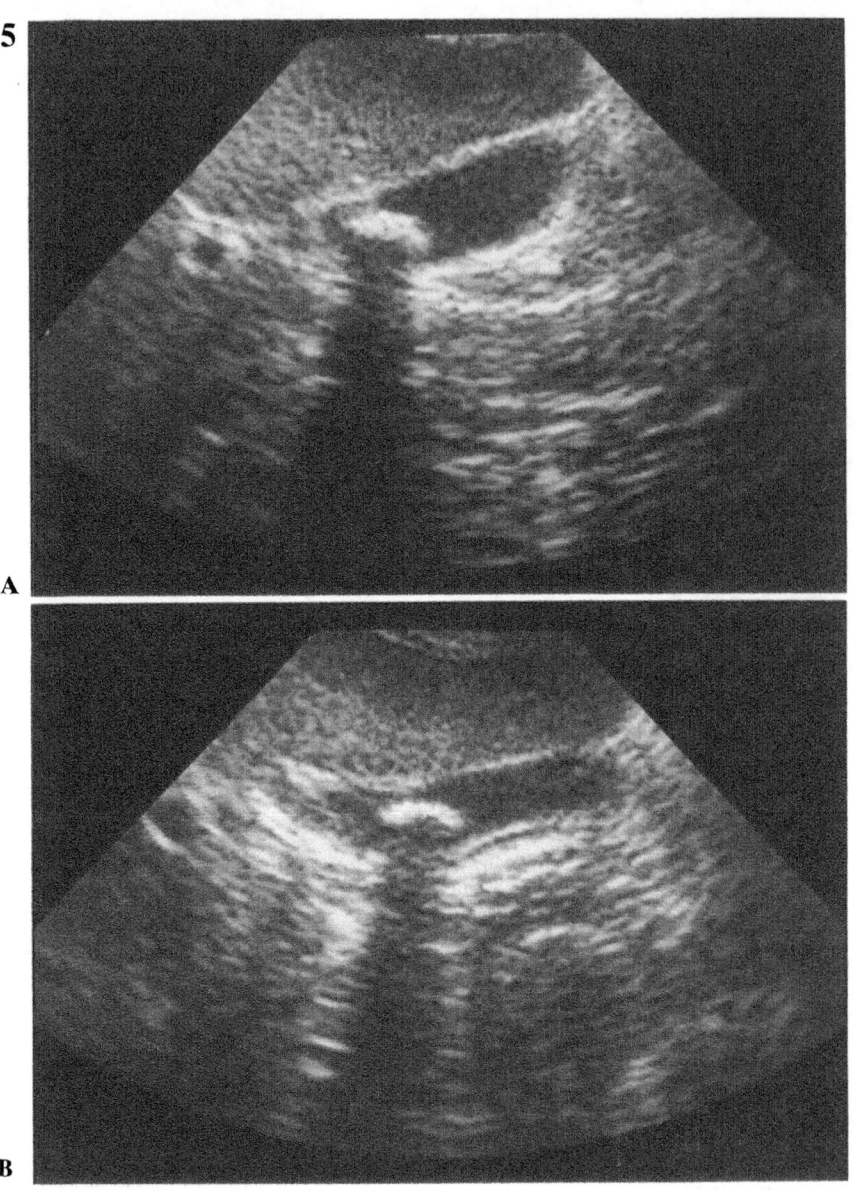

A

B

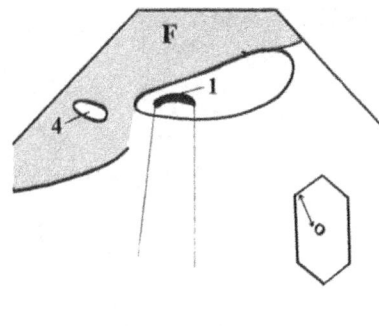

F liver   **5**
1 cholelithiasis, direct sign
2 acoustic shadowing, indirect sign
3 duodenal gas
4 portal vein

Case 5

Clinical data: A 40-year-old woman was referred for poorly defined abdominal pain.

Description: There is an arciform echogenic structure within the gallbladder, with an acoustic shadow. The gallbladder wall has a normal thickness. Endoscopic sonography demonstrates an absence of pain on passage of the transducer, and mobilization of the stone when the patient lies in the left lateral decubitus position (Scan B). Also note the superior displacement of the gallbladder body by duodenal gas.

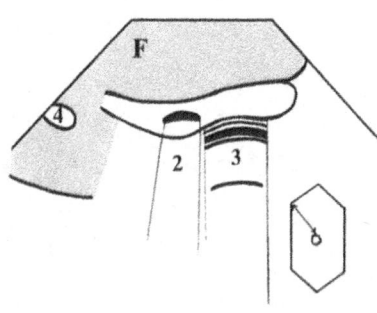

Diagnosis: The patient has gallstones.

Comment: The diagnosis of gallstones is based upon two sonographic elements:
- The *direct sign* is a regular arciform echo-producing structure. This will always be visible when the stone measures more than 5 mm. The limit of visualization is 2 mm.
- The *indirect sign* is the acoustic shadow caused by total reflection of the ultrasound beam. The acoustic shadow opposite the gallbladder neck (Case 4) is due to a refraction artefact of the beam, which is tangential to the gallbladder wall. It must never be confused with acoustic shadowing cast by stones (Case 15B).

The acoustic shadow does not depend on the chemical constitution or the morphology of stones, but on their acoustic impedance. It is determined by the size of the stone and by its location with respect to the focal zone. One must therefore use a frequency compatible with the depth of the structure to be explored. However, an overly small stone (i.e. one smaller than the lateral resolution of the transducer) or a larger stone that is eccentrically placed (i.e. not entirely located within the beam) will not cast a shadow. It is therefore necessary to utilize several approaches, hence the importance of the recently developed real-time scanners.

A cluster of small stones my cast an aggregate acoustic shadow.

The sensitivity of sonography in diagnosing calculi is great (2%–3% are false-negative results), and its specificity is even greater (under 1% are false-positive results).

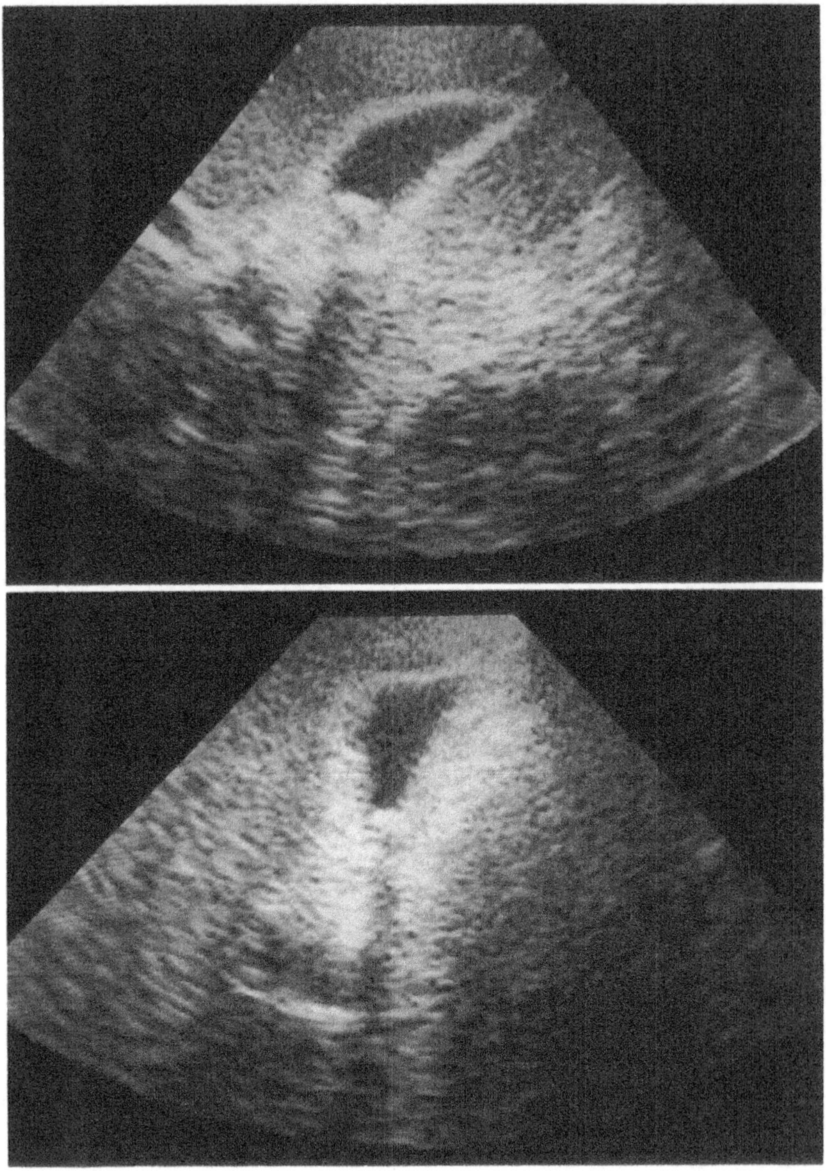

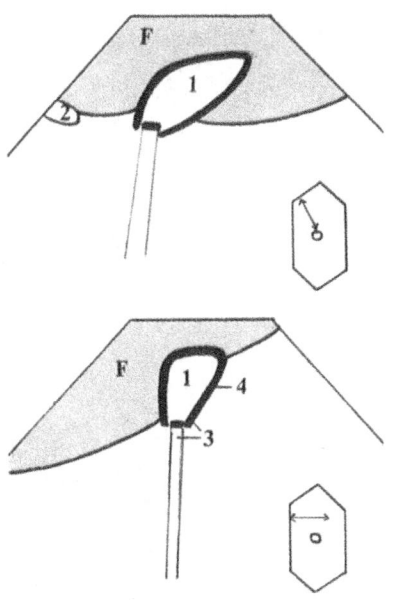

F liver **6**
1 gallbladder
2 portal vein
3 cholelithiasis, direct and indirect sign
4 thickened gallbladder wall

Case 6

Clinical data: A 40-year-old woman was referred for investigation of a urinary tract infection. She had no hepatobiliary symptoms.

This *Description* is easy: There is a 1-cm-long arciform echogenic image at the junction of the body and neck of the gallbladder, with acoustic shadow. The gallbladder wall is thickened; it measures 3.5 mm.

Endoscopic sonography shows motion of the stone when the patient is placed in the left lateral decubitus position, and absence of pain on passage of the transducer. The patient confirmed that she was really fasting.

Diagnosis: This is easy: gallstones.

Comments: Contraction of the gallbladder causes diminution of its size and thickening of its walls and even sometimes disappearance of the gallbladder lumen.

In patients with calculi the gallbladder walls may be slightly thickened even if there are no inflammatory changes. The normal thickness is 3–4 mm. The pathophysiology of thickened walls in the absence of cholecystitis is poorly understood. Two associated phenomena are lowering of the intravesicular osmotic pressure and increased pressure in the portal vein.

Gallstones is a very common condition – 15% of the population is affected. The stones are composed of cholesterol crystals, which are calcified in only 15% of cases and are then visible on routine radiographs. The clinical data are variable – gallstones may be asymptomatic, slightly symptomatic or accompanied by acute or chronic complications.

Ultrasound investigation should always be preceded by a plain radiograph of the abdomen. In some cases this is very informative.

7

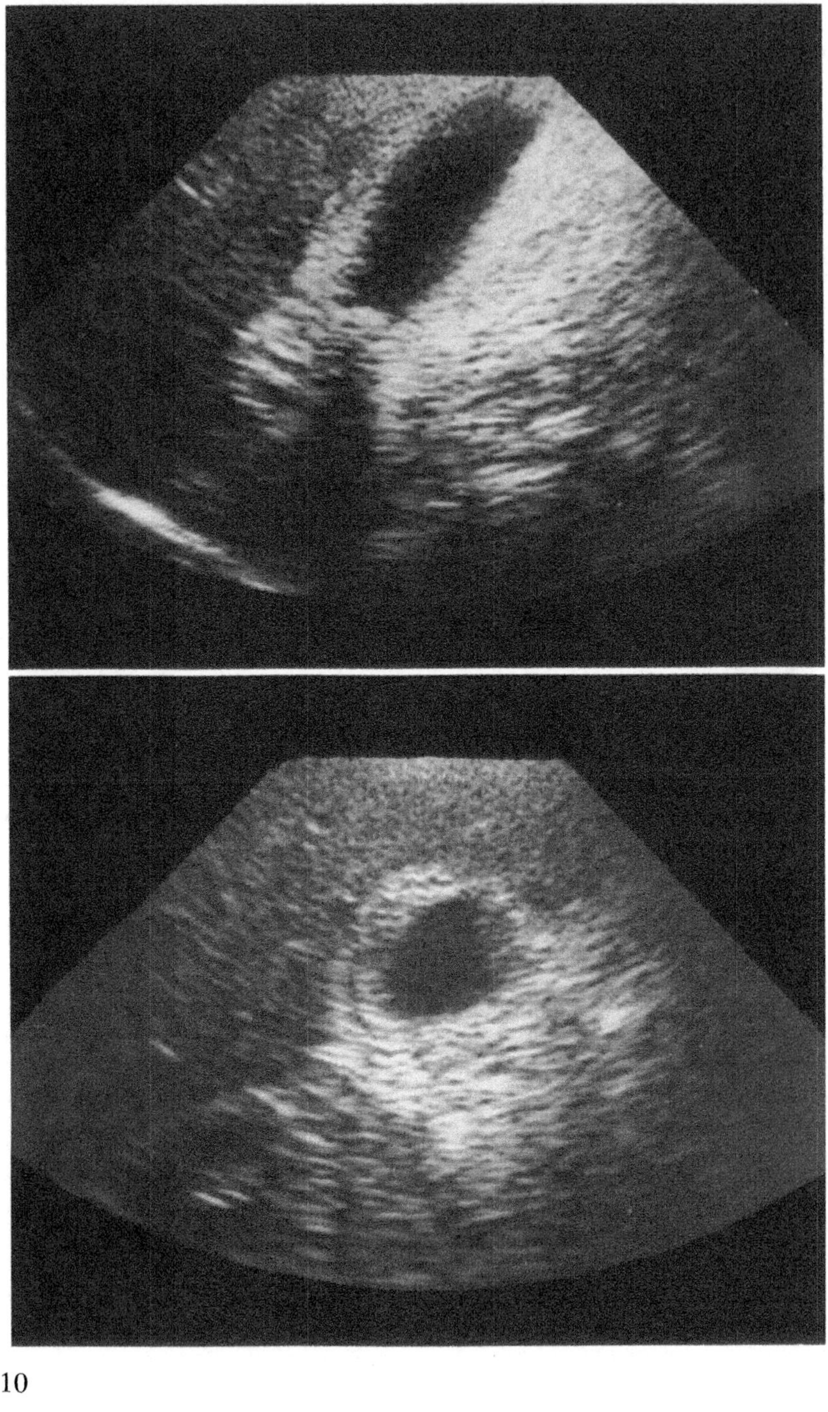

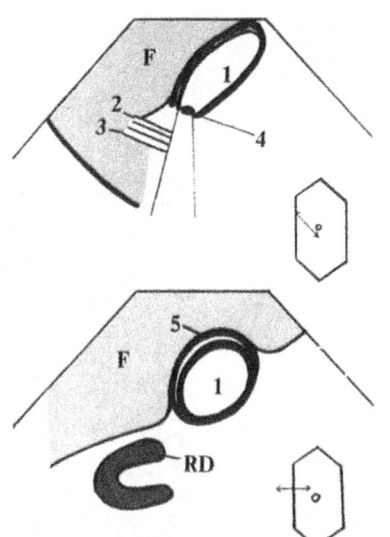

F liver
RD right kidney
1 gallbladder
2 main bile duct
3 portal vein
4 cholelithiasis
5 thickened gallbladder wall

Case 7

Clinical data: A 45-year-old man, hospitalized because of a threatened myocardial infarct, has had unexplained pyrexia for 2 days.

Description: There are three pathological signs:
– Moderate dilatation of the gallbladder.
– At the level of the neck, an arciform echogenic image (direct sign) with acoustic shadow (indirect sign), representing a stone in the gallbladder.
– Thickening (1 cm) and hyperechogenicity of the gallbladder wall, with a discontinuous hypoechogenic layer.

The sonographer has searched for the following signs:
– Presence of a "sonographic Murphy's sign" (pain caused by the passage of the transducer, with inhibition of respiration; this was absent in this case, because the patient had been given analgesic medication.
– Absence of calculus movement in response to changes in the patient's position.

Diagnosis: The patient has acute cholecystitis with gallstones. All signs are present, except retention of biliary deposits or sludge.

Comments: According to some authors, a hypoechogenic layer within the gallbladder wall is a *specific* but inconstant sign of acute cholecystitis. Whether this layer is continuous or not, it is a sign of early inflammation. It disappears rapidly as soon as medical treatment is applied. It corresponds to submucosal oedema. There is a risk of confusing it with perivesicular effusion and thus of underestimating the gallbladder wall's thickness. Parietal thickening is *not* *specific* to acute cholecystitis.

The inner margin of the gallbladder wall is regular. The outer margin is irregular and poorly demarcated from the hepatic parenchyma. This corresponds to cellular infiltration of the serosa.

Acute cholecystitis without stones is uncommon (3%–10%) and severe; it occurs after trauma or surgery.

8

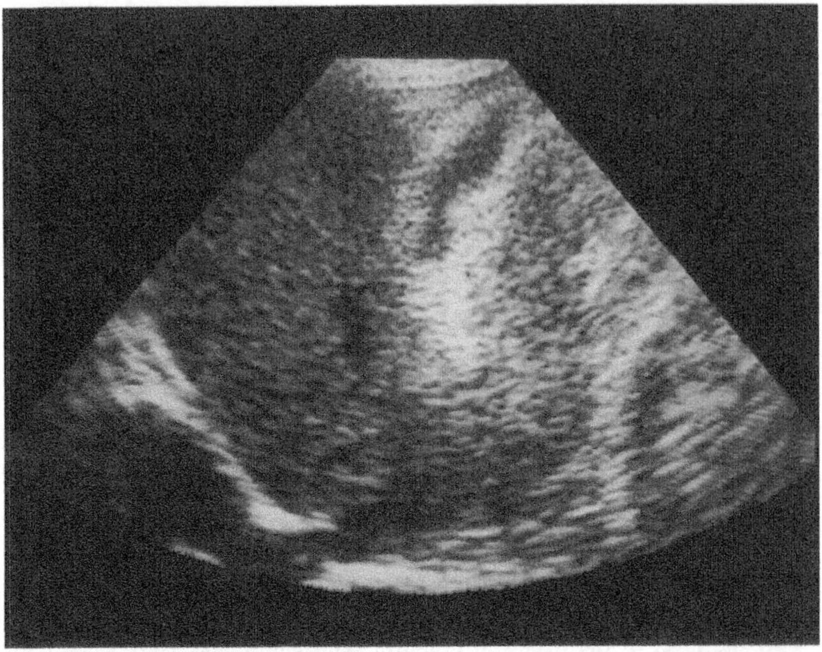

9

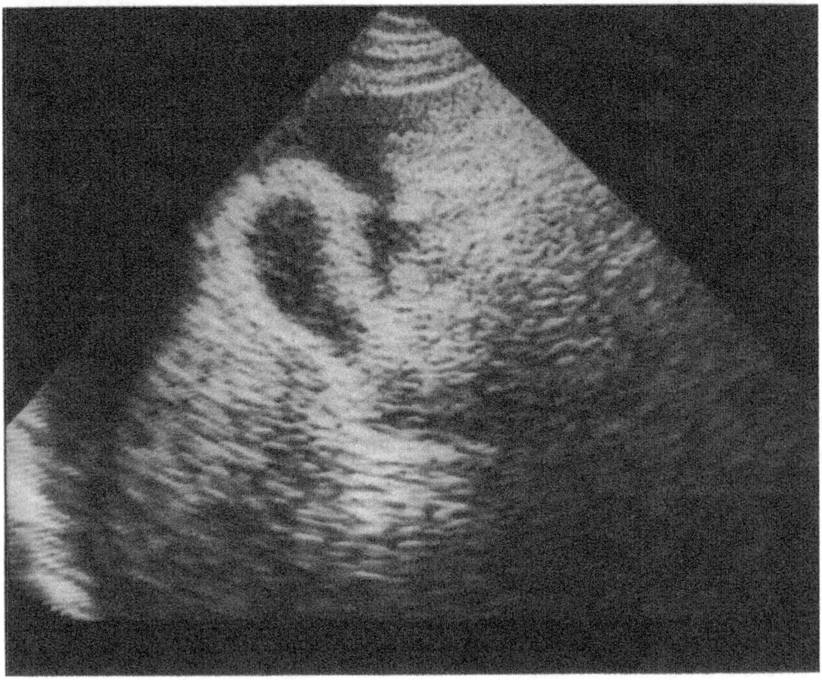

12

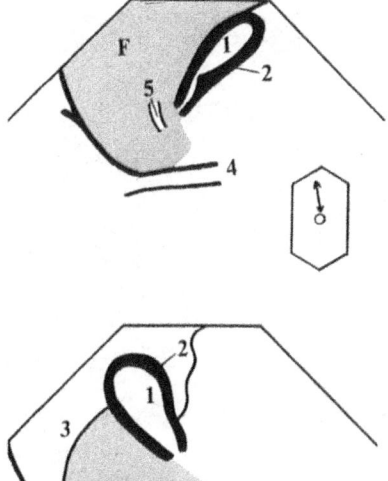

F liver
1 gallbladder
2 thickened gallbladder wall
3 ascites
4 inferior vena cava
5 branch of portal vein

Cases 8 and 9

Clinical data: These two patients were referred for different reasons. The first case concerns the assessment of acute alcoholism, the second shows decompensated cirrhosis with abundant ascites.

Description: The two cases show thickening of the gallbladder wall. This is a frequent sonographic finding. The first mistake which should not be committed is to examine a patient who has been eating (Case 8). As a matter of fact, an even partially contracted gallbladder normally has a thickened wall. Questioning the patient usually permits one to make the diagnosis.

Comments: The other classical causes of gallbladder-wall thickening are intraperitoneal effusion of any origin (Case 9) and hypoalbuminaemia secondary to renal failure, cirrhosis, cardiac insufficiency or multiple myeloma. The mechanism of thickening is oedema of the wall due to a decrease in osmotic pressure.

Viral hepatitis deserves particular attention. Most of these patients have thickened gallbladder walls sometimes with sludge, whatever the type of hepatitis. Thickening is commonly very marked, over 5 mm. Duplication of the wall may occur. Studies have shown a correlation between the degree of thickening and the degree of albuminaemia and of bilirubinaemia. Inflammation of the gallbladder wall by direct viral invasion has also been considered.

We also point out the possibility of gallbladder collapse caused by stress or by shock conditions.

10

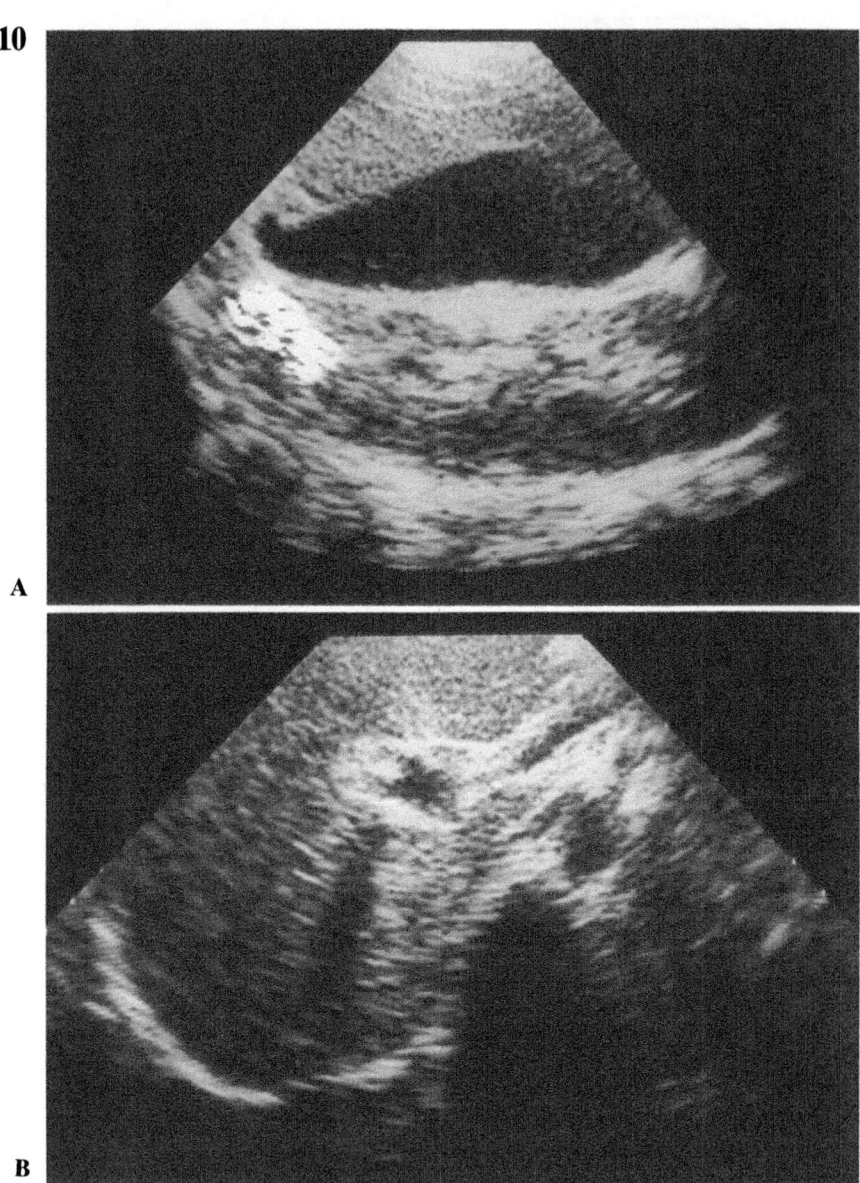

A

B

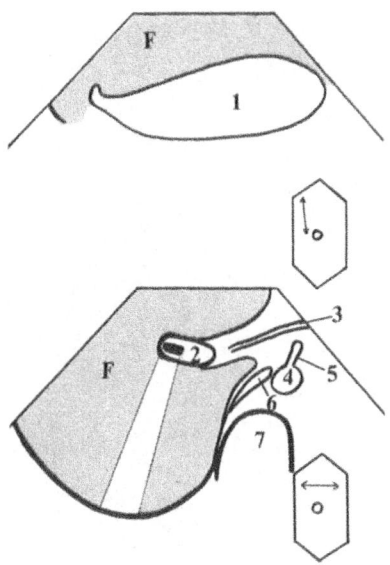

F liver
1 gallbladder
2 gallbladder neck
3 splenic vein
4 aorta
5 origin of the superior mesenteric artery
6 right crus of the diaphragm
7 body of vertebra

Case 10

Clinical data: A 25-year-old Turkish woman experienced sudden intense pain in the right upper quadrant of the abdomen. She was afebrile.

Description: The images are easy to analyse:
– The gallbladder is large (11 cm long, 5 cm in diameter) with normal walls.
– There is a 1.5-cm-wide hypoechogenic image, casting a shadow, in the gallbladder neck.

The endoscopic sonogram demonstrates pain caused by passage of the transducer and no positional migration of the stone (in the lateral decubitus and upright positions).
   Note the normal image of the right crus of the diaphragm (Scan B).

Diagnosis: The pain was due to biliary colic.

Comments: Because of its subjectivity the value of the sonographic Murphy's sign (pain caused by the passage of the transducer, with inhibition of respiration) is disputable. The sensitivity of this sign is good (85%) but its specificity for the diagnosis of acute cholecystitis is questionable, since it is also present in chronic conditions.
   The normal cystic duct is not usually visible.
   When there is a small stone impacted in the cystic duct, the diagnosis is difficult; even if the duct is dilated above the obstacle, the small amount of bile present prevents visualization of the stone.
   When a stone is impacted in the gallbladder neck, only the absence of mobilization in the erect position can confirm the impaction. In fact, an uncomplicated stone situated in the gallbladder neck will not move when the patient is placed in the left lateral decubitus position.

11

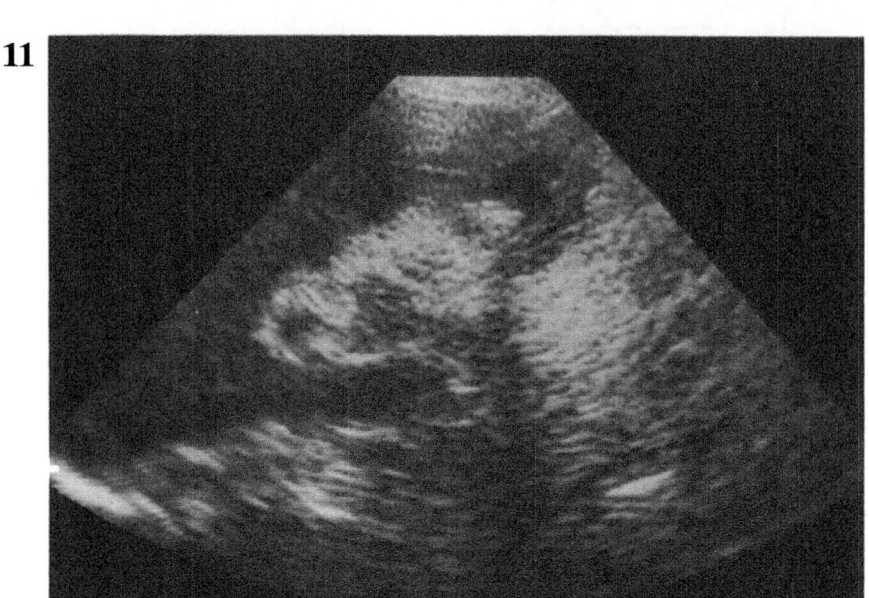

12

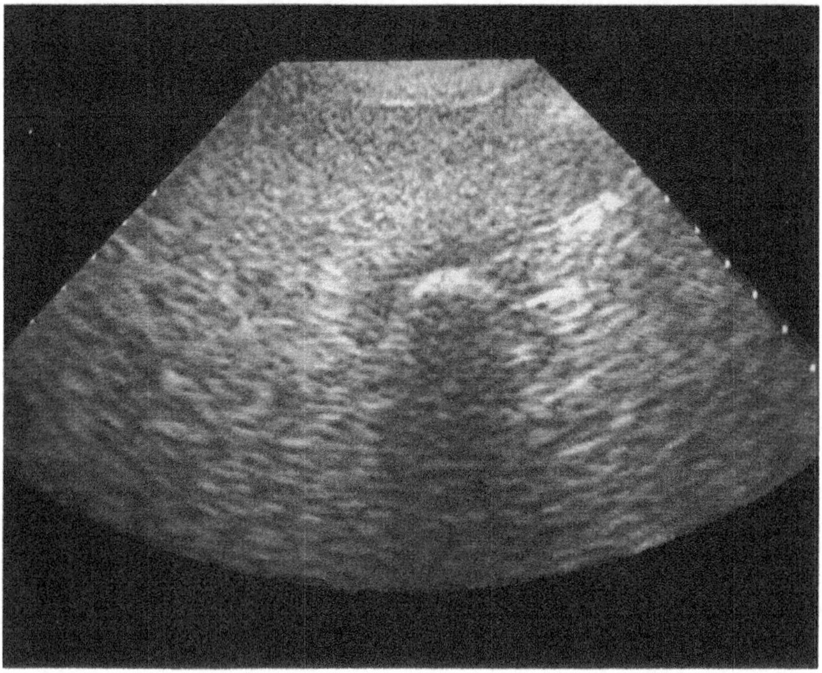

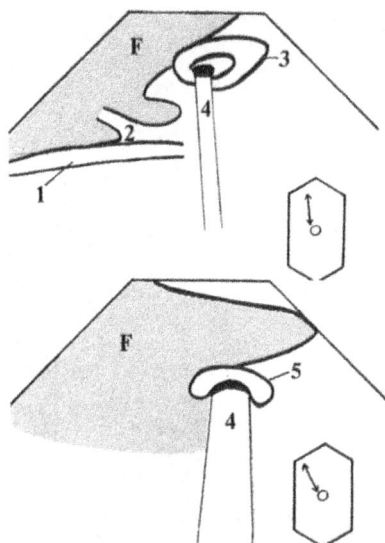

F liver
1 inferior vena cava
2 portal vein
3 thickened gallbladder wall
4 cholelithiasis
5 superior wall of gallbladder

Case 11

Clinical data: A 55-year-old woman was hospitalized for diffuse abdominal pain.

Description: The presence of stones is obvious. The gallbladder wall is markedly thickened (8 mm) and hypoechogenic, with well-defined limits. The gallbladder is very small and retracted. Passage of the transducer did not cause pain, and the stone could not be mobilized. The patient was fasting.

Diagnosis: This is easy: chronic cholecystitis with stones.

Comments: The classical appearance comprises the three following signs: gallstones, marked thickening of the wall, tendency to retraction.

You should not make the gross error of confusion this appearance with that of gastrointestinal structure (in which brownian movements will be present). Calcification of the inferior hepatic border will also be easily ruled out.

Case 12

Clinical data: A corpulent 60-year-old woman was admitted for hyperglobulonaemic purpura.

Description: The classical image of gallstones is now well known; the gallbladder is, however, not recognizable. It is reduced to merely a hypoechogenic layer above the stones. There was no pain on passage of the transducer. The patient was fasting.

Diagnosis: is easy: scleroatrophic gallbladder with gallstones.

Comments: Sometimes it is difficult to show the gallbladder. When you have verified that there is no cholecystectomy scar and made sure that the patient is fasting, you must persist in searching for the gallbladder, since agenesis of this organ is uncommon.

Absence of a visible gallbladder lumen exists in 15%–25% of cases. There are two possibilities. In the first the diagnosis is suggested by the presence of a hyperechogenic arc with an acoustic shadow, occupying the gallbladder bed: it is calcification of the gallbladder wall. Sometimes the diagnosis is suggested by the presence of a "double arc": this consists of two echogenic, arciform lines separated by a thin hypoechogenic layer. The proximal arc represents the superior wall of the gallbladder; the distal arc represents the gallstones.

13

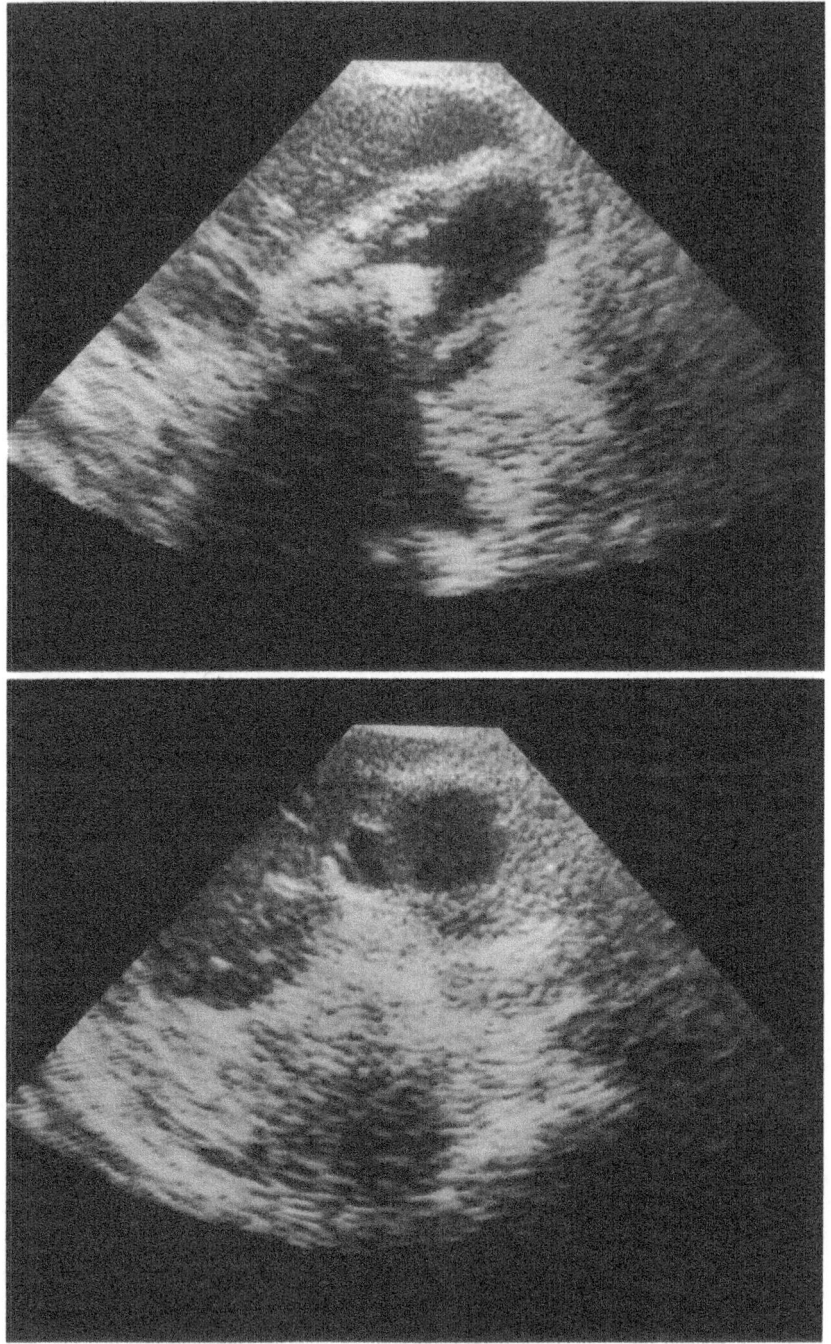

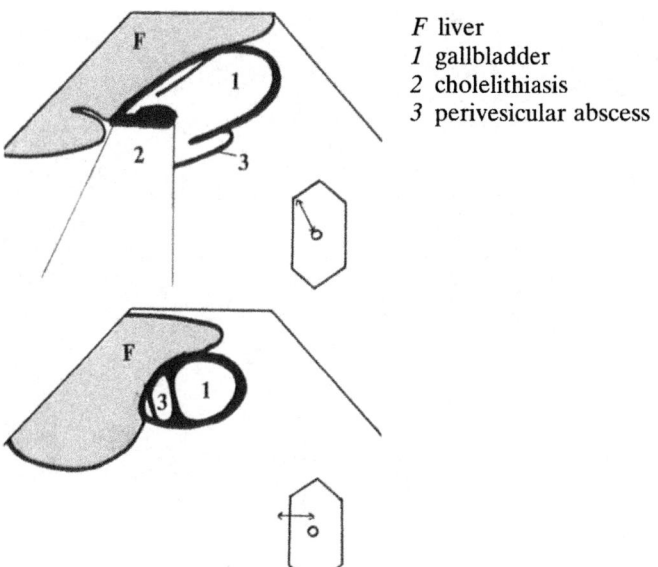

F liver **13**
1 gallbladder
2 cholelithiasis
3 perivesicular abscess

Case 13

Clinical data: This 86-year-old woman was subfebrile, with abdominal pain, predominantly on the right side.

Description: You are already familiar with some of these images a hyperechogenic image with an acoustic shadow, signifying marked lithiasis; thickening of the gallbladder wall. Note, moreover, the presence of a discontinuous large hypoechogenic area around the gallbladder. Endoscopic sonography demonstrates immobility of the stone, and pain caused by passage of the transducer.

Diagnosis: This is a perivesicular abscess secondary to acute cholecystitis.

Comments: Perforation of the gallbladder is seen in 5%–10% of patients with acute cholecystitis, predominantly in older patients. The mechanism of perforation is impaction of a stone in the cystic duct with distension, oedema of the wall, ischaemia, subsequent necrosis and rupture.

There are three types of gallbladder perforation: acute, with free peritoneal rupture (the sonogram lacks specificity and shows intraperitoneal effusion); subacute, with localized effusion in the gallbladder bed (the most common form); and chronic, with fistulous communication with a hollow viscera (search for the presence of air in the biliary tree).

An effusion surrounding the gallbladder appears after perforation. Its ultrasound appearance varies – an anechogenic collection in the beginning, it may become more heterogeneous after a few days.

Some conditions may mimic perforation – localized ascites; pancreatitis (with associated sonographic signs at the level of the pancreas, and effusion in the anterior pararenal space); ulcerous perforation in the omenta.

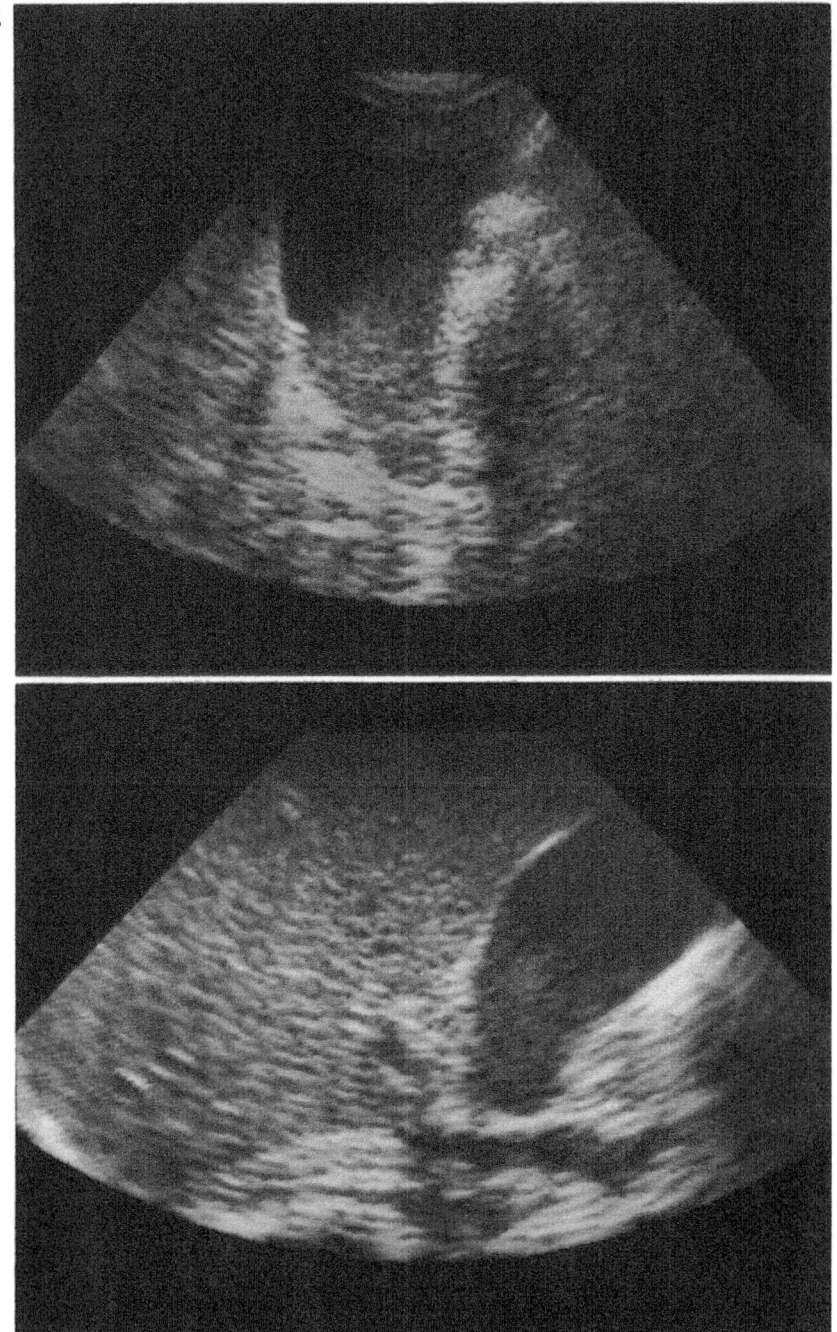

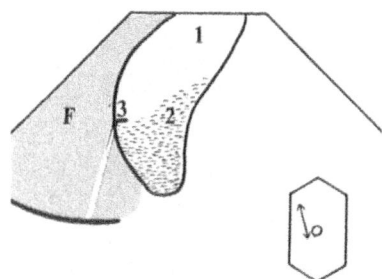

F liver
1 gallbladder
2 "sludge"
3 small gallstones
4 portal vein
5 inferior vena cava
6 right hepatic artery

14

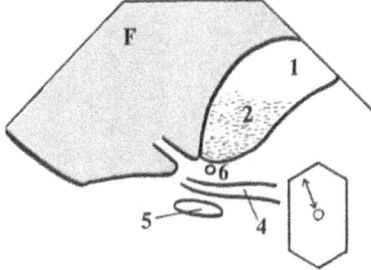

Case 14

Clinical data: This 55-year-old man had axillary lymph-node metastases from an undifferentiated epithelioma of unknown origin. There was marked alteration of the patient's general status.

Description: There are numerous identical low-amplitude echoes in the lower part of the gallbladder. The superior limit is irregular and indistinct. When the patient is placed in the lateral decubitus position this echogenic layer moves slowly to the most downward-sloping portion of the gallbladder. The size of the gallbladder is normal, and its walls are thin. Note the small stones in the upper part of the layer.

Diagnosis: Again, this is easy: echogenic fluid within the gallbladder, indicating viscous bile or biliary sludge.

Comments: Sludge consists mainly of calcium bilirubinate and a small amount of cholesterol crystals. Pus and blood may also be present. Stones are found in 40% of cases, which suggests a possible correlation between sludge and lithogenous bile. However the sonographic appearance does not depend upon the nature of the sludge.

Sludge indicates failure of the gallbladder to empty; it is due to a clinical condition apart from disease of the gallbladder. Its most frequent cause is prolonged fasting or a fat-poor diet. Sludge is also present in any obstruction of the extrahepatic bile ducts, in inflammation of the gallbladder, in haematological diseases and in all conditions causing haemolysis.

Its configuration is variable. Case 14 represents the most common form. The deposits may have a hypo- or even hyperechogenic nodular form, mimicking a tumoural process (Case 19). If the gallbladder is completely filled, identification of the sludge is difficult. In some cases scanning artefacts must be ruled out. They are identically located in transverse and longitudinal scans and disappear when the gain setting is changed.

15

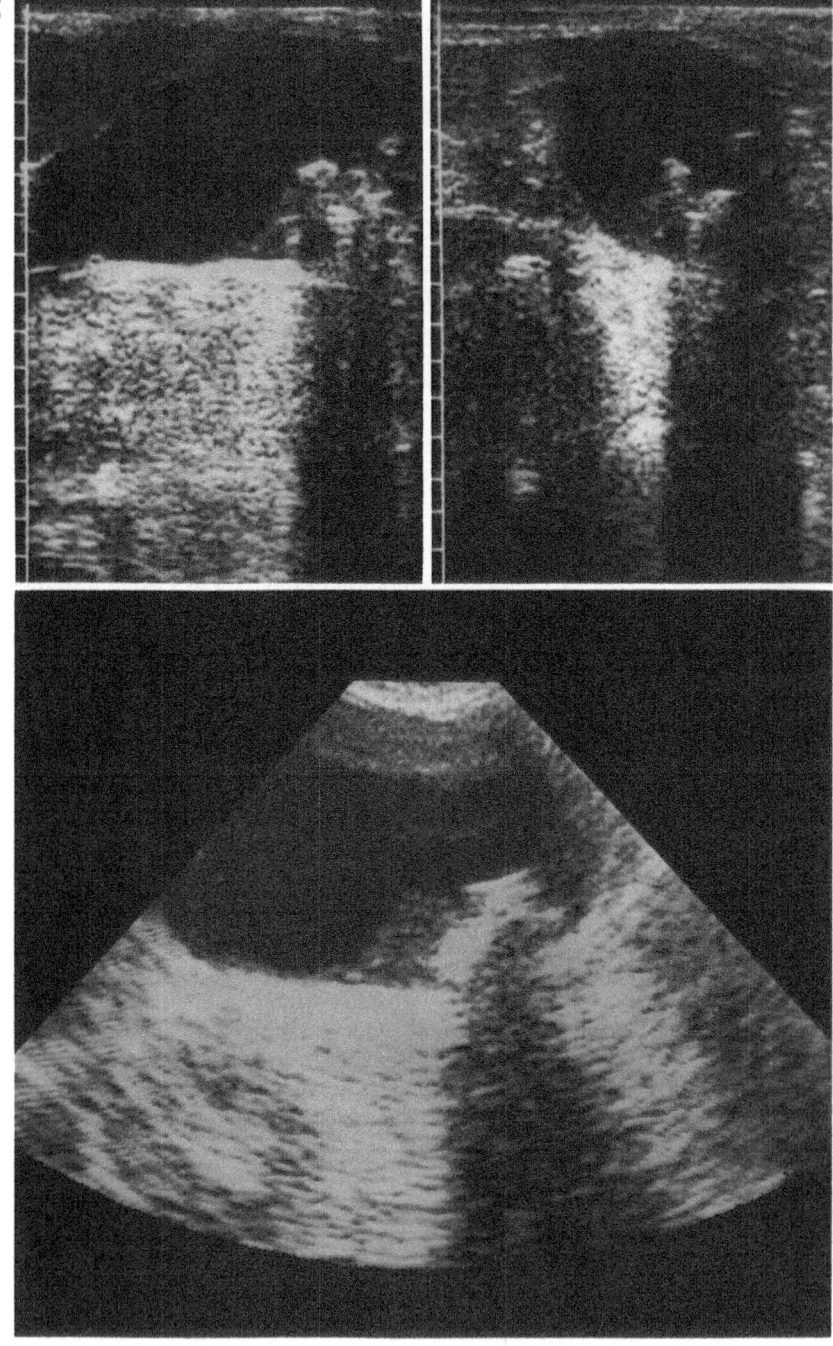

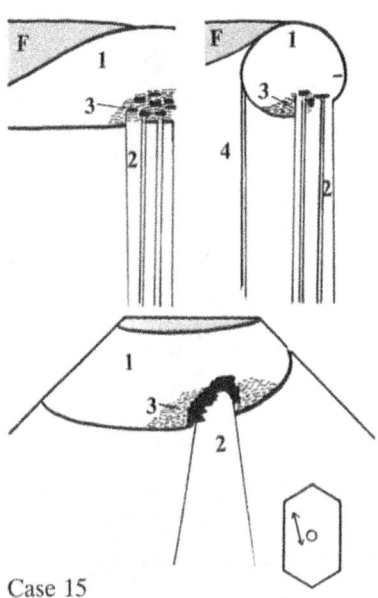

F liver **15**
1 gallbladder
2 cholecystolithiasis
3 sludge
4 acoustic shadowing of the gallbladder wall

Case 15

Clinical data: A 75-year-old woman was investigated for an inflammatory syndrome, and poorly defined abdominal pain.

Description: You will have already noticed the large size of the gallbladder (13.5 cm in longitudinal section, 6 cm in transverse section), as well as the presence of gallstones. These are confined in a cluster of low-intensity echoes with an irregular upper margin. The gallbladder wall is thin, and the investigation is otherwise normal. The cluster of stones shifts when the patient is placed in the lateral decubitus position.

Diagnosis: This is hydrocholecystis with stones and sludge in the gallbladder.

Comments: Hydrocholecystis is primarily a clinical diagnosis. Its ultrasound imaging is very easy.

This condition is an indirect sign of transient or chronic obstruction of the cystic duct, most often by a stone. There are sometimes other stones in the gallbladder. One should always make sure that there is no obstruction of the extrahepatic bile ducts.

The ultrasound criteria of hydrocholecystis concern mainly the transverse diameter (more than 5 cm). When there is doubt, a gallbladder-contraction test can be performed. It is often impossible to visualize a stone impacted in the cystic duct. Because of its small size, it may be confused with echoes from the porta hepatis. In the classical form the gallbladder walls are thin and its content is solely liquid.

Sludge can take on a polypoid appearance and therefore risks being confused with a malignant tumoural process, the more so as the latter is clearly hypoechogenic. One should think of carrying out two tests – mobilization to the most inferior part and repetition of the investigation 1 or 2 days later.

16

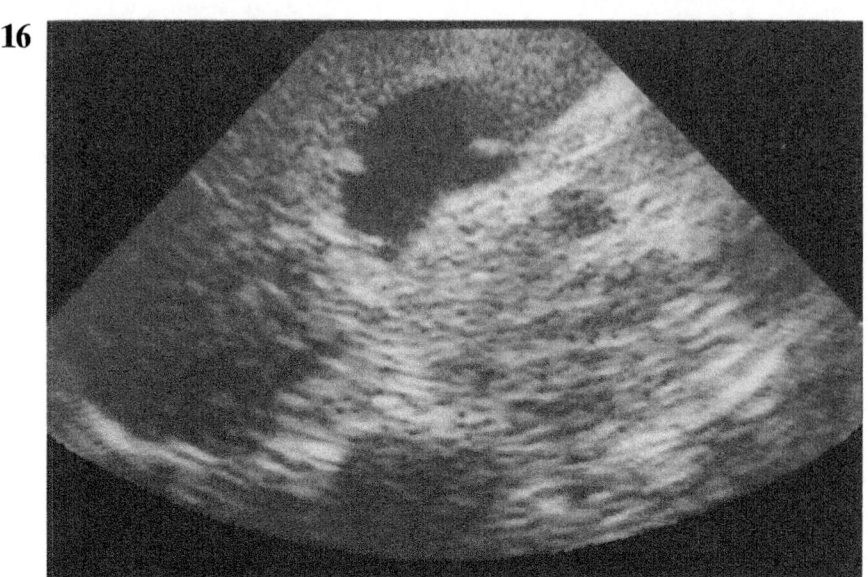

17

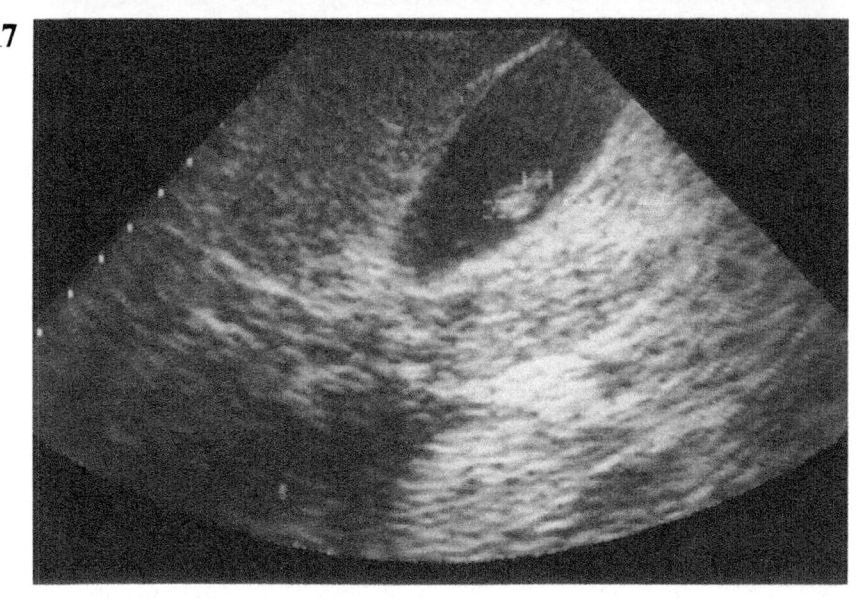

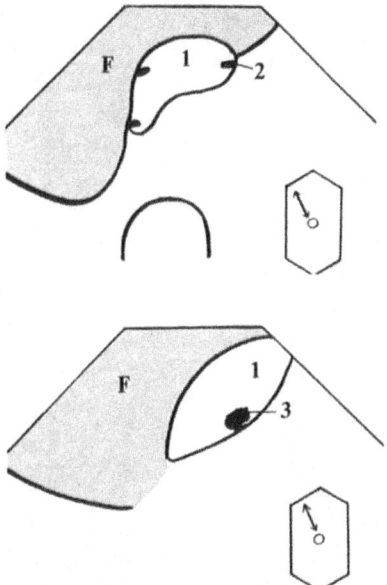

F liver
1 gallbladder
2 cholesterolosis
3 benign tumour of the gallbladder

Case 16

Clinical data: A 25-year-old woman was hospitalized for evolving systemic lupus erythematosus.

Description: There are several polypoid masses of 3–4 mm diameter, which are fixed, not casting shadow, and attached to the otherwise-normal gallbladder wall.

Diagnosis: This is easy: cholesterolosis.

Comments: This uncommon condition is poorly described in sonographic literature. The polyps consist of voluminous cholesterol deposits; they represent the major form of the disease and are always associated with microscopic lesions. They are usually situated in the fundus or in the body of the gallbladder. They may be single or multiple and are always small (1–5 mm). Functional signs of gallbladder dyskinesia are frequently associated.

Case 17

Clinical data: A 30-year-old man was hospitalized for right renal colic.

Description: There is a rounded area of increased echogenicity attached to the gallbladder, without shadows; this area is large (1 cm). A transverse section of the gallbladder shows it to be attached to the lateral wall.

Diagnosis: This is a benign adenomatous tumour of the gallbladder.

Comments: Benign epithelial tumours (adenoma and papilloma) are much more frequent than mesenchymatous tumours.

The adenoma is a well-circumscribed tumour of glandular origin, often located in the gallbladder neck. It is large, more than 5 mm in diameter; it never degenerates. Papilloma, which is more rare, is an endoluminal villous tumour which may degenerate. Moreover, it is rarely encountered in patients under 30 years of age. Benign tumours of the gallbladder are asymptomatic. Benign masses are usually more echogenic than malignant processes.

Adenomyomatosis is rarely visualized, since the investigation is performed in a fasting patient. In fact, it is easier to display when the gallbladder is contracted.

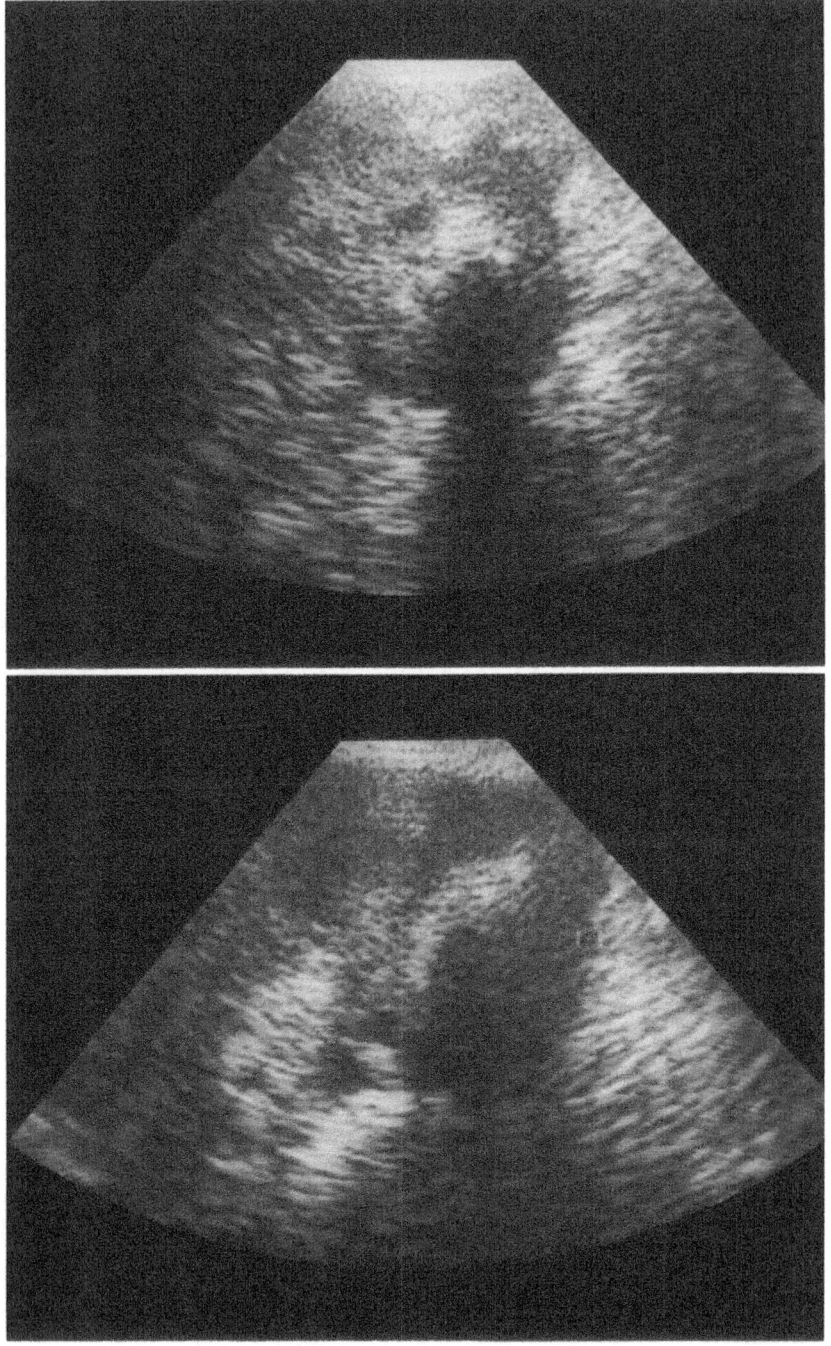

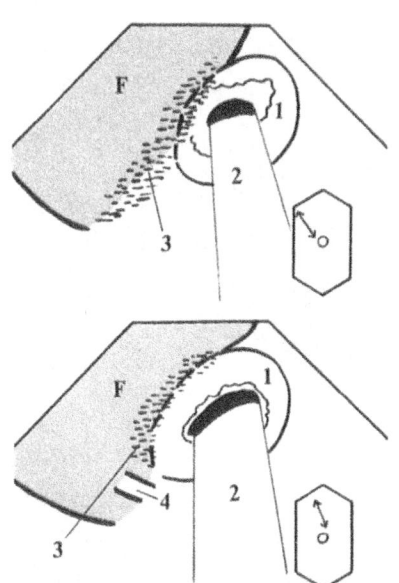

F liver

1 irregular thickening of the gallbladder wall

2 cholecystolithiasis

3 poor demarcation between liver and
   gallbladder

4 portal vein

Case 18

Clinical data: This 65-year-old woman
was hospitalized because of pain. A
mass was palpated in the right upper
quadrant of the abdomen. There is a
history of surgery for breast cancer.

Description: There is a large oval mass (9 cm in the longer axis) occupying the
gallbladder bed. It is composed of two parts – an eccentric hyperechogenic area
casting a shadow (a sign of the presence of stones), surrounded by a hypoechogenic layer 1–3 cm thick, with an irregular external limit. Note the poor
delimitation of the mass with regard to the hepatic parenchyma. The intra- and
extrahepatic bile ducts are not dilated. The investigation was otherwise normal.

Diagnosis: This is cancer of the gallbladder with gallstones.

Comments: Cancer of the gallbladder is the fifth on the list of gastrointestinal
cancers. It accounts for 50%–80% of bile-duct cancers, is found in 0.2%–0.4% of
postmortem examinations, and is a peroperative or chance pathological finding
in 2% of cholecystectomies performed for simple lithiasis. In fact, stones
predispose to cancer of the bile duct; only 10% of cancers are found in
gallbladders without stones. Although the exact pathology is still unknown,
three factors have been implicated: mechanical irritation, infection and biliary
stasis.

    Cancer of the gallbladder is mainly encountered in elderly women. It is a
severe condition with a 5-year-survival rate of 10%. It is asymptomatic or poorly
symptomatic and, in any case, the clinical signs are nonspecific and diversely
associated – fever, pain in the right upper quadrant, mass in the right upper
quadrant, progressive jaundice.

    In 70%–90% of cases there is an adenocarcinoma (15% are fungating
papillary carcinomas and 65% are infiltrating carcinomas). More rarely, the
tumour is a colloid carcinoma or a metaplastic epidermoid carcinoma. Polymor-
phism, and the frequent occurrence of associated inflammatory changes,
account for the fact that it is often undetected, even preoperatively.

19

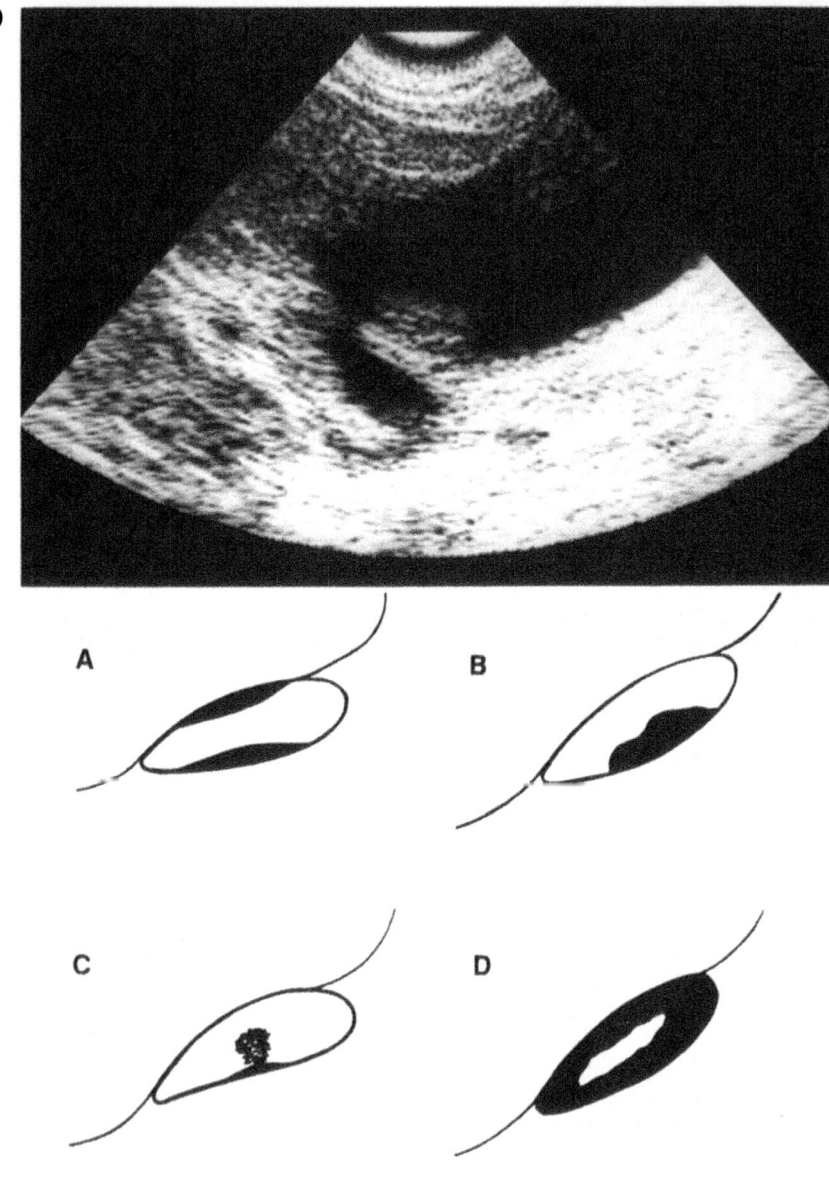

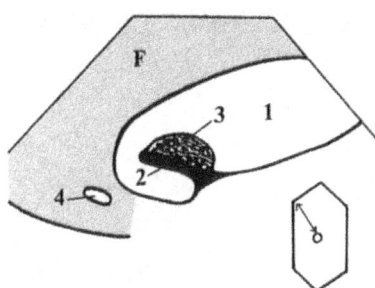

F liver **19**
1 gallbladder
2 fold of infundibulum
3 tumoural mass
4 portal vein

Case 19

Clinical data: A 20-year-old man with a malignant melanoma was investigated for re-evaluation.

Description: Analysis of the image is easy. There is a regular hypoechogenic and homogeneous mass situated within the gallbladder at the junction of the neck and body. Endoscopic sonography demonstrates no mobilization during changes in position. Two investigations carried out 3 days apart show this mass to be unchanged.

Diagnosis: This is difficult, as the lesion was a metastasis in the gallbladder. It is necessary to repeat this investigation with the patient in the left lateral decubitus position and in the erect position and also to perform an investigation some days later in order to rule out sludge. This superficially placed gallbladder was studied using a 5 MHz transducer.

Comments: There have been few descriptions of metastases in the gallbladder. Such metastases are not uncommon and are sometimes found on postmortem examination. There are four sonographic types:
A. Localized thickening of the gallbladder wall
B. Mass in the gallbladder
C. Polypoid mass with localized thickening of the wall
D. Global thickening of the gallbladder wall

Cancers of the stomach, the pancreas and of the bile ducts involve the gallbladder by direct retrograde spread. Cancers of the lungs, kidneys or oesophagus and malignant haematomas show vascular dissemination. Malignant melanoma is the most frequent primary cancer (two-thirds of cases). The initially submucous nodules becom pediculate. Type A anomaly corresponds to the first stage. It is most often asymptomatic, but can also be revealed by chronic or acute inflammation.

The differential diagnosis includes benign tumoural processes (usually more echogenic) and carcinoma of the gallbladder (especially when there are also gallstones). This condition must absolutely not be mistaken for sludge.

20

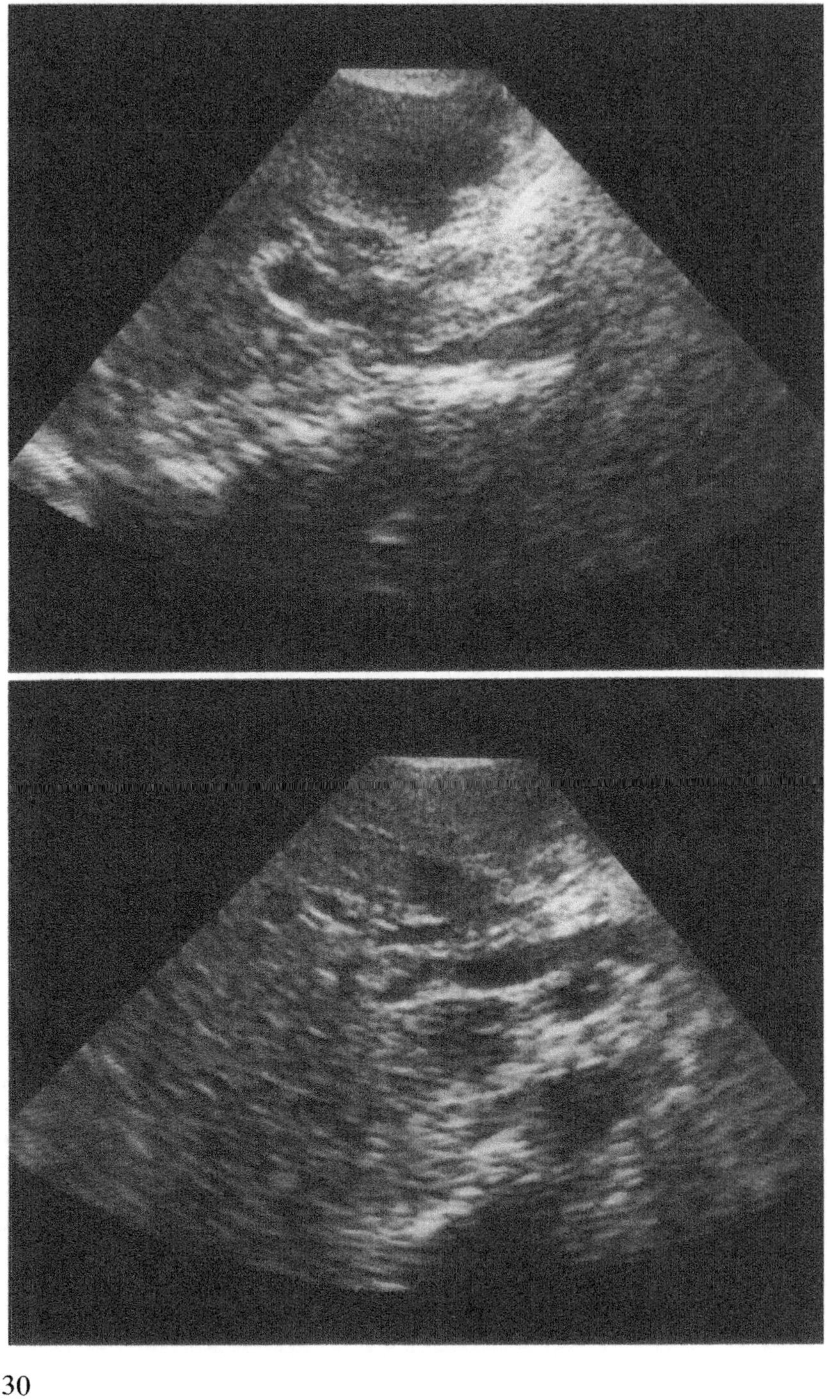

A

B

30

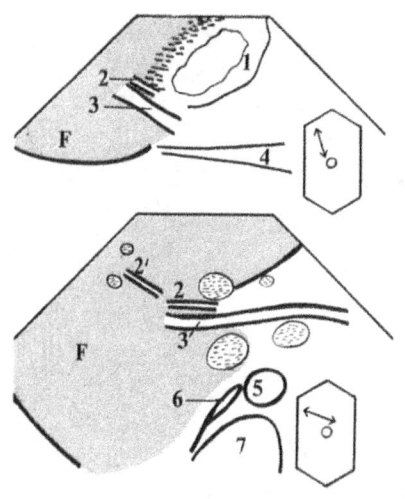

F liver
1 gallbladder with thickened walls
2 bile duct
2' left hepatic duct
3 portal vein
4 inferior vena cava
5 aorta
6 right crus of diaphragm
7 body of vertebra

Case 20

Clinical data: This 70-year-old woman had abdominal pain, predominantly in the right iliac fossa, and fever.

Description: You must notice two abnormalities:

– The gallbladder has irregularly thickened and globally hypoechogenic walls. The gallbladder lumen is reduced but present. Note the poor differentiation from the hepatic parenchyma (Scan A).
– There are intrahepatic hypoechogenic areas around the porta hepatis. The hypoechogenic structure below the portal vein corresponds to an adenopathy. There is no clear dilatation of the bile ducts (Scan B).

Diagnosis: You are wrong if you suspected cholecystitis with abscess of the liver. Surgery showed a carcinoma of the gallbladder invading the hepatic parenchyma, the porta hepatis and the transverse colon.

Comments: Cancer of the gallbladder has several sonographic appearances. The diffuse form is the most common. There can be a mass which occupies the entire gallbladder bed and is hypoechogenic and poorly delimited, with dense central echoes and acoustic shadow (Case 18), or a hypoechogenic irregular thickening of the wall, with a still-visible lumen (Case 20). The localized forms are more rare; they show a hypoechogenic regular thickening of the wall or a hyperechogenic polypoid image. There are also misleading forms – hydrocholecysts with tumours localized at the gallbladder neck; pyocholecysts.

Dilatation of the intrahepatic bile ducts is frequent and reflects extension to the porta hepatis. Involvement of the liver occurs either by contiguity at the level of the gallbladder bed, or by haematogenous metastasis. In the latter case detection is difficult when there is concurrent dilatation of the intrahepatic bile ducts.

In the localized forms differentiation from a benign tumour (usually more echogenic) is difficult. It is also difficult to differentiate the diffuse forms from a scleroatrophic gallbladder or from cholecystitis (chronic or acute). It may sometimes be difficult to rule out a tumour of the liver or a tumour of the right colic angle. Finally, a voluminous mass with bile-duct dilatation can also mimic cancer of the head of the pancreas.

21

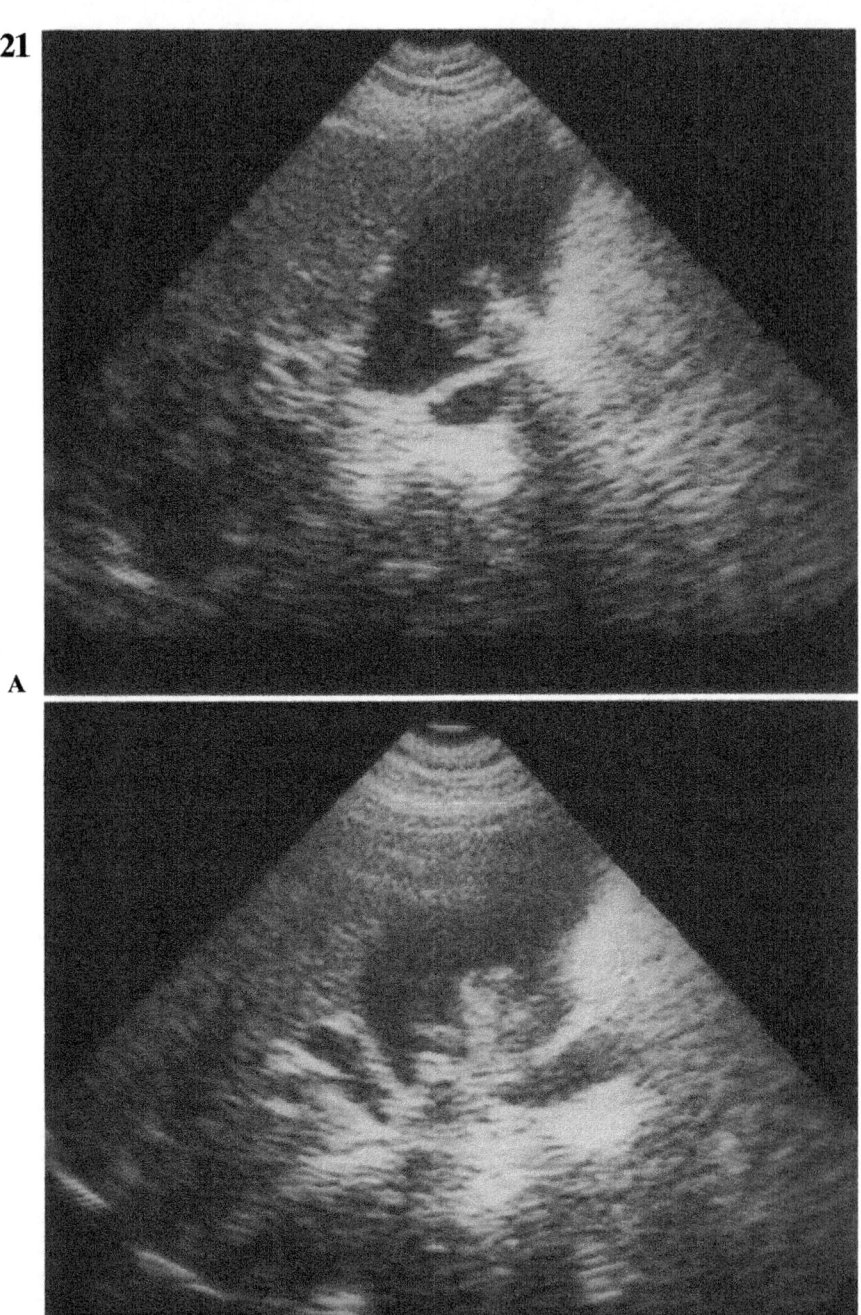

A

B

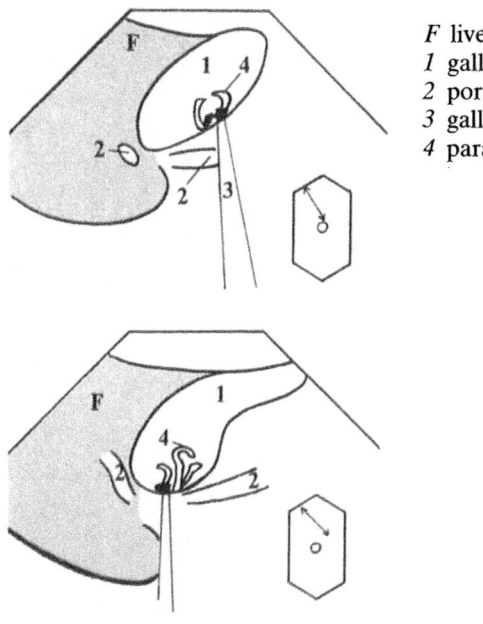

F liver
1 gallbladder
2 portal vein
3 gallstones
4 parasites

Case 21

Clinical data: A 45-year-old man, a native of Eastern Africa, had been suffering from spontaneously regressive subicteric episodes.

Description: You should have noticed two types of abnormality in the gall-bladder:
– There are small hyperechogenic areas with acoustic shadows cast by stones.
– There is also a less-echogenic curved structure, 3 mm thick and 3.5 mm long, the upper part of which is hook – shaped. On Section B this image is flanked by two smaller, identical images.

Diagnosis: This is parasitosis in the gallbladder associated with stones. The parasites proved to be ascarides.

Comments: Ascaris lumbricoides is a large roundworm of man. In the adult stage is measures 15–20 mm length and 3–4 mm in diameter. After ingestion the eggs hatch in the small intestine or colon. The worms may penetrate Vater's ampulla and proceed towards the common bile duct. However, only young individuals, because of their small size, are liable to enter the cystic canal and the gallbladder and to grow there. This occurs in the case of abundant infestion.

The clinical symptomatology is variable – benign: of the subicteric type, or spontaneously regressive biliary colic with diverse gastrointestinal disorders; or severe: retention jaundice, abscess of the gallbladder or liver, and cholangitis.

The association of ascarides with gallstones is described in the literature. Parasitosis seems to be a lithogenic factor.

22

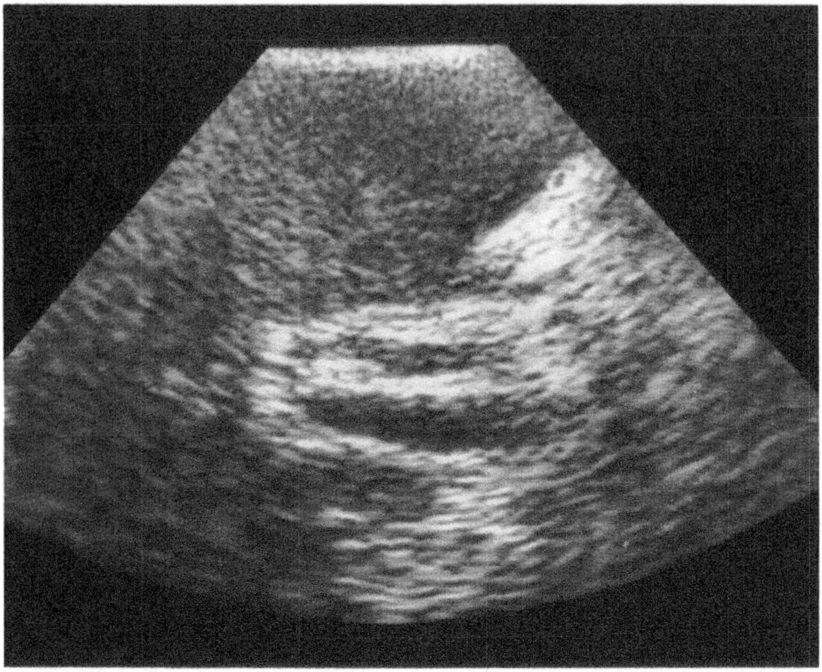

23

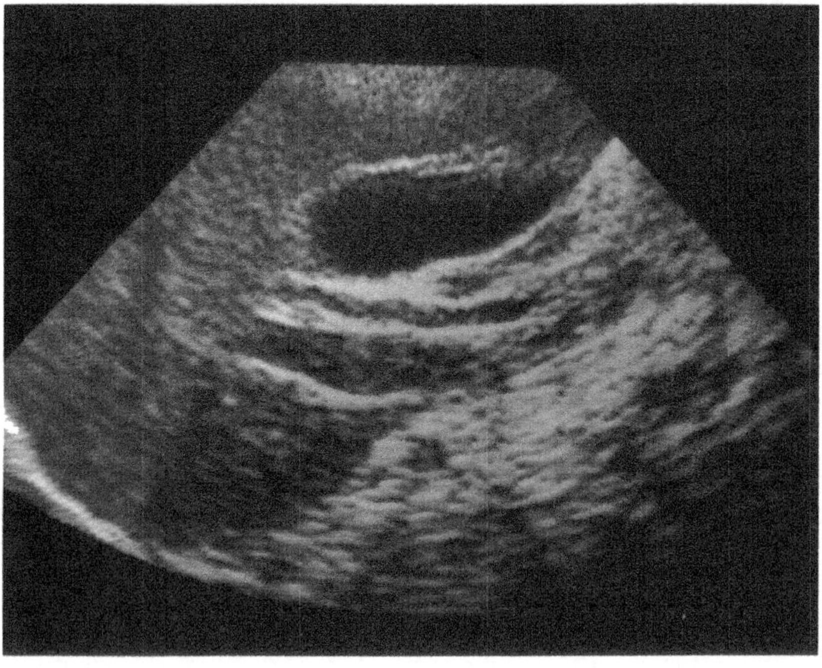

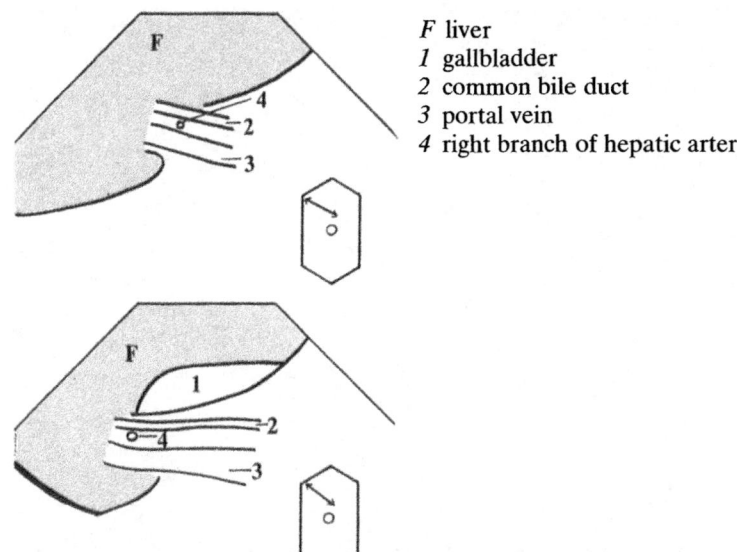

F liver   **22**
1 gallbladder   **23**
2 common bile duct
3 portal vein
4 right branch of hepatic artery

Cases 22 and 23 show normal findings. You must accurately identify the different structures of the porta hepatis.

The main bile duct must always be visualized. It is first roughly identified with the patient in the dorsal decubitus position, with a subcostal recurrent-oblique scan; it appears as an annular or oval structure anterior to the portal vein. The transducer must then be rotated some degrees to show the duct in its long axis as a tubular structure. Finally, the patient is placed in the left lateral decubitus position. It is indispensable to ask the patient to suspend breathing.

The main bile duct has two parts – the common hepatic duct, formed by the junction of the right and left hepatic ducts at the porta hepatis, and the common bile duct, formed by the junction of the common hepatic and cystic ducts. The common bile duct first runs inferiorly, to the left and backwards; it passes behind the superior part of the duodenum, crosses the posterior surface of the head of the pancreas and opens into the descending part of the duodenum. At the level of the pancreas the bile duct must be differentiated from the gastroduodenal artery which runs along the anterior surface of the pancreatic head. The biliary confluence is situated between the quadrate lobe in front and the caudate lobe behind. The term "bile duct" is in fact used for the entire main biliary duct since the junction with the cystic duct is not visualized in ultrasonography.

The diameter of the bile duct varies from 3 to 7 mm, with a mean value of 4 mm. A diameter above 7 mm is considered pathological when there is no lesion in the gallbladder. Sometimes the bile duct is very thin; even when reduced to 1 or 2 mm it must be considered as normal. The diameter of the portal vein is 9–13 mm. Do not make the gross error of confusing the bile duct with the portal vein, or the portal vein with the inferior vena cava, leading to a wrong diagnosis of bile-duct dilatation.

24

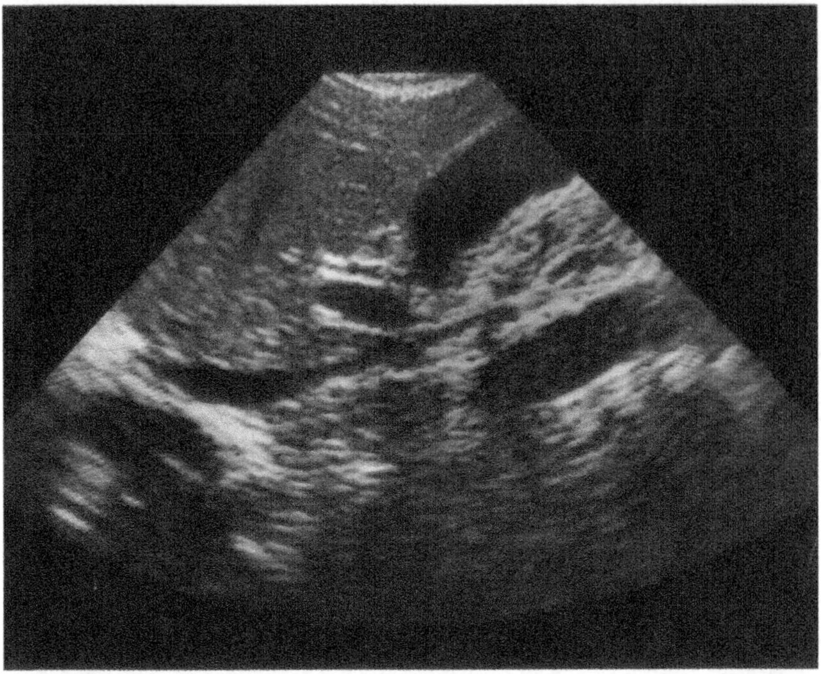

25

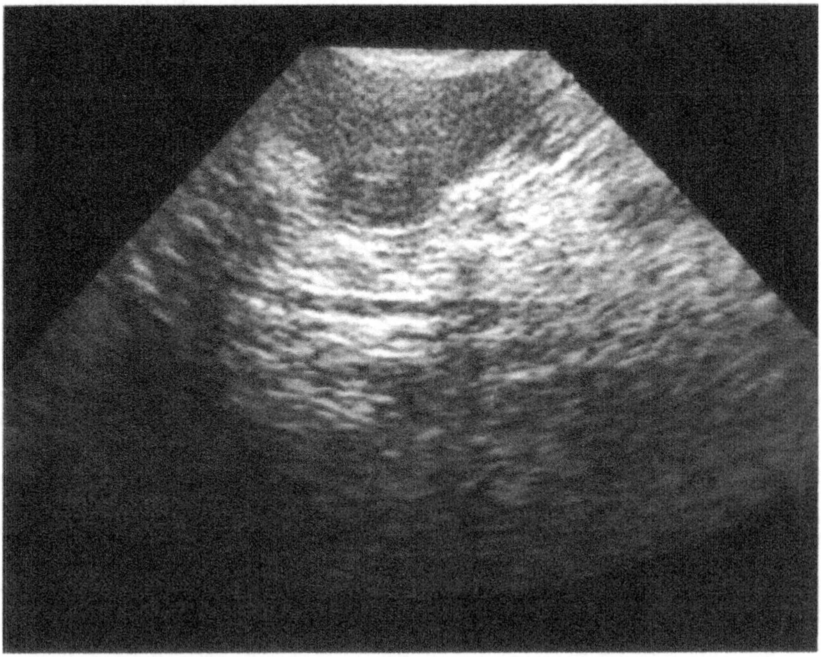

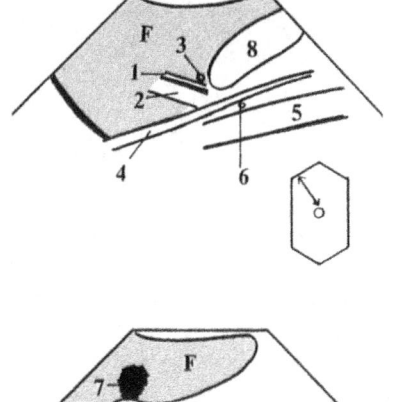

F liver
1 common bile duct
2 portal vein
3 right branch of hepatic artery
4 inferior vena cava
5 aorta
6 right renal artery
7 round ligament of the liver
8 gallbladder

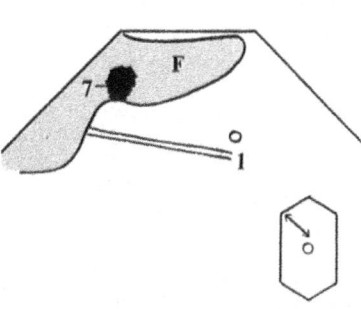

Cases 24 and 25

The bile duct is usually seen on the right anterior and lateral aspect of the portal vein; it can sometimes be seen on the right. To simplify, the bile duct is divided into two parts – proximal and parallel to the portal vein; distal and parallel to the inferior vena cava. The angle formed by the two parts is termed the genu. The proximal part can always be visualized, whereas the genu and distal part are frequently obscured by bowel gas. Therefore it may be difficult to indicate the exact site and nature of a low-situated obstacle. Note also that retrograde cholangiography shows the bile duct to have slightly larger dimensions than does ultrasonography. This is due to increased pressure in the main bile duct caused by the injection of contrast. On the other hand, with ultrasonography the biliary system is always examined in inspiration, which slightly increases the real diameter of the main bile duct, and also there is a risk of measuring the diameter on an oblique section. Despite these slight magnification factors, ultrasonography remains the investigation that best preserves the normal physiology.

The hepatic artery proper ascends along the left aspect of the portal vein but divides early so that the right hepatic branch usually passes inferior to the bile duct (Case 22), sometimes superiorly (Case 24). It is seen as a ring-shaped structure between two tubular structures. The hepatic artery may be tortuous; if it is seen longitudinally it is difficult to distinguish it from the bile duct in such cases.

We have described the three main elements of the porta hepatis. Other structures can be distinguished. The right and left hepatic ducts may unite later or even remain separate. The cystic duct, usually not visualized, may also be very large.

26

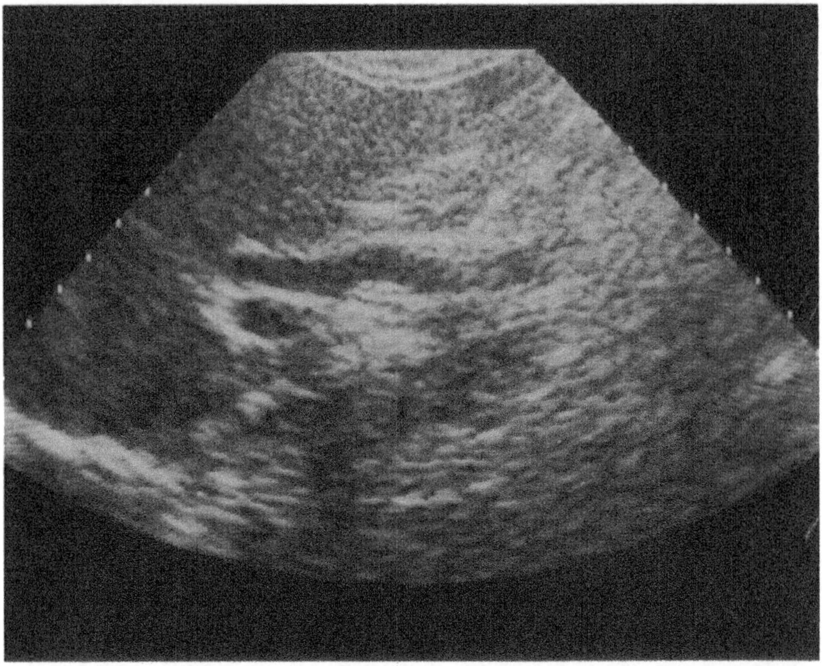

27

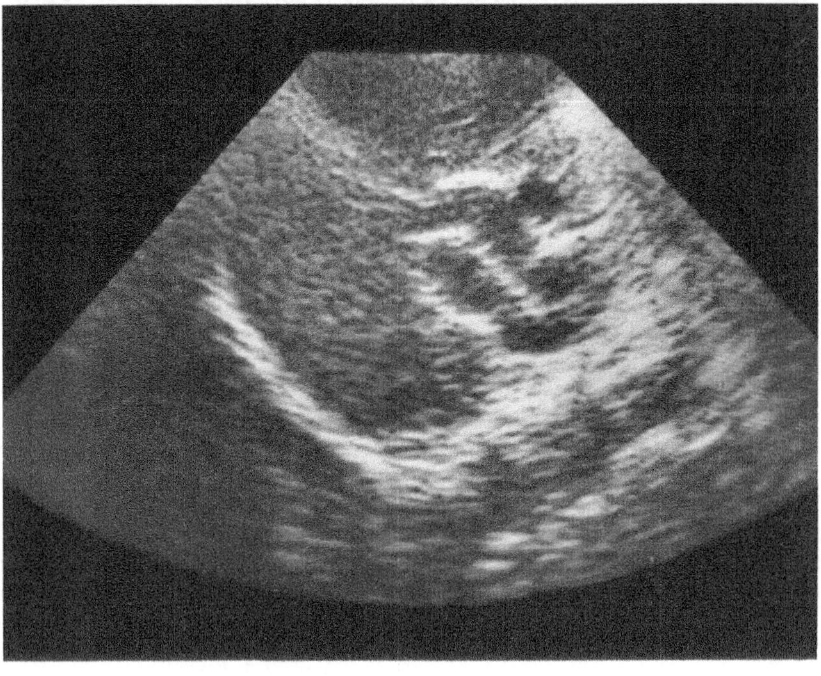

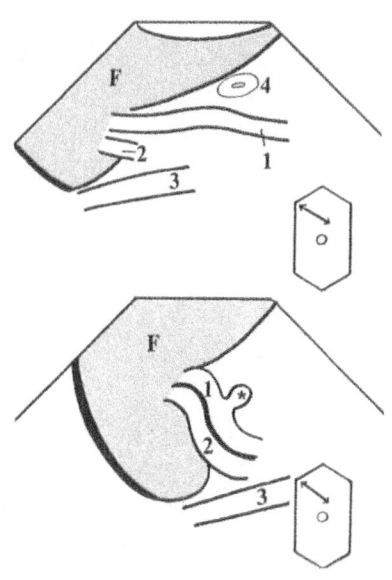

F liver
1 common bile duct
2 portal vein
3 inferior vena cava
4 duodenum

Case 26

Clinical data: A 60-year-old woman has poorly defined abdominal pain and a history of cholecystectomy.

Description: The bile duct measures 8 mm and is visible up to the head of the pancreas.

Diagnosis: These are normal findings.

Comments: Dilatation of the main bile duct after cholecystectomy (7–10 mm) is a classical notion. There is, however, some controversy. It was first described in dogs, by Oddi in 1890, but cholangiographic studies proved it to be pathological and due to the presence of an obstacle. Ultrasound studies have confirmed the existence of dilatation after cholecystectomy but been less definite about it. Moreover, dilatation is inconstant.

Case 27

Clinical data: A 92-year-old woman was hospitalized with alteration of general status. Cholecystectomy had been performed 20 years earlier.

Description: The bile duct measures 10 mm and is traced up to the pancreas. Intravenous cholangiography did not show an obstruction. Note the small rounded, hypoechogenic structure, terminating in the bile duct. It corresponds to the also-dilated stump of the cystic duct (*).

Comments: A bile duct which was normal before cholecystectomy must remain so after.

A bile duct which was dilated before cholecystectomy may become normal again. The bile duct contains some oblique muscle fibres and elastin fibres. When these are not ruptured by marked and/or prolonged distension, the diameter may become normal again. If that is not the case, it remains dilated.

The frequency of asymptomatic dilatation in old patients is explained by the poor contractility of the muscle fibres.

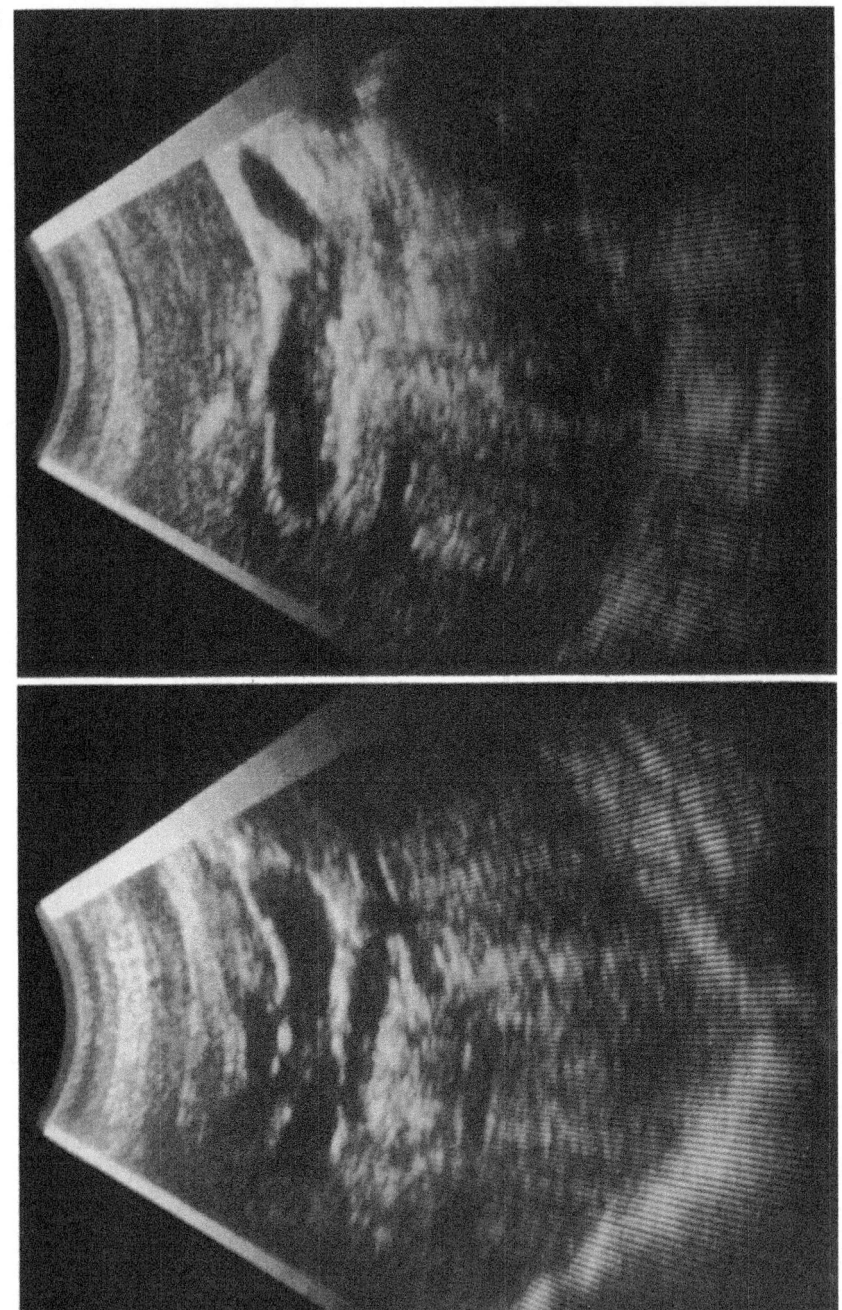

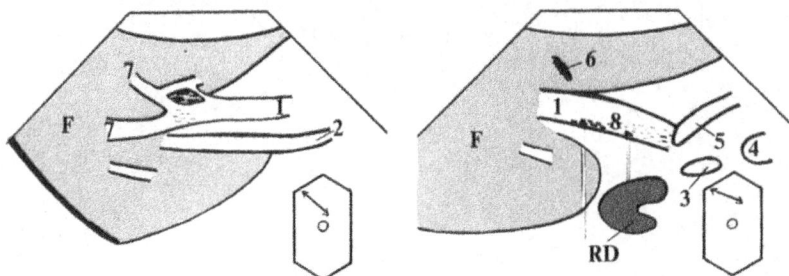

RD

F liver
RD right kidney
1 dilated main bile duct
2 portal vein
3 inferior vena cava

4 aorta
5 splenic vein
6 round ligament
7 dilatation of the intrahepatic bile ducts
8 intracholedochal calculi and sludge

Case 28

Clinical data: A 60-year-old woman has jaundice.

Description: There is obvious dilatation of the intrahepatic bile ducts (tortuous tubular structures in the vicinity of the porta hepatis). The bile duct is markedly dilated (2 cm). There are two types of endoductal hyperechogenic image in the most inferior part of the bile duct. The very dense ones against the posterior wall, with thin acoustic shadows, corresponds to stones; the others, situated below, are less echogenic and correspond to bile of abnormally high viscosity. The gallbladder is scleroatrophic.

Diagnosis: There are stones within the bile duct.

Comments: Diagnosing stones in the bile duct can be difficult because the acoustic shadow is often absent and also because there are false images (Case 31). When the bile duct is filled with stones the absence of a bile-stone interface renders identification difficult. The presence of stones in the bile duct remains the main cause of dilatation of the main bile duct (50% of cases). It is, moreover, the most frequent complication of chronic cholecystitis and affects 15% of the patients who have stones in the gallbladder. The sensitivity of the ultrasound method is considered to be 55%, but its specificity is higher.

On the other hand, there are intraductal calculi with a subnormal main bile duct.

Jaundice may also be absent. Blockage of a stone can be intermittent; also, a small stone can remain asymptomatic for a long time. This is particularly the case when stones develop in the main bile duct, thus allowing its progressive dilatation and adaptation to the stone. In such cases ultrasonography is positive even before the appearance of clinical signs.

29

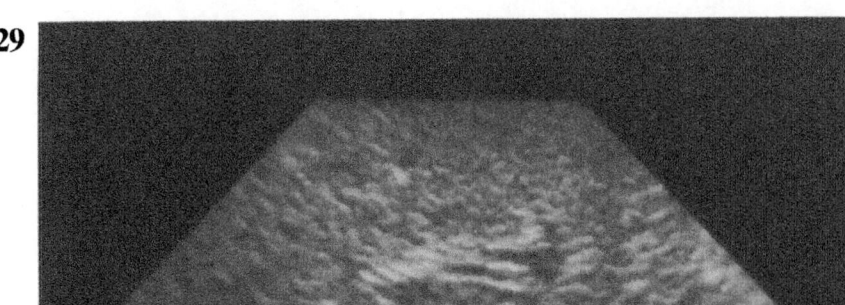

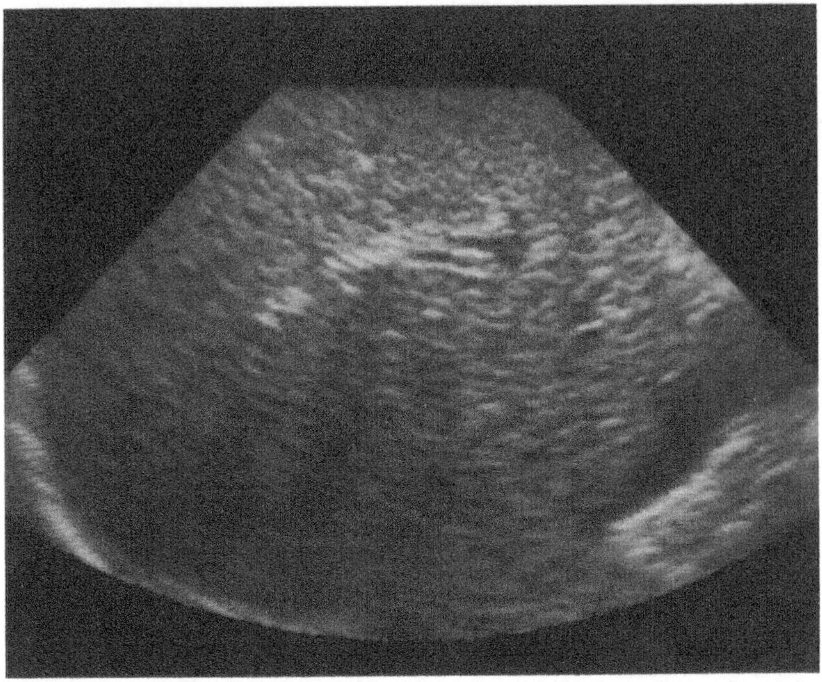

30

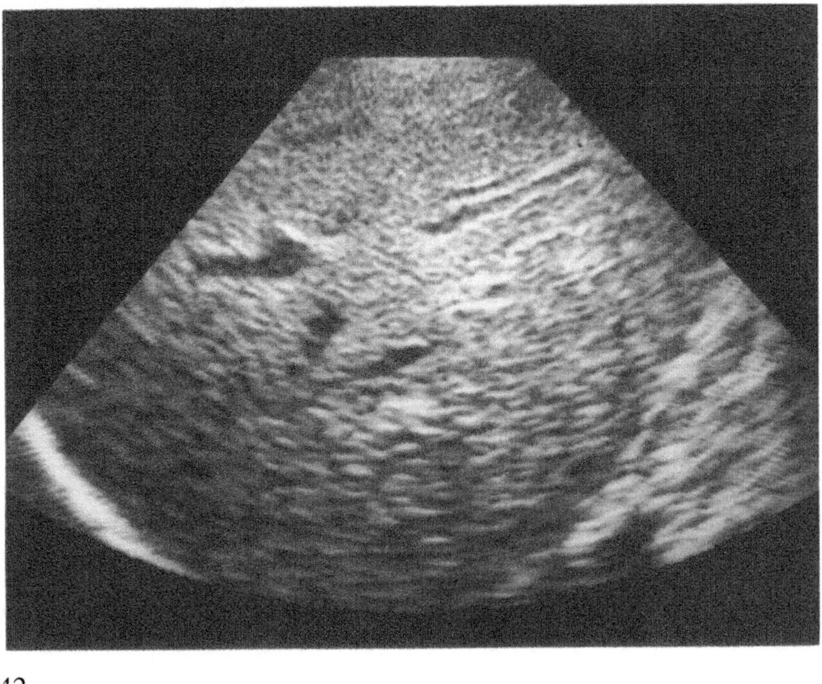

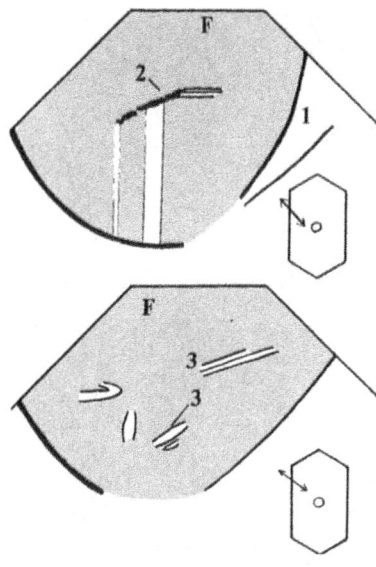

F liver
1 inferior vena cava
2 air in the intrahepatic bile duct
3 dilatation of the intrahepatic bile ducts

Case 29

Clinical data: A 60-year-old man with long-standing fever has a history of cholecystectomy with biliary-digestive anastomosis.

Description: Tubular, hyperechogenic structures are disseminated throughout the parenchyma of the liver. There is acoustic shadowing. The shape and number of the structures depend on the inclination of the transducer, and they follow the course of the portal system. This is the classical image of air in the biliary system.

Comments: This is most often a chance finding during ultrasound investigation in patients who have been operated several times. Otherwise it strongly suggests gallstone ileus. Acoustic shadows and strong echoes are parallel to the vascular axis. It should be noted that the presence of air prevents sonographic evaluation of the biliary system's dimensions. It is also of importance not to confuse this process with a lithiasic pathology of the intrahepatic bile ducts.

Case 30

Clinical data: A 40-year-old man has jaundice.

Description: Note the image of the "shotgun sign" formed by an intrahepatic bile duct above and parallel to the corresponding portal branch. It is a sign of dilated intrahepatic biliary ducts.

Diagnosis: There is a stone in the main bile duct.

Comments: When they are normal, the intrahepatic biliary ducts are not visible. In some cases however, one can visualize the right and left hepatic duct along the corresponding portal branches. They are the more anterior structures.

Dilatation of the intrahepatic biliary ducts at some distance from the porta hepatis is a sign specific to extrahepatic obstruction, which can precede hyperbilirubinaemia.

If moderate bile-duct dilatation is common in old patients, intrahepatic dilatation of the biliary ducts is abnormal in young as well as in old patients. Also, marked dilatation of the intrahepatic bile ducts impedes correct sonographic study of the liver parenchyma because of the posterior reinforcement behind the fluid-filled structures.

31

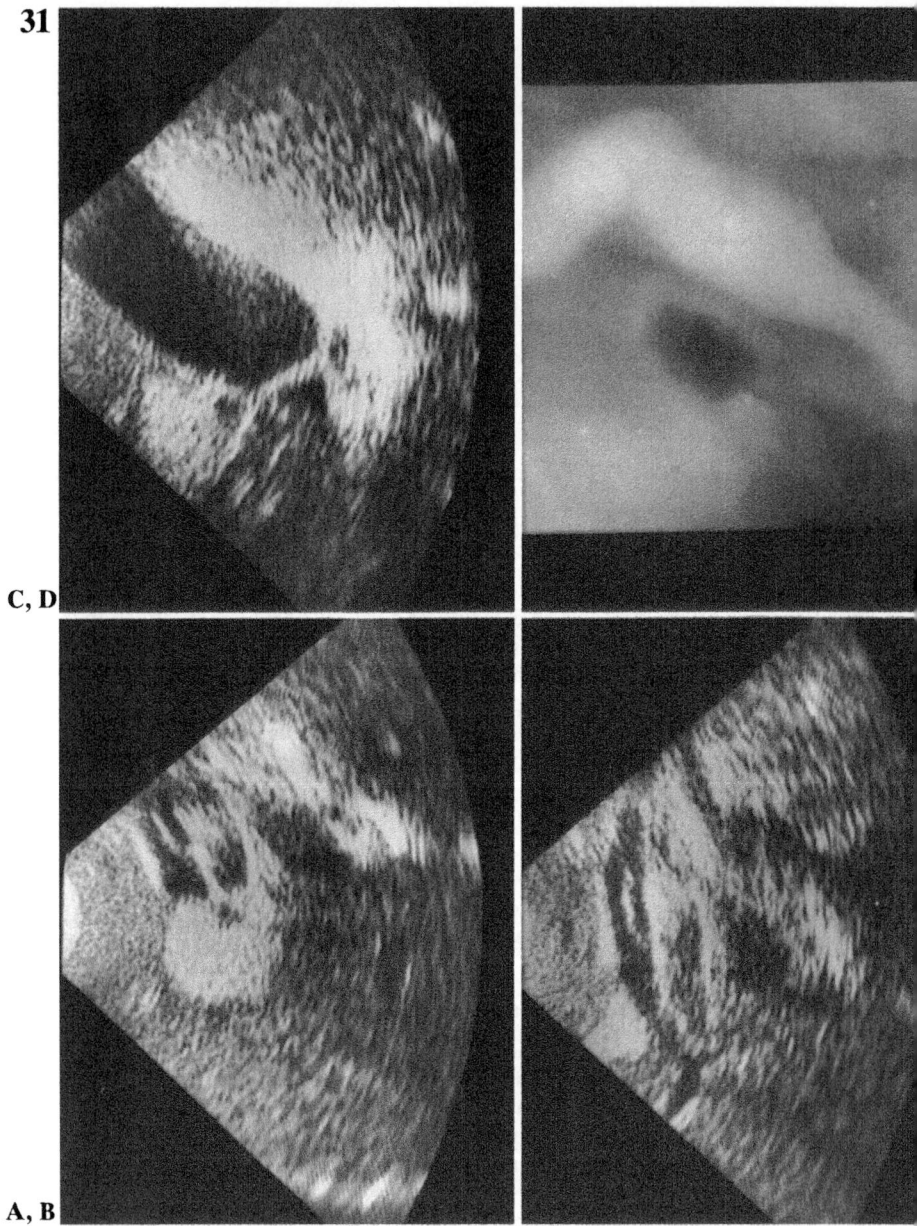

C, D

A, B

44

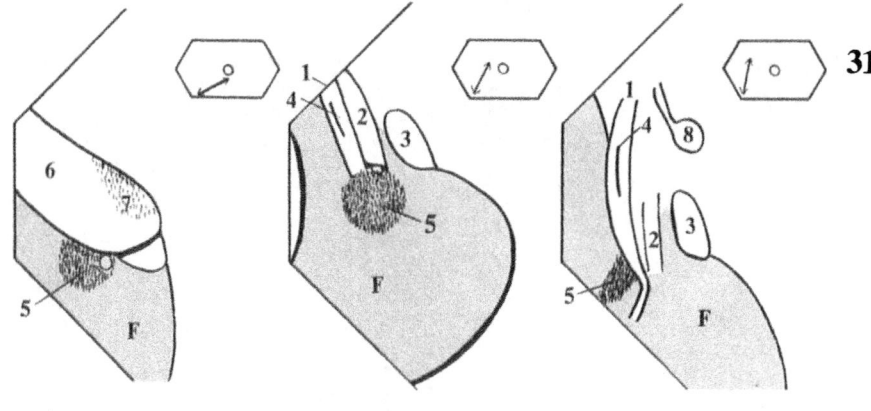

F liver	*4* right hepatic artery	*8* aorta and origin
1 dilated bile duct	*5* hepatic angioma	of superior mesen-
2 portal vein	*6* gallbladder	teric artery
3 inferior vena cava	*7* sludge	

Case 31

Clinical data: A 60-year-old woman has persistent epigastric pain and subicterus. There are disturbances in the biochemical data.

Description: There are four striking points:
- A clearly-defined, homogeneous hyperechogenic structure, just above the porta hepatis. Note the posterior attenuation of the echoes (Scan A).
- Dilatation of the main bile duct (11 mm). The duct may be traced as far as the head of the pancreas, where it becomes more narrow and stops abruptly (Scan B).
- The gallbladder is large and contains sludge. The left and the right hepatic ducts are dilated, but their distal parts are not visualized.
- A hyperechogenic linear structure situated in the bile duct (Scans A and B).

Diagnosis: This is facilitated by intravenous cholangiography, which shows a stone lodged in Vater's ampulla. The hyperechogenic structure corresponds to a huge angioma.

Comments: The linear structure which seems intracholedocal is a pitfall. It is in fact the right hepatic artery which crosses the bile duct. If this is particularly protuberant it produces an indentation in the form of a hyperechogenic line, more visible when the bile duct is dilated. It should not be confused with lithiasis, the more so in that absence of acoustic shadow is not an absolute criterion (Case 28).

In older patients and after cholecystectomy the problem is to affirm organic dilatation, especially when intrahepatic participation is lacking. The clinical data provide the clue. If the ultrasound investigation does not afford definite evidence of lithiasis, and when biochemistry allows it, intravenous cholangiography must be carried out.

Stones lodged in the sphincter of Oddi are difficult to diagnose.

32

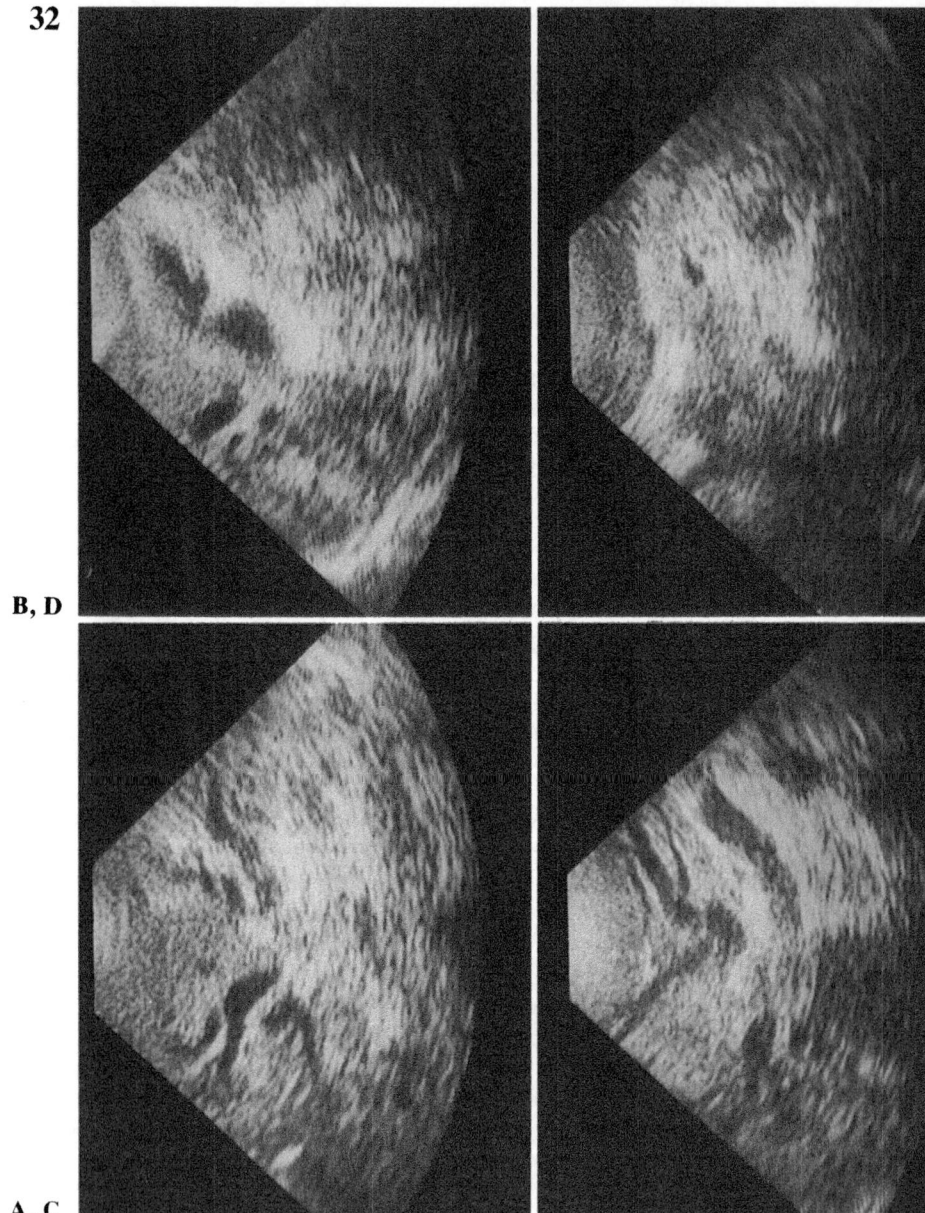

B, D

A, C

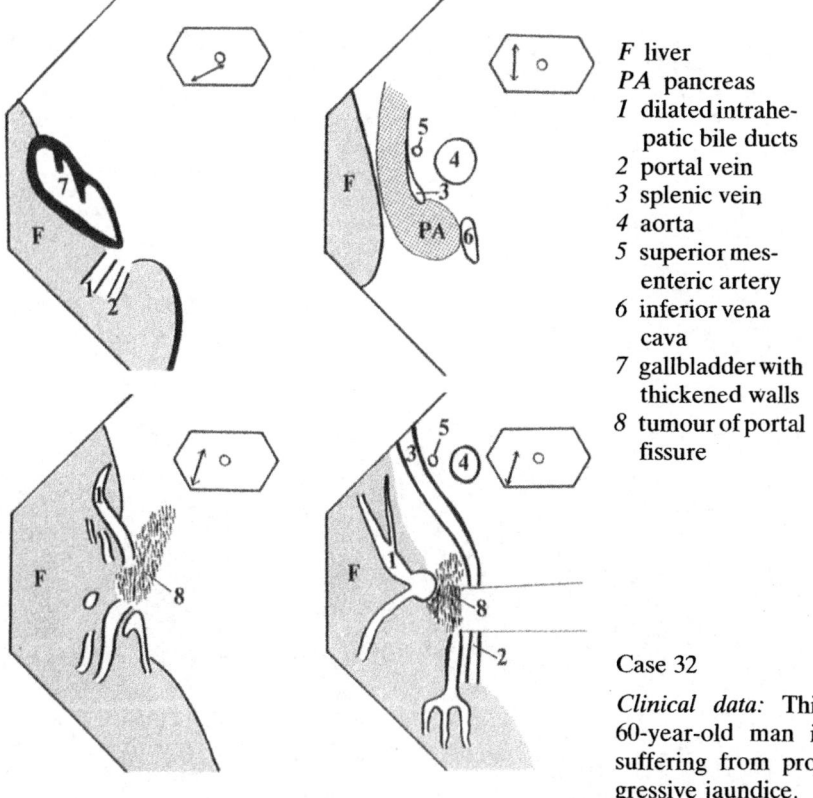

F liver
PA pancreas
1 dilated intrahe-
   patic bile ducts
2 portal vein
3 splenic vein
4 aorta
5 superior mes-
   enteric artery
6 inferior vena
   cava
7 gallbladder with
   thickened walls
8 tumour of portal
   fissure

Case 32

Clinical data: This 60-year-old man is suffering from progressive jaundice.

Description: Analysis of the images is easy. There is significant dilatation of the right and left hepatic ducts (10 mm) as well as of the intrahepatic biliary ducts. The bile duct is not visible, but at the level of the hilar junction there is a poorly delimited hyperechogenic formation, at which the dilated hepatic ducts terminate. The gallbladder is small and has thickened walls. Since the patient has fasted, this is a sign of gallbladder dysfunction. Note the presence of gallstones (Scan C). The portal vein shows normal shape and calibre (Scan B); the pancreas is also normal (Scan D).

Diagnosis: This is carcinoma of the main bile duct.

Comments: Carcinomas of the bile duct in man classically occur between the ages of 60 and 80 years. They are less frequent than carcinomas of the gallbladder and do not seem to depend upon the presence of gallstones. They are mainly well-differentiated adenocarcinomas. The preferential site is the bile duct, then comes the cystico-choledocal region, and then the hepatic duct. There exists a peculiar form in which the process involves the entire extra- and intrahepatic biliary system. The state of the gallbladder depends upon the site of the cancer. When the lesion is located in the bile duct, the gallbladder is voluminous and distended; in the other cases it is small, has thickened walls, or is entirely contracted.

32

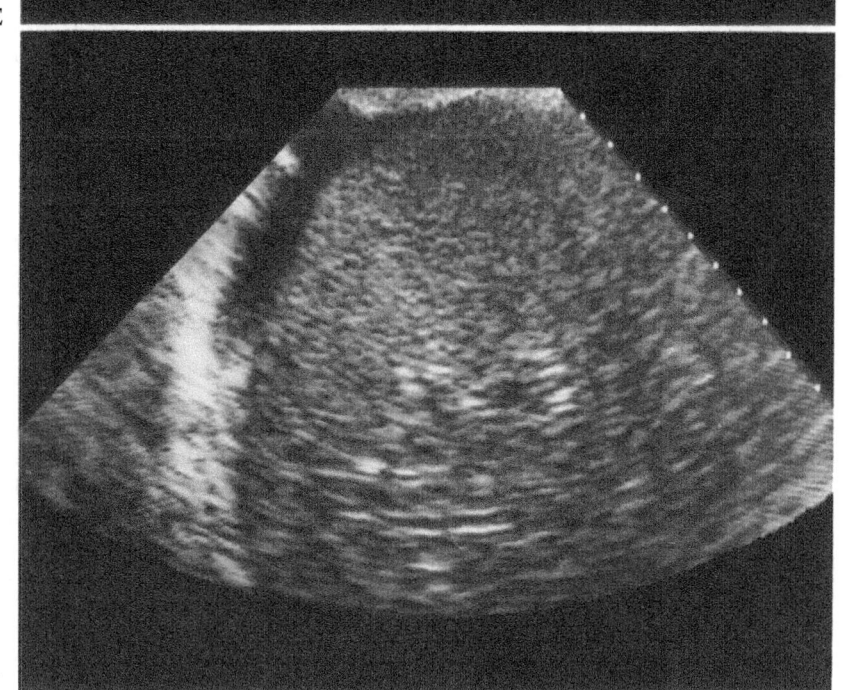

E

F

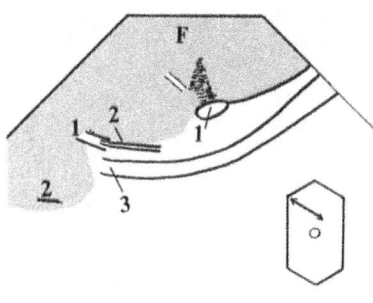

F liver   **32**
1 bile duct
2 internal drainage catheter
3 portal vein
4 interhepatodiaphragmatic fluid
5 diaphragm

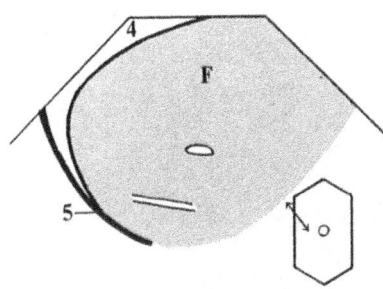

Case 32 (continue)

Clinical data: The same patient is shown, 3 weeks later.

Description: You must have noted the following three points:
– The biliary duct dilatation is reduced.
– There is a layer of fluid between the liver and the diaphragm (Scan F).
– Most importantly, there is a tubular structure above the portal vein. It corresponds to the internal biliary drainage catheter (Scan E).

Comments: Local and regional extension is rapid, with ascending propagation towards the intrahepatic bile ducts, effraction of the wall, invasion of the hepatic pedicle and metastases in the liver parenchyma.

    Although the ideal treatment is still exeresis, this is often impossible due to extension of the tumour or the patient's poor general status. Palliative treatment is then undertaken. Transtumoural drainage under endoscopic sonographic control with placement of a multiperforated catheter joining the dilated bile ducts and the duodenum is performed. This is combined with external bile drainage allowing repeated lavage. This method ensures anicteric survival. Complications occur frequently, however – contamination of the biliary tract, cholangitis, and bile leakage around the catheter.

33

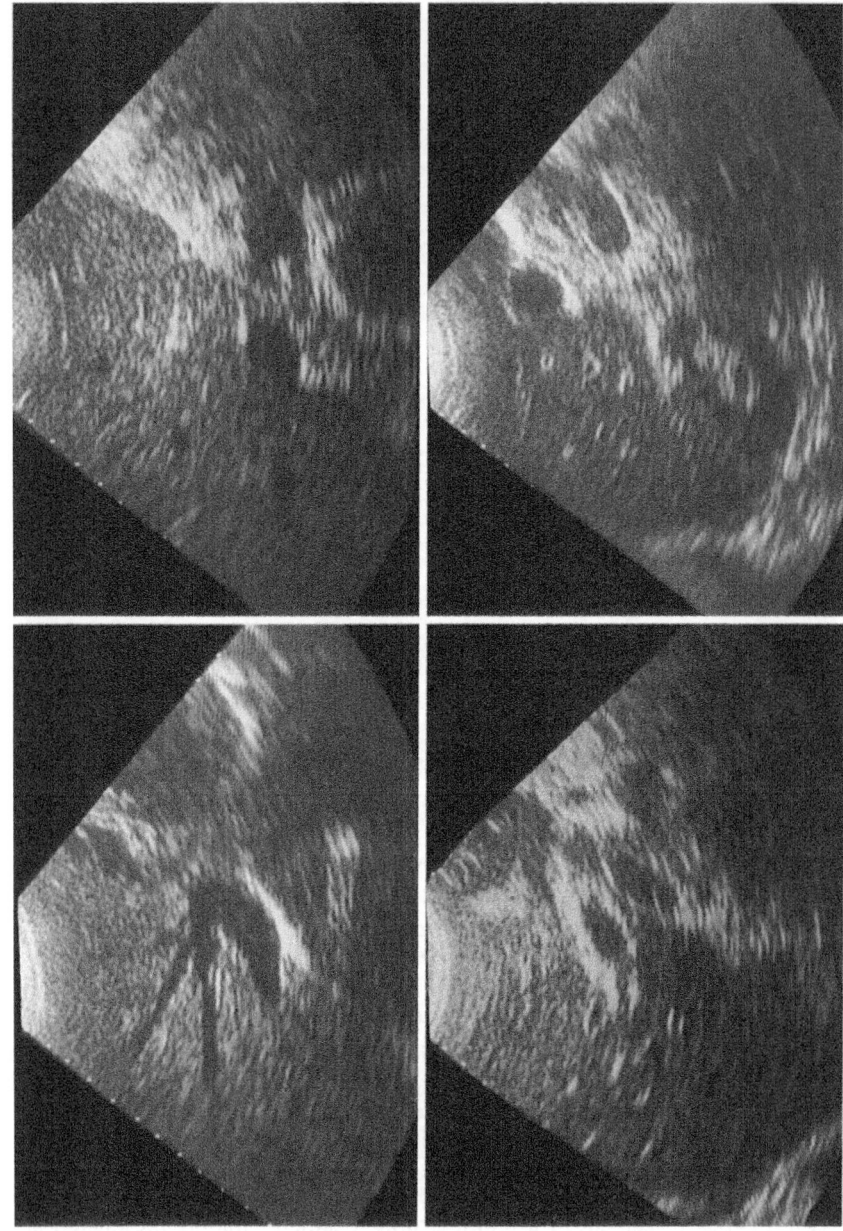

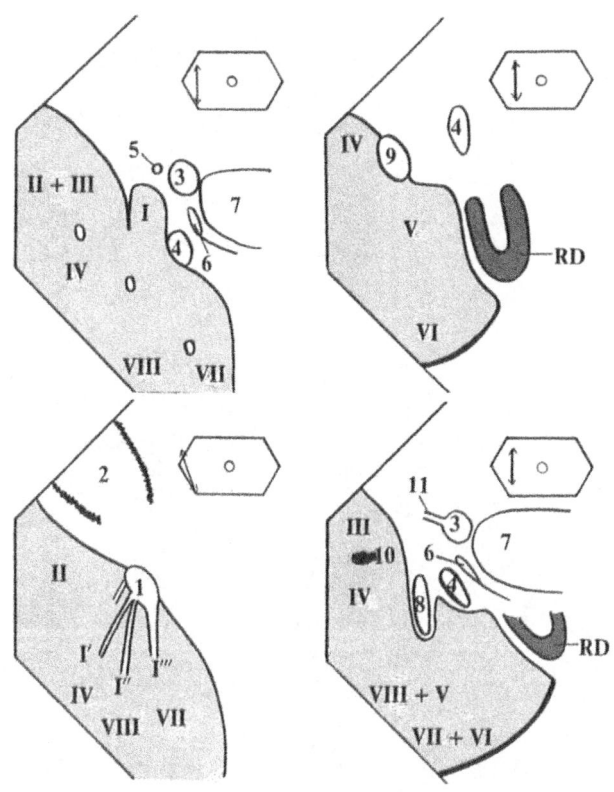

RD right kidney
Segment I is the caudate or Spigelian
   lobe
The anterior and inferior part of *seg-*
   ment IV is the quadrate lobe
1 inferior vena cava
1' left hepatic vein
1" middle hepatic vein
1''' right hepatic vein
2 cardiac cavities

3 aorta
4 inferior vena cava
5 origin of the coeliac trunk
6 right crus of diaphragm
7 vertebral body
8 portal vein
9 gallbladder
10 round ligament
11 origin of superior mesenteric
   artery

34

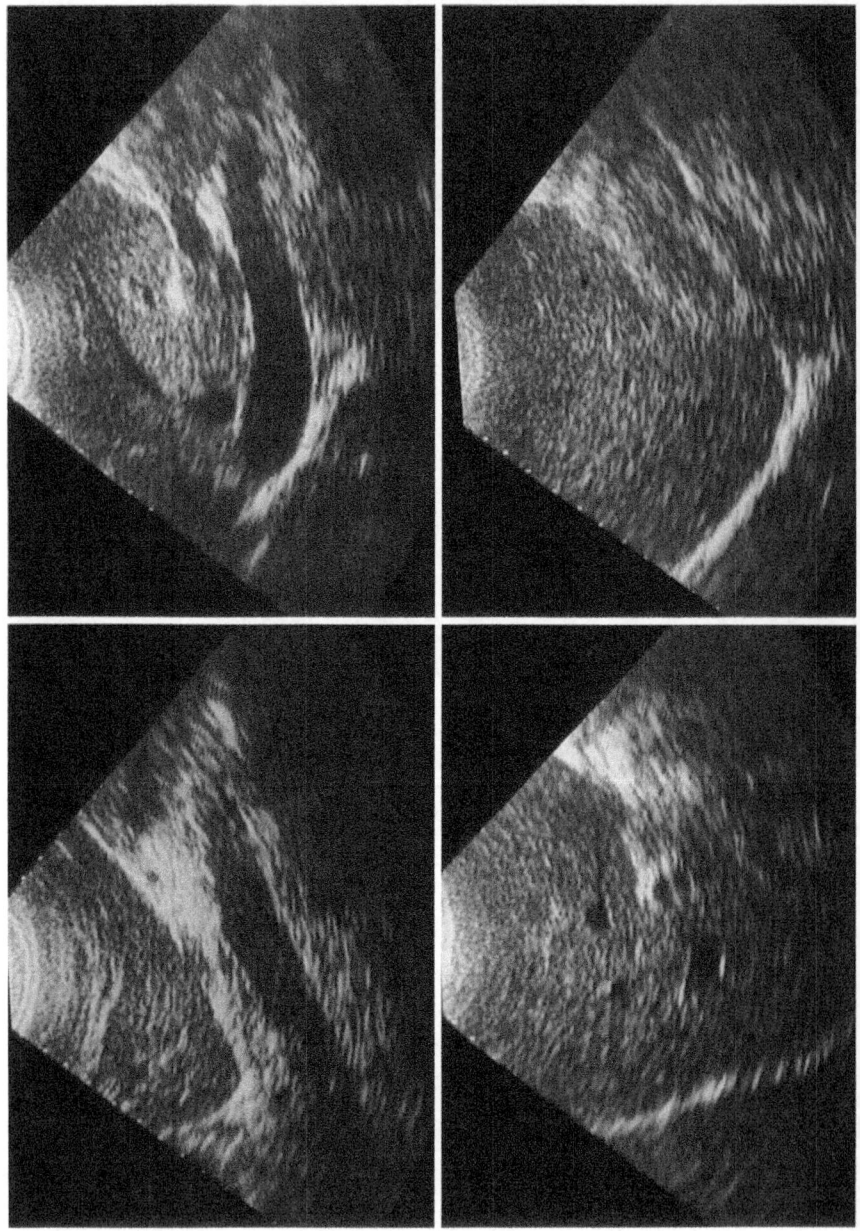

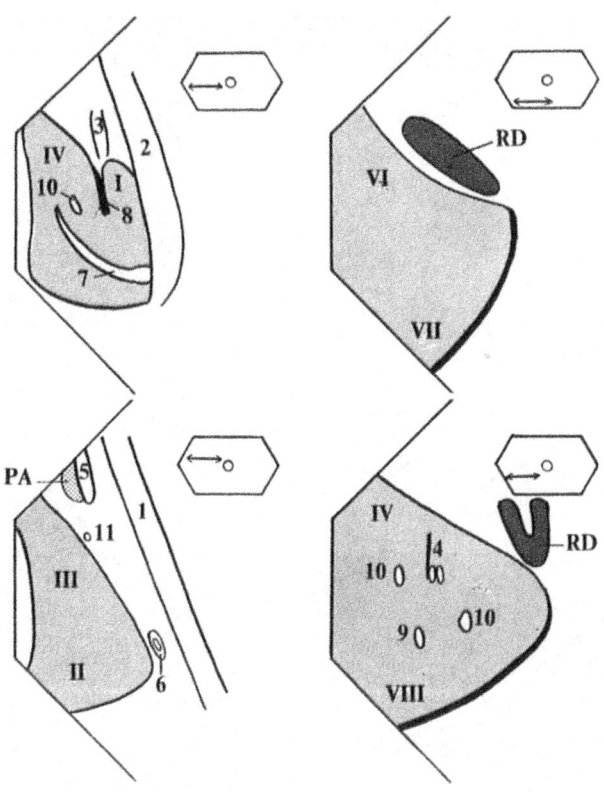

RD right kidney
PA pancreas
1 aorta
2 inferior vena cava
3 portal vein
4 hepatic pedicle (portal vein + common bile duct). Note the normal size of the common bile duct after cholecystectomy

5 superior mesenteric vein
6 lower portion of oesophagus
7 left hepatic vein
8 hyperechogenicity of portal fissure
9 right hepatic vein
10 branches of the portal vein
11 hepatic artery

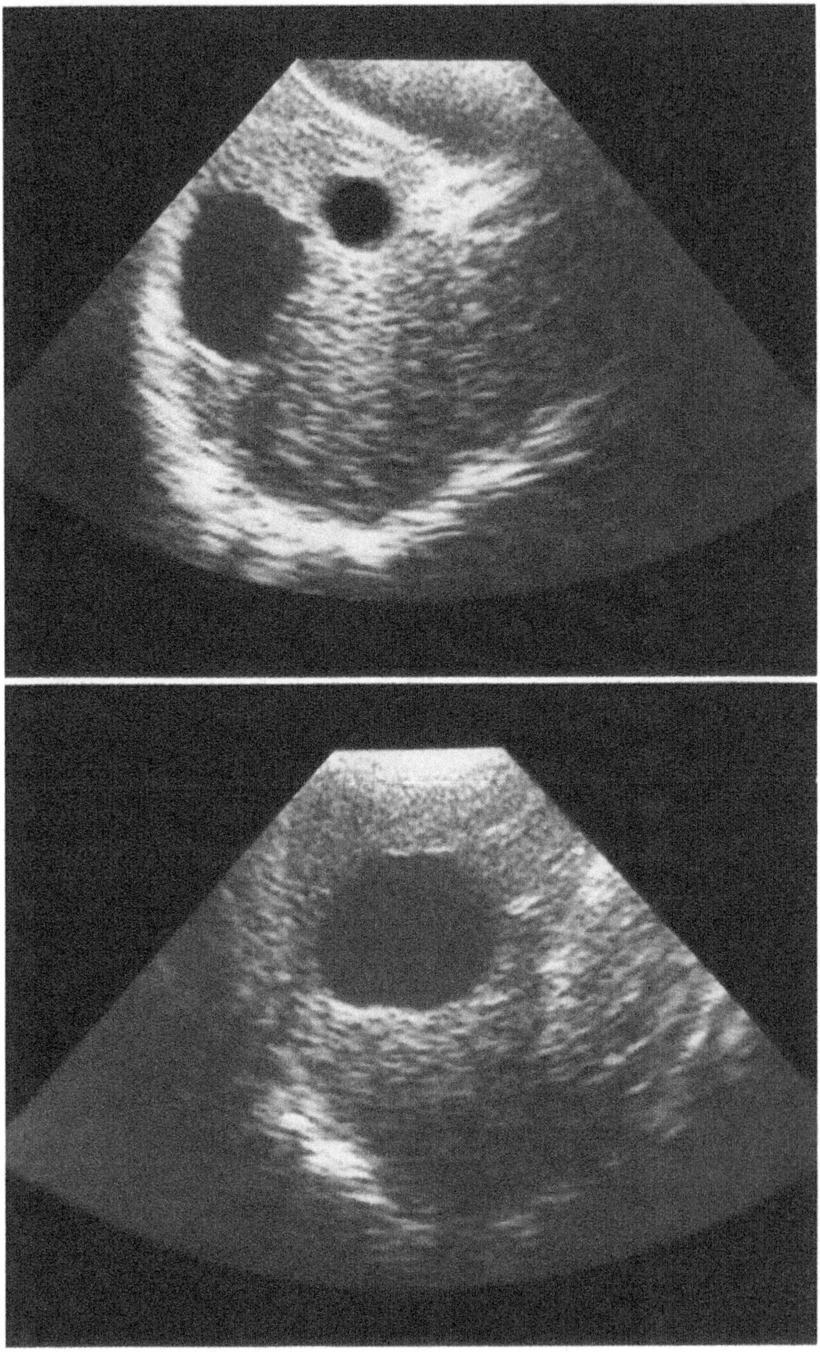

A

B

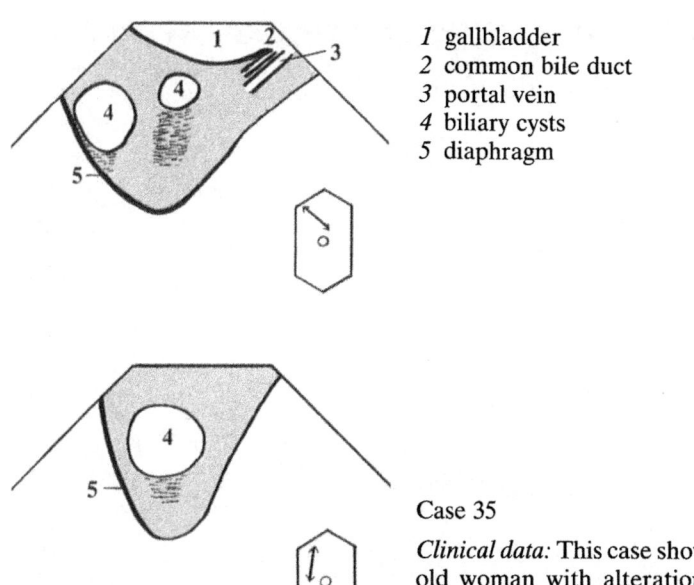

1 gallbladder
2 common bile duct
3 portal vein
4 biliary cysts
5 diaphragm

35

Case 35

Clinical data: This case shows a 70-year-old woman with alteration of general status.

Description: There are three rounded echo-free masses with a zone of relative echo enhancement. They measure respectively 4, 3 and 1.5 cm, and are located in segments VI and VII. They have smooth, sharply defined walls. The absence of internal echoes is affirmed by increasing the gain, a sign that the mass contains fluid. Note the different shape of the gallbladder (Scan A).

Diagnosis: This is easy: simple biliary cysts.

Comments: Biliary cysts are common (4% of liver sonograms) and are mainly encountered in middle-aged women. They may be congenital or, more rarely, acquired (post-traumatic, parasitic or inflammatory). They are usually solitary, but there can be several of them. The cyst is asymptomatic and is usually a chance finding; the mean size is 4 cm; however, there are also large cysts, up to 15 cm, that compress the bile ducts. Anatomically the cyst is a closed cavity which does not communicate with the biliary tree, is lined with biliary epithelium, and contains a clear liquid. The typical appearance described here does not require differential diagnosis. Sometimes, however, the walls are not smooth and the content is echogenic, possibly with septations, reflecting infectious or haemorrhagic complications. Such cases are difficult to differentiate from a necrotic metastasis, hydatid cyst or abscess.

Renal polycystosis is a rare autosomal dominant condition. In one third of cases there is hepatic and/or pancreatic polycystosis. Caroli's disease is different; it is a congenital condition characterized by cystic dilatation of the intrahepatic bile ducts, which may or may not be associated with dilatation of the extrahepatic bile ducts.

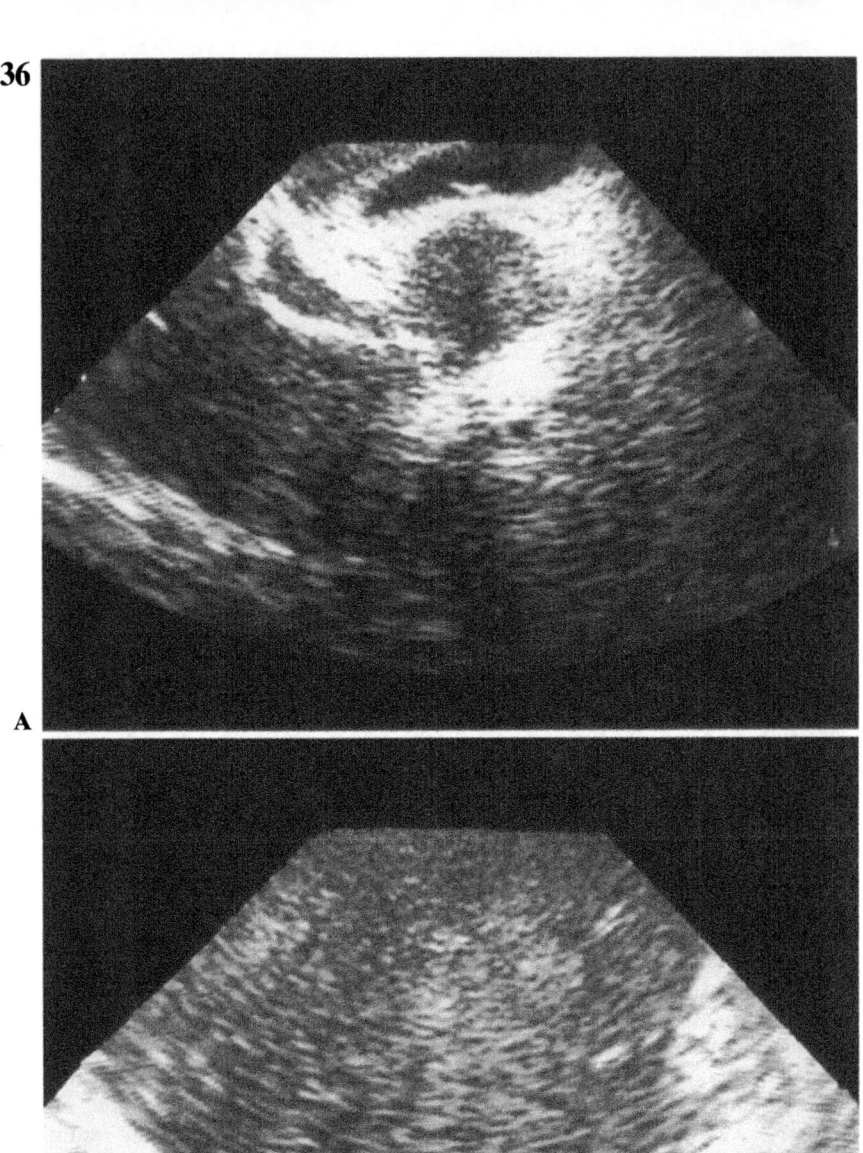

A

B

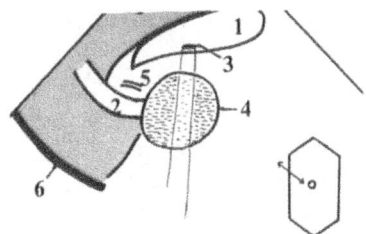

F liver **36**
1 gallbladder
2 portal vein
3 cholecystolithiasis
4 marked adenopathy
5 common bile duct
6 diaphragm

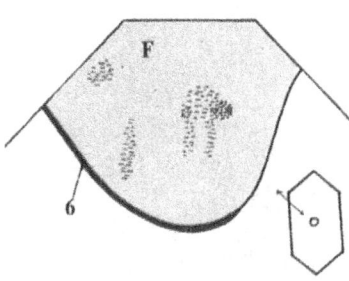

Case 36

Clinical data: A 55-year-old man requires re-evaluation of a bronchial neoplasm.

Description: You should see three pathological elements.

– A hilar mass is situated at the level of the initial portion of the portal vein (Scan A). It is rounded, solid, of homogenous echostructure, hypoechogenic and clearly delineated. Its diameter is 3 cm. You have easily diagnosed lithiasis of the gallbladder.

– In hepatic segments VI and VII there are two irregularly shaped hyperechogenic areas, which are poorly delimited and of the infiltrative type. There ist no hepatomegaly, and the rest of the hepatic parenchyma is normal.

Diagnosis: This is the classical appearance of hepatic metastases with hilar adenopathy.

Comments: Hepatic metastases are the most frequent tumours of the liver (18 times more frequent than primary tumours).
The sonographic appearance is very variable, and the observed lesions are not specific. We shall see several cases. The form described here is common (30%–37%, depending on the authors). Hepatomegaly is inconstant. It depends upon the site and, mainly, the extent of the lesion.
  The most frequent secondary locations of bronchial neoplasms are the adrenal glands. The liver is the third most common location, after lymph-node invasion.

37

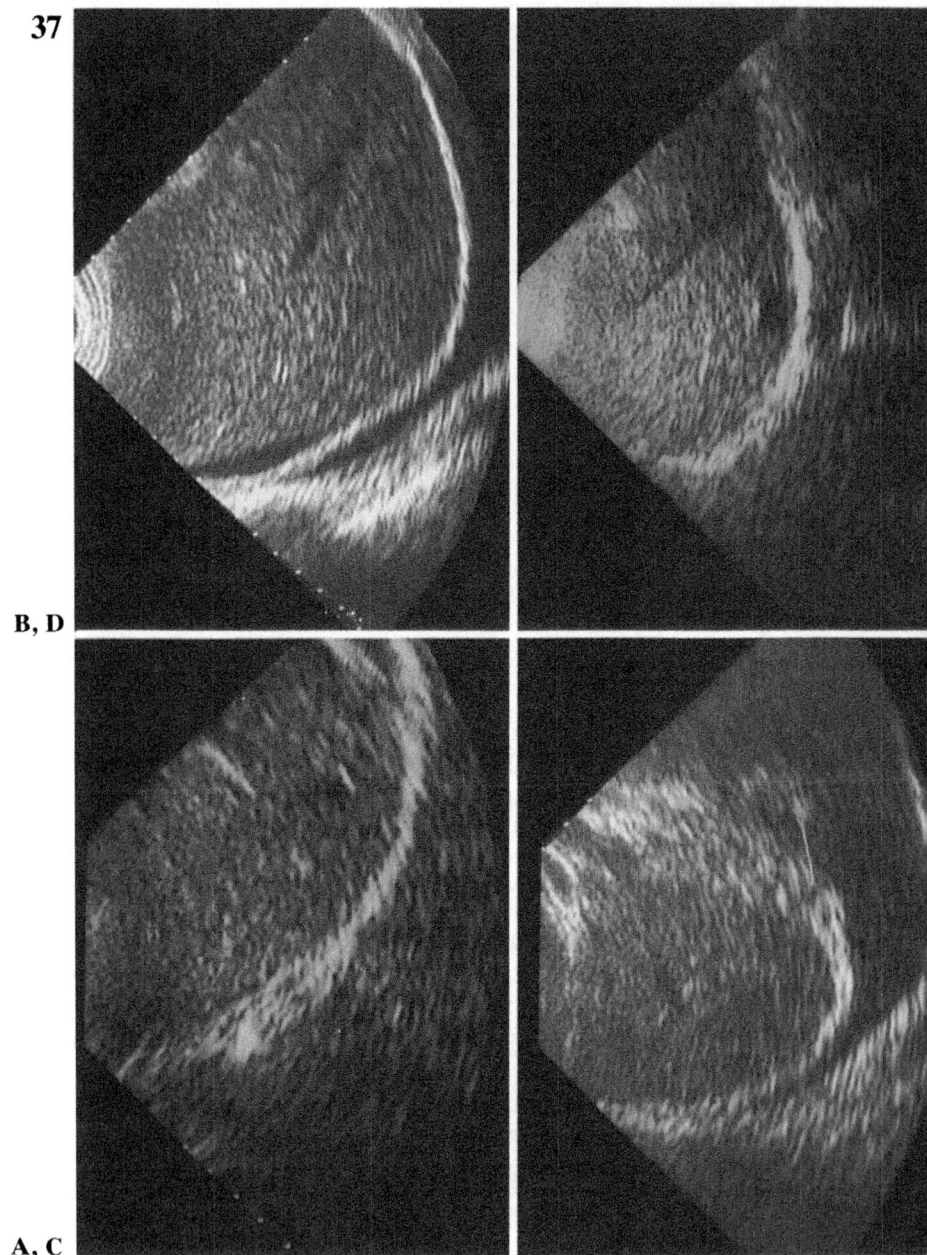

B, D

A, C

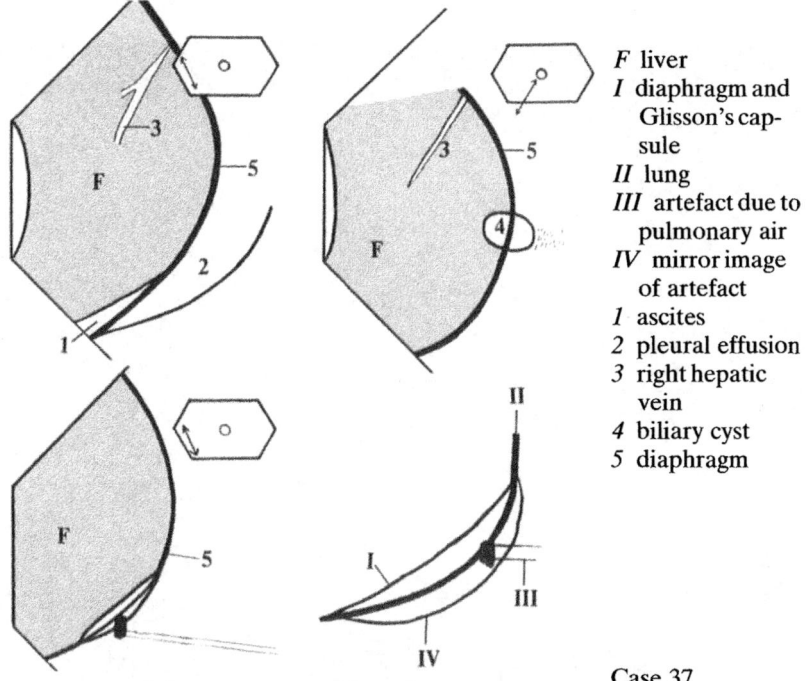

F liver
I diaphragm and Glisson's capsule
II lung
III artefact due to pulmonary air
IV mirror image of artefact
1 ascites
2 pleural effusion
3 right hepatic vein
4 biliary cyst
5 diaphragm

Case 37

In all abdominal sonograms, the diaphragm is visualized as a single thick hyperechogenic, curvilinear image above the liver. In 80% of normal patients one can actually distinguish three hyperechogenic lines in the posterosuperior and right lateral portion, especially when the patient has been instructed to take a deep breath. These three lines are seen over a variable length; they unite at each extremity (Scan A). The hyperechogenic image with posterior shadowing, or "reverberation artefact" is due to air in the lungs and comes from the median line; it is inconstant. In vitro studies have shown that the internal line corresponds to the liver capsule-diaphragm complex, and the median line to the pleura-lung complex. The external line is unreal: it is the mirror-image artefact. The median line acts as a mirror reflecting the internal line. This artefact may result from interposition of pleural fluid in the subpulmonary space due to increased negative intrathoracic pressure and/or to the shape of the diaphragm. It occurs only in the vicinity of strongly reflective interfaces such as diaphragm and pulmonary air.

When there is pleural effusion alone (Scan C) the lung is shifted, as is the reverberation artefact. Only one line or two parallel lines will remain. The mirror-image artefact disappears.

When there is pleural effusion and ascites (Scan B), there is then only one thick, hyperechogenic line corresponding to the diaphragm. The same is seen when there is ascites alone.

The mirror-image artefact can be responsible for a pseudomass. It results from the supradiaphragmatic projection of an infradiaphragmatic mass. (Scan D shows a biliary cyst which appears to be situated on both sides of the diaphragm.)

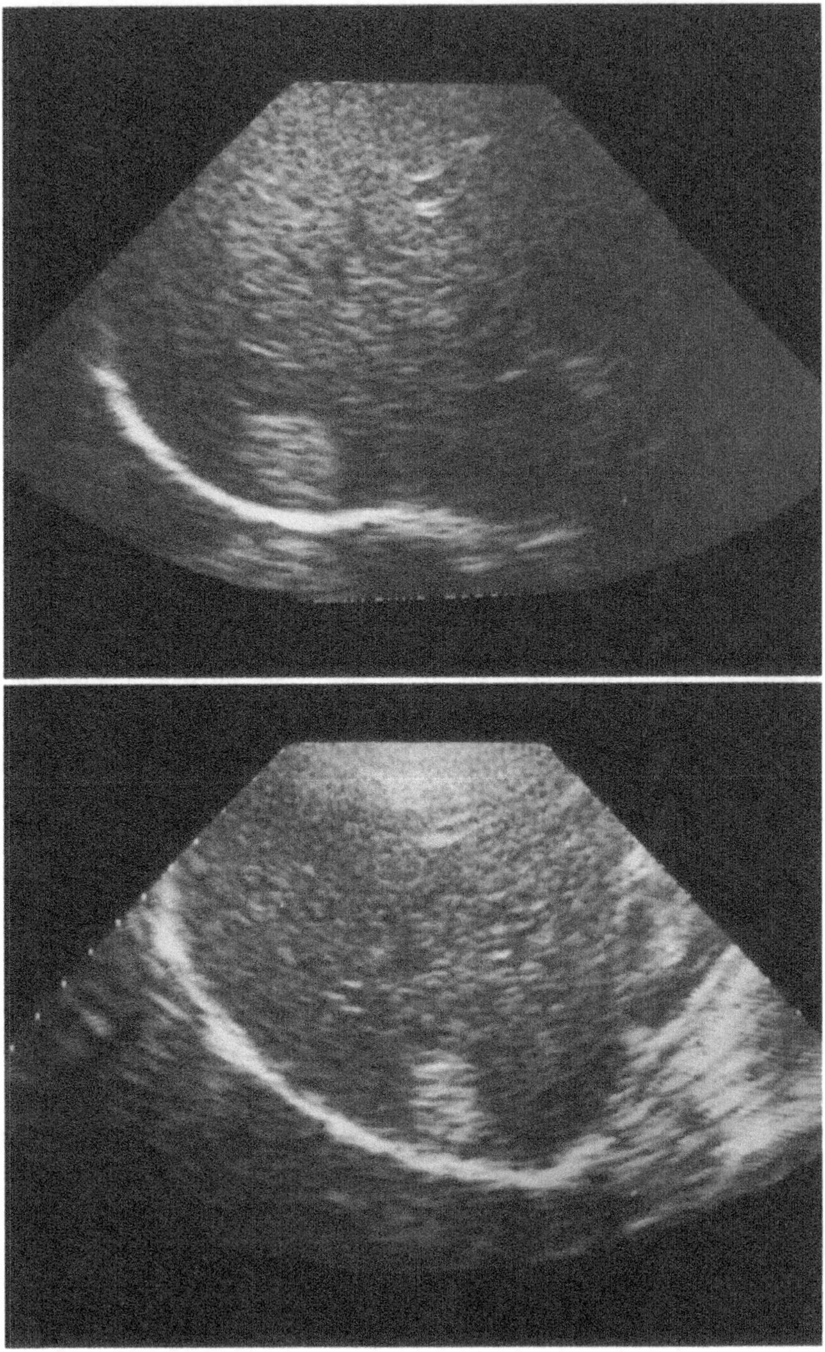

A

B

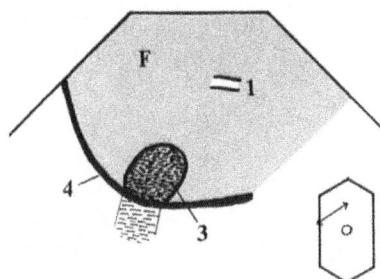

F liver **38**
RD right kidney
1 portal vessel
2 hepatic vessel (note there is no visualization of the walls)
3 angioma
4 diaphragm

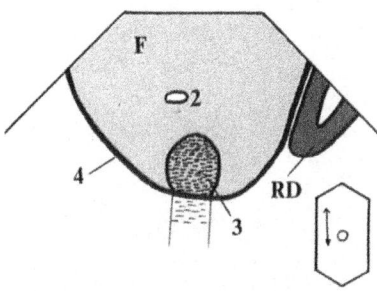

Case 38

Clinical data: This 35-year-old woman
has poorly defined abdominal pain.

Description: Analysis of the sonograms is easy. There is a hyperechogenic, homogeneous, rounded mass with sharp borders, measuring 2 cm in diameter. It is located against the dome of the diaphragm, in segment VII. It is isolated, and the surrounding hepatic parenchyma is normal. Note the presence of the mirror-image (Scan A).

Diagnosis: This is easy: haemangioma of the liver.

Comments: Haemangioma of the liver is the most frequent benign liver tumour. It is found in about 0.4%−7% of postmortem examinations. It occurs most often in women, and in three out of four cases the angioma is situated in the right hepatic lobe. Three sonographic patterns are described:
− This typical case taken as an example shows the most frequent pattern. The hyperechogenicity of the lesion is due to the numerous vascular interfaces. The presence of acoustic enhancement is described as supporting the diagnosis of angioma, but it is not specific. As a matter of fact, it is also found with small hepatocarcinomas. It is also inconstant, being visible only in haemangiomas of at least 2.5 cm diameter. Acoustic enhancement is due to the low attenuation factor of this fluid mass. In this form the angiomas are 1−5 cm in size. Some nodules are strongly reflective and may cast shadow, even in the absence of calcifiation (Case 31 A)
− In 20% of cases the angioma is heterogeneous with echogenic and echo-poor areas and poorly delineated borders. It is larger, 5−12 cm in size.
− Uncommonly there are anechogenic, rounded areas, of small or medium size, which mimic simple cysts.

39

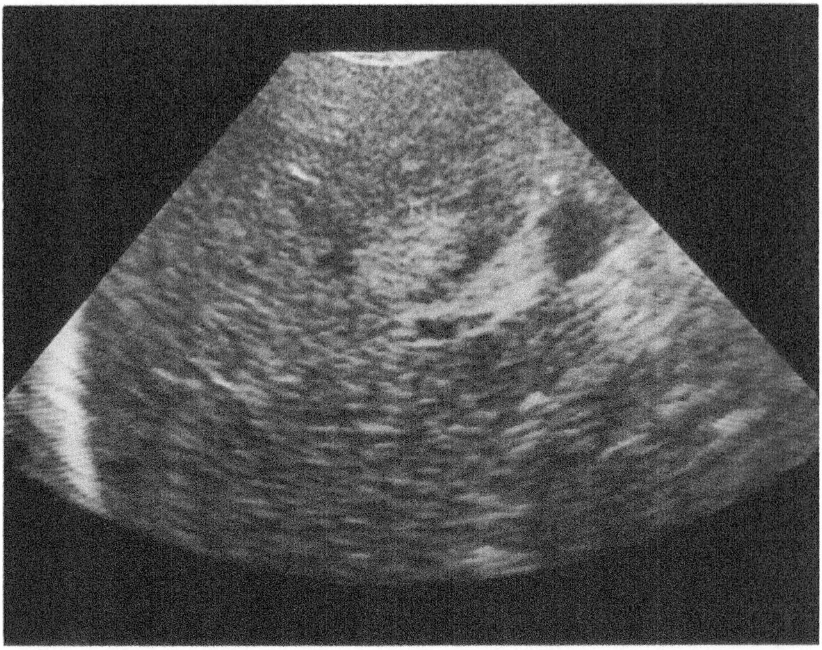

40

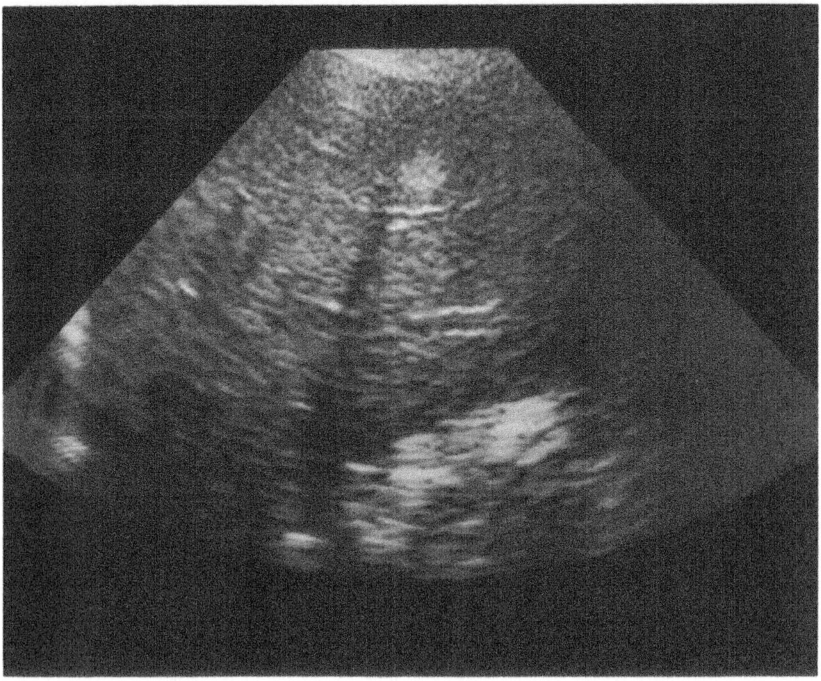

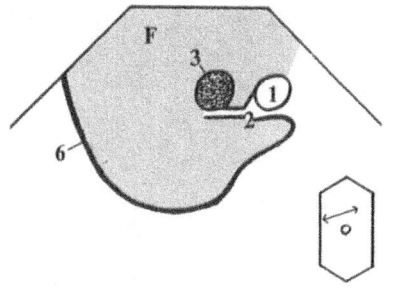

F liver **39**
RD right kidney **40**
1 gallbladder
2 portal vein
3 hepatic angioma
4 distal branches of portal vein (note
    visualization of the walls)
5 diaphragm

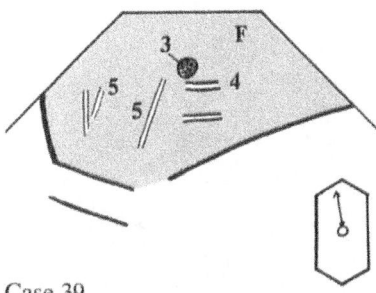

Case 39

Clinical data: A 40-year-old woman has axillary adenopathy.

Case 40

Clinical data: A 50-year-old man has unexplained pyrexia.

Description: In both cases there is a hyperechogenic image with well-delineated borders, which is homogeneous and shows an identical appearance to Case 38.

Diagnostic: This is haemangioma of the liver. Note the absence of relative echo enhancement in both cases. In fact, the lesions are small, 2 cm and 1 cm respectively.

Comments: Small haemangiomas are asymptomatic and are usually chance findings. Most often isolated, they are multiple in 10% of cases. Larger haemangiomas are usually revealed by pain in the hypochondrium subsequent to haemorrhage or to intratumoural thrombosis. The heterogeneous pattern of large haemangiomas is due to the presence of blood-filled cystic pouches.

When there is a typical pattern but no particular clinical data, the diagnosis is easy and must be definite. Sonographic survey can be proposed.

When there is a history of neoplasia, or when the image is atypical, one should rule out a primary or secondary malignant tumour, focal nodular hyperplasia, and adenoma.

Angiography seems superior to computed tomography for visualization of abnormal vessels. When there is an extensive haemangioma, embolization seems advisable.

41

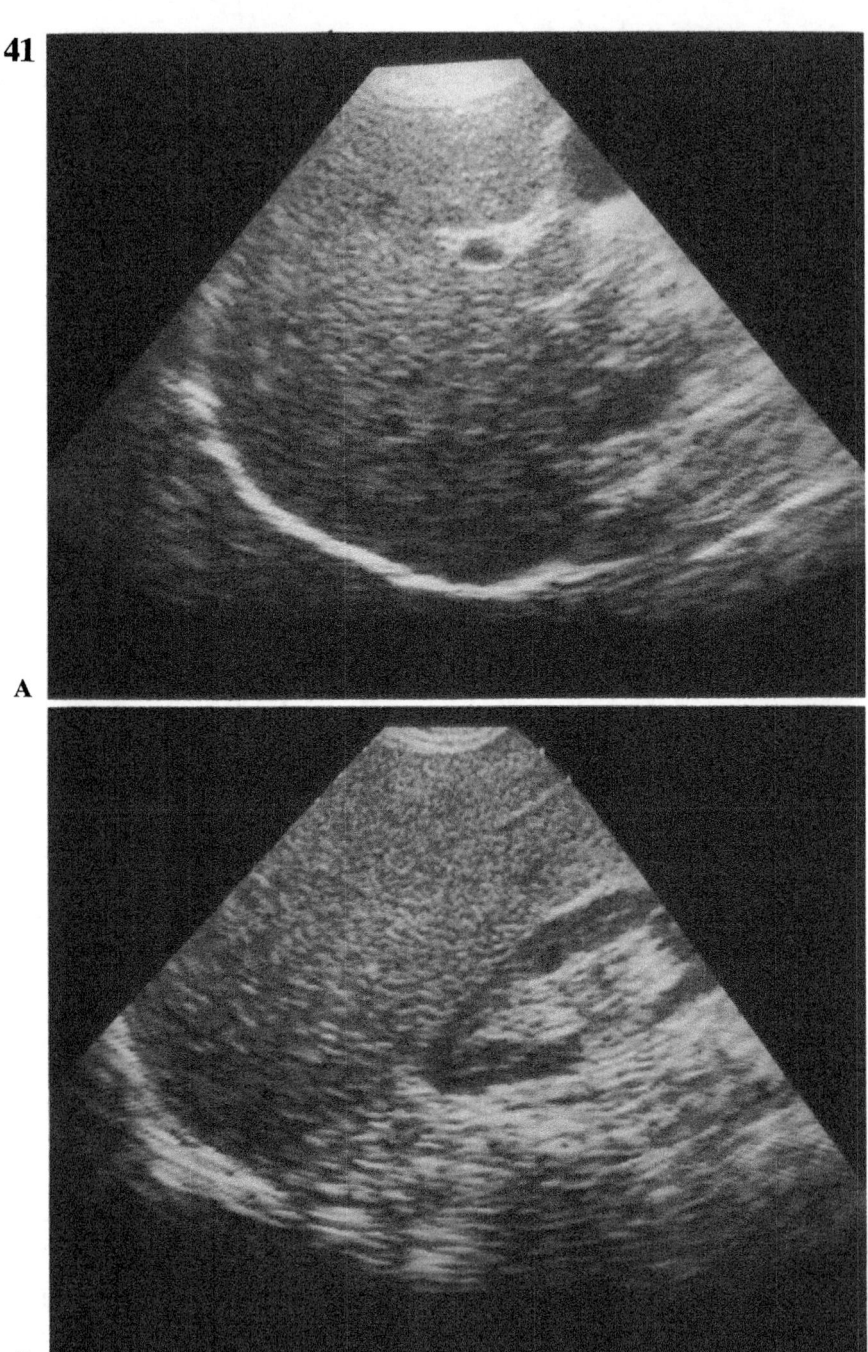

A

B

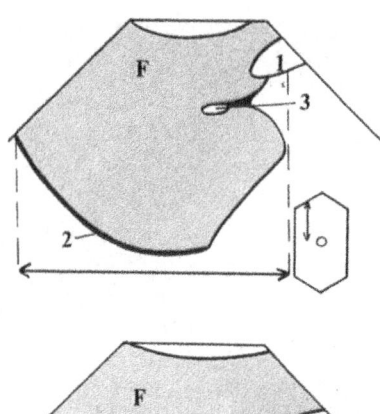

F liver   *2* dome of diaphragm **41**
RD right kidney   *3* portal vein
1 gallbladder

Case 41

The notion of hepatomegaly is clinico-pathologic, based upon the weight of the liver at postmortem examination, and upon the patient's age, weight and sex. The size of the liver diminishes with age.

Assessment of hepatomegaly is one of the most frequently requested studies in sonography. Several authors have proposed that assessment be based upon multiple landmarks, and measurements and calculations of volume, which are difficult to carry out in routine practice. An easy and reliable method must be found.

Correlations with postmortem ultrasound studies have yielded the most precise value from a parasagittal scan passing through the midclavicular line. The distance between the highest point of the diaphragmatic dome and the antero-inferior border of the liver must be below or equal to 13 cm in the dorsal and in lateral decubitus positions. Values above 15 cm are pathological. This measurement is unreliable when there is ascites or a tumour in the antero-inferior part of the liver (Scan A).

There are also other criteria which are easier to utilize:
– On transverse scans, the thickness of the hepatic parenchyma on the antero-posterior line tangential to the left aspect of the vertebral bodies must be below or equal to 5 cm.
– The antero-inferior extremity of the right hepatic lobe must not extend beyond the right kidney. In practice this criterion is not reliable, since in thin and old women the right liver extends beyond the kidney, without this having pathological significance (Scan B).
– Finally, there is a useful criterion: the exploration field measures 16 cm, and the whole of the normal liver can be shown on the screen.

The liver has numerous anatomical and topographical variants. The most frequent are aplasia of the left lobe and hypoplasia of the right lobe. Riedel's lobe is often seen in thin and old women. It is a process extending from the right lobe, distinct from the accessory lobe and from segments V and VI. It is attached to the liver by a parenchymatous neck or by a fibrous pedicle. Its etiology is uncertain. Its identification is usually easy, since the echostructure is the same as that of the liver. It may sometimes be difficult to differentiate from a vertical liver.

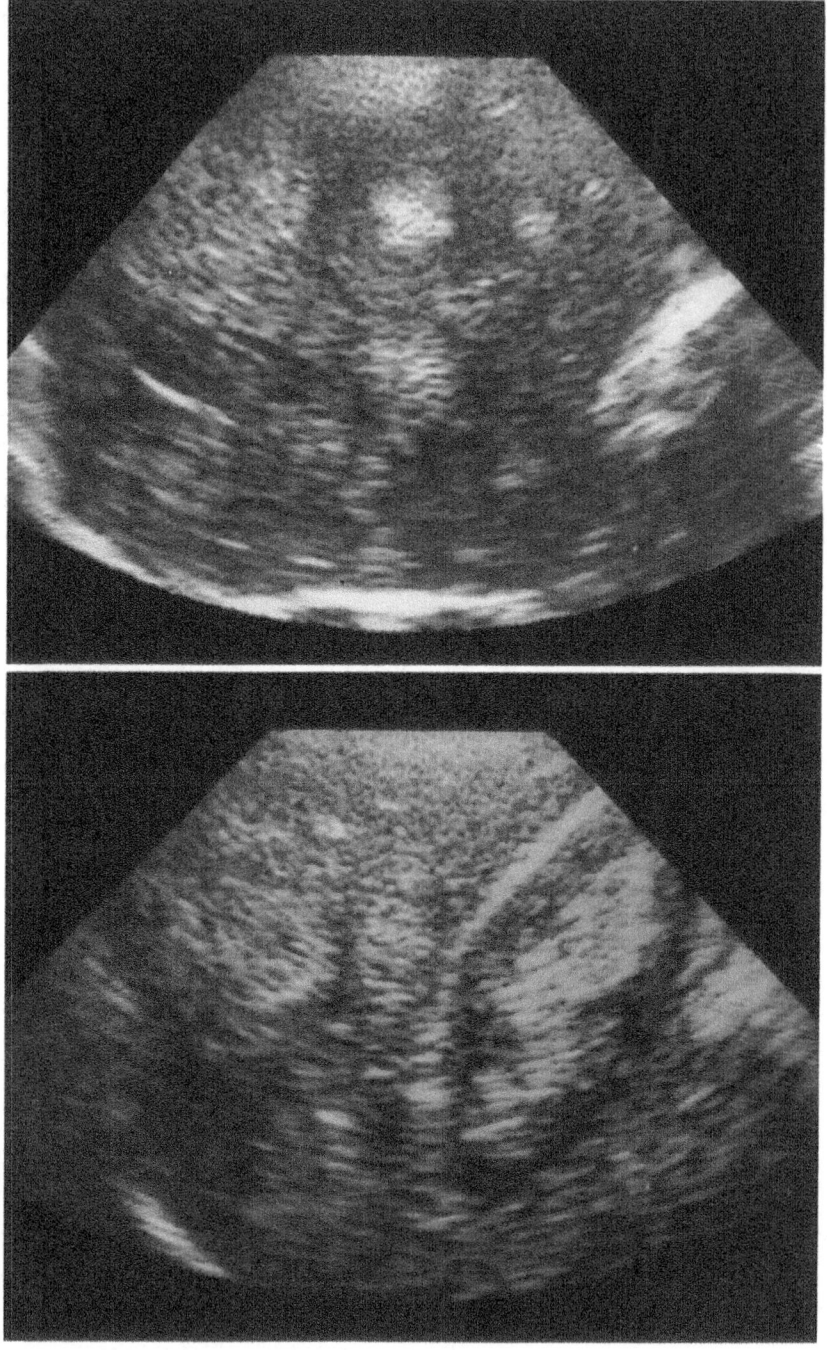

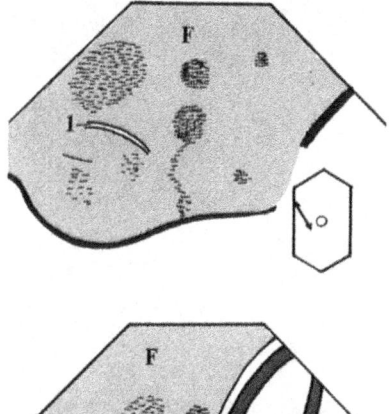

F liver
RD right kidney
1 branch of hepatic vein

42

Case 42

Clinical data: A 60-year-old man who had had surgery for carcinoma of the sigmoid colon 1 year before, is undergoing investigations for reassessment.

Description: Note the numerous hyperechogenic areas, homogeneous or heterogeneous, more or less well-delineated, invading the entire right hepatic lobe. The left lobe is normal; there is no hepatomegaly.

Diagnosis: The lesion is obvious: hepatic metastases.

Comments: This hyperechogenic pattern of multiple metastases is classically known as the "snow-storm" appearance. Some tumours – colorectal, hepatocarcinoma and digestive carcinoid – have hepatic sites which remain isolated for a long time. The location of the lesions does not depend upon the type of primary cancer. Usually, the size of the metastases is inversely proportional to their number. It is necessary to point out the importance of hepatic metastases; although they are not the direct cause of death, they are a necessary stage for tertiary spread of the cancer via vascular dissemination (diffuse carcinomatosis).

Intratumoural calcifications are rare. They are seen in colloid cancers, in colonic and in gastric carcinomas, in endocrine tumours of the pancreas and in carcinomas of the ovary. They can also be seen after chemo- and radiotherapy. They appear as intense echoes with acoustic shadowing.

43

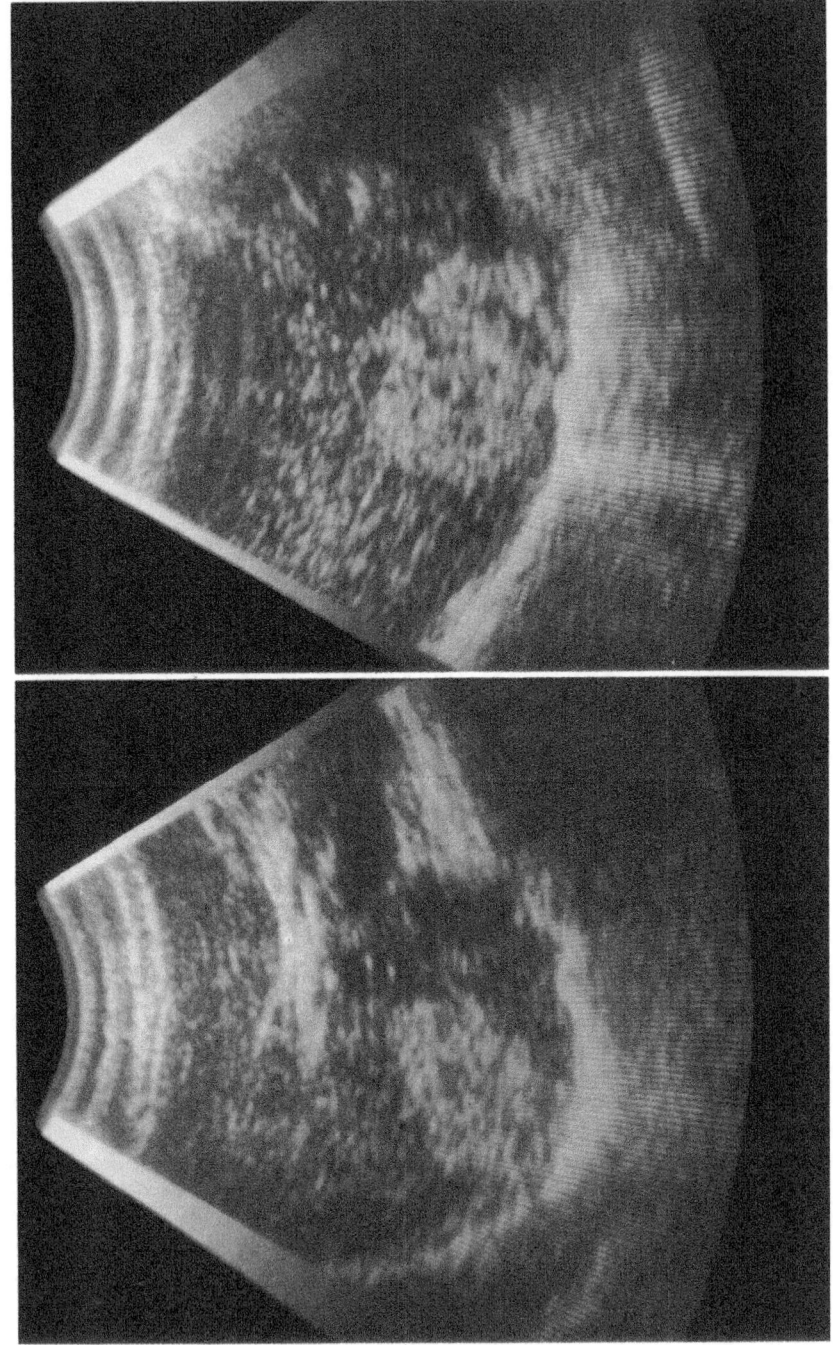

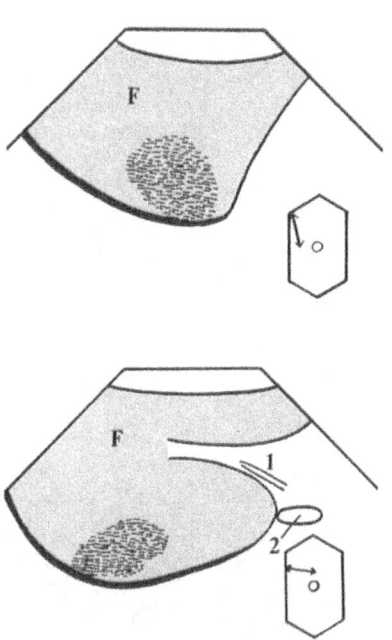

Case 43

Clinical data: A 35-year-old woman, suffering from sudden pain in the right hypochondrium, has no remarkable history.

Description: There is a large, hyperechogenic, heterogeneous mass with sharp but irregular borders in segment VI. There is no deformation of the diaphragm. The sonogram is otherwise normal.

Diagnosis: With ultrasound alone, diagnosis is impossible. Several benign tumours can be suggested: adenoma, focal nodular hyperplasia, haemangioma. A secondary lesion cannot be definitely excluded. It was a hamartoma of the liver.

Comments: Hamartomas of the liver are uncommon benign primary tumours. They include all elements of the hepatic parenchyma to variable degrees. Their echo-patterns are numerous and misleading. In some cases even the pathologist hesitates with the diagnosis of adenoma when the hepatocytes predominate. Hamartomas with biliary predominance show a liquid pattern. Hamartomas of the mesenchymatous type have cystic formations.

There is no specific sonological sign. These tumours are usually large, uni-or multifocal, hyperechogenic and heterogeneous. Angiography may be helpful.

Hamartomas are usually asymptomatic and present in two ways: with an abdominal mass, or with abdominal pain secondary to intratumoural bleeding.

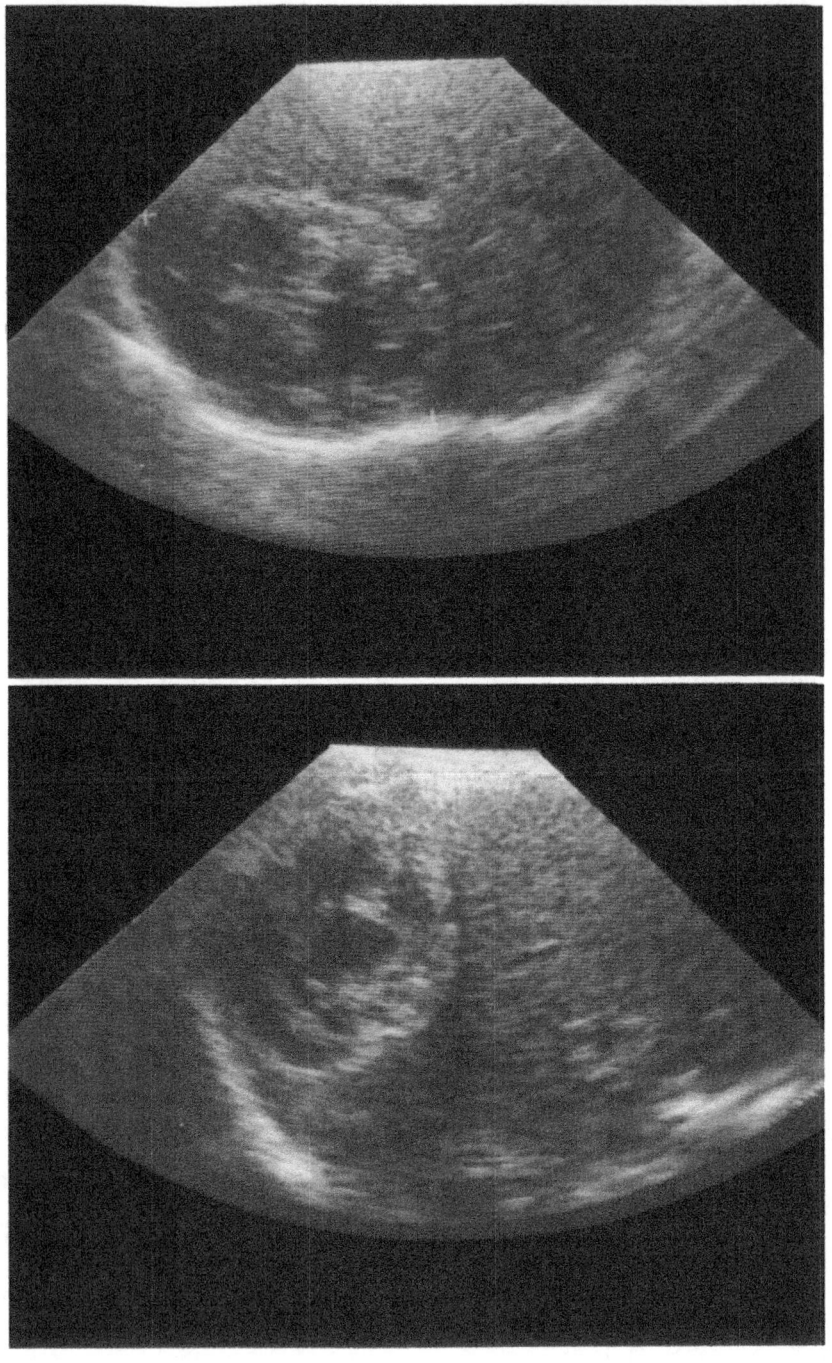

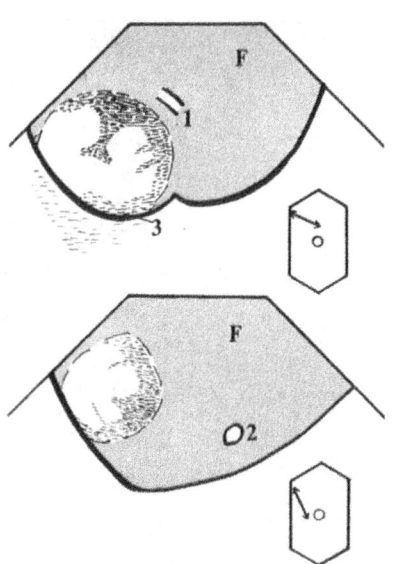

F liver
1 hepatic branch
2 portal branch
3 deformation of the diaphragm

44

Case 44

Clinical data: This 30-year-old Algerian woman is suffering from pain in the right hypochondrium.

Description: The lesion is obvious. There is a large mass of 10.5 cm diameter situated in segment VIII, causing deformation of the diaphragm. Its echostructure is heterogeneous – It is a fluid structure (note the relative echo-enhancement), containing hyperechogenic areas, especially in the periphery, anarchically distributed towards the centre of the lesion.

Diagnosis: This is easy: hydatid cyst of the liver, type IV.

Comments: Let us recall the five echo-patterns of hydatid cysts. Type I corresponds to the early form, with a purely fluid type image. The presence of localized thickening of the wall permits one to exclude a simple hepatic cyst. Type II corresponds to localized or complete duplication of the capsule, which appears as a "floating membrane". Type III ist a septated cyst. Type IV is polymorphous and most misleading, sometimes having an intensely echogenic structure, or a mixted-type structure (shown here). This appearance is due to the detachment of the proligerous membrane in the lumen of the cyst, producing several folds. The liquid areas within the solid masses correspond to daughter cysts. Type IV is a calcified cyst.

Only visualization of the capsule, with or without daughter cysts, allows definite ultrasound diagnosis. Otherwise, serologic tests are indispensable.

In countries where the disease is not endemic, there is a risk of false-negative diagnoses, whereas in countries where it is endemic false-positive diagnoses are common.

Do not forget that with very large cysts it may be difficult to indicate the organ of origin.

45

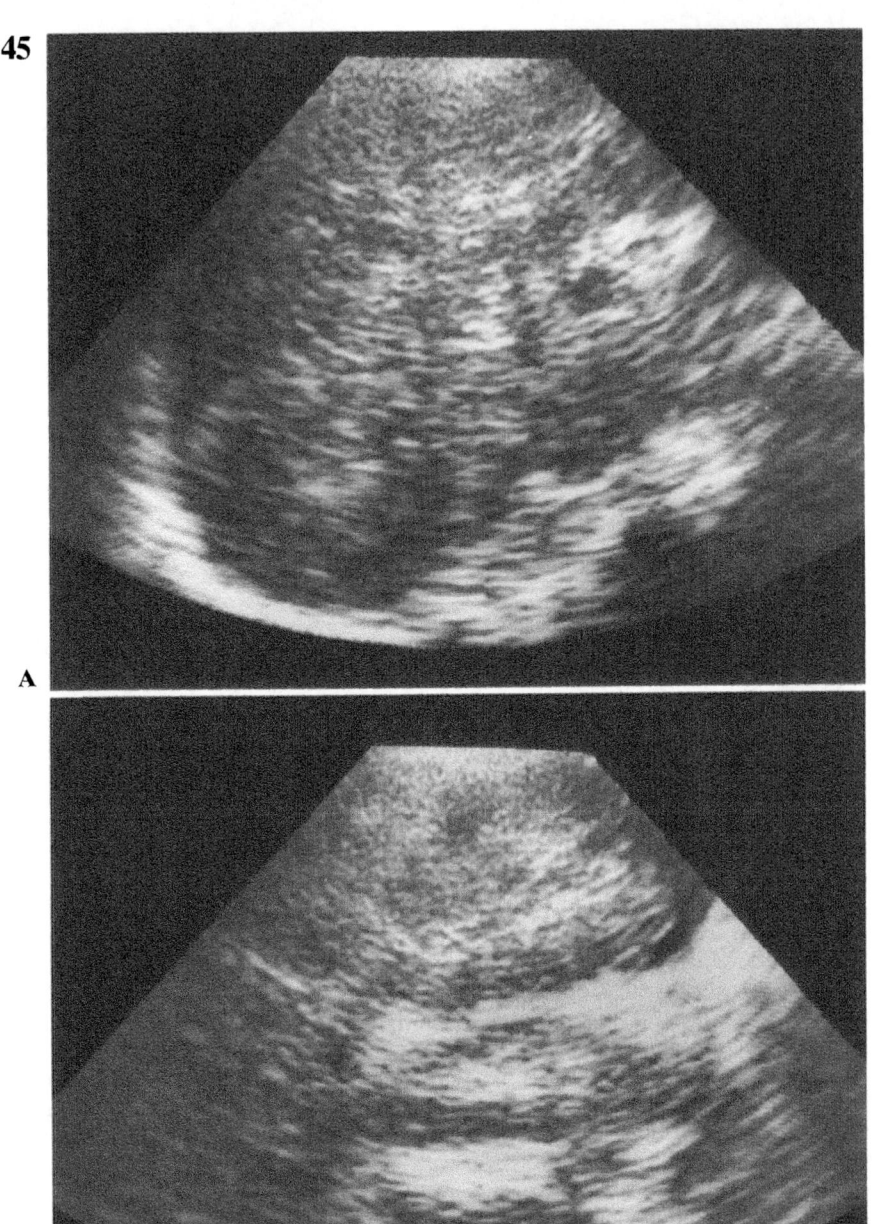

A

B

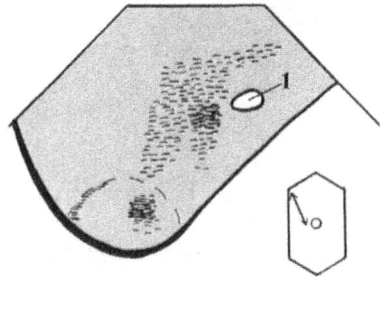

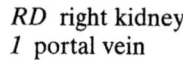
RD right kidney
1 portal vein

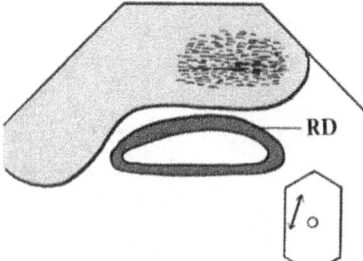

Case 45

Clinical data: A 70-year-old man has alteration of general status, pain in the right hypochondriac region and hepatomegaly with pain on palpation.

Description: Analysis of the scans is simple. There is remodelling of the entire right hepatic lobe, with poorly defined hyperechogenic areas. There is obviously hepatomegaly, since the right border of the liver is seen to be far up under the ribs and to compress the right kidney (Scan B). There is no anomaly in the left lobe.

Diagnosis: These images suggest two hypotheses: hepatoma or metastases. In fact, it was a diffuse hepatoma of the right hepatic lobe.

Comments: The hepatoma is the most common primary liver tumour. It is rare in Europe (3% of all cancers), and occurs in men with a history of alcoholism. It may however occur in normal livers in 25% of cases. All types of cirrhosis can be complicated by hepatoma: in decreasing order of frequency, post-hepatitic, haemochromatosic and ethylic.

The ultrasound patterns are not specific: hypo, hyperechogenic or mixed. There are sometimes calcifications. The tumour may be localized, and then poorly delimited, or invade the entire liver (in the latter case, diagnosis using ultrasound is very difficult). In the localized forms, there are very often intrahepatic metastases. Usually, sonography underrates the exact extent of the lesions.

Angiography shows a hypervascularized structure of tumoural type and demonstrates that ultrasound-guided fine-needle biopsy is contraindicated, which permits one to avoid haemorrhagic complications.

Sonography alone does not permit definite diagnosis. The clinical context and, especially, significantly increased serum alpha foeto-protein levels should always be taken into account.

46

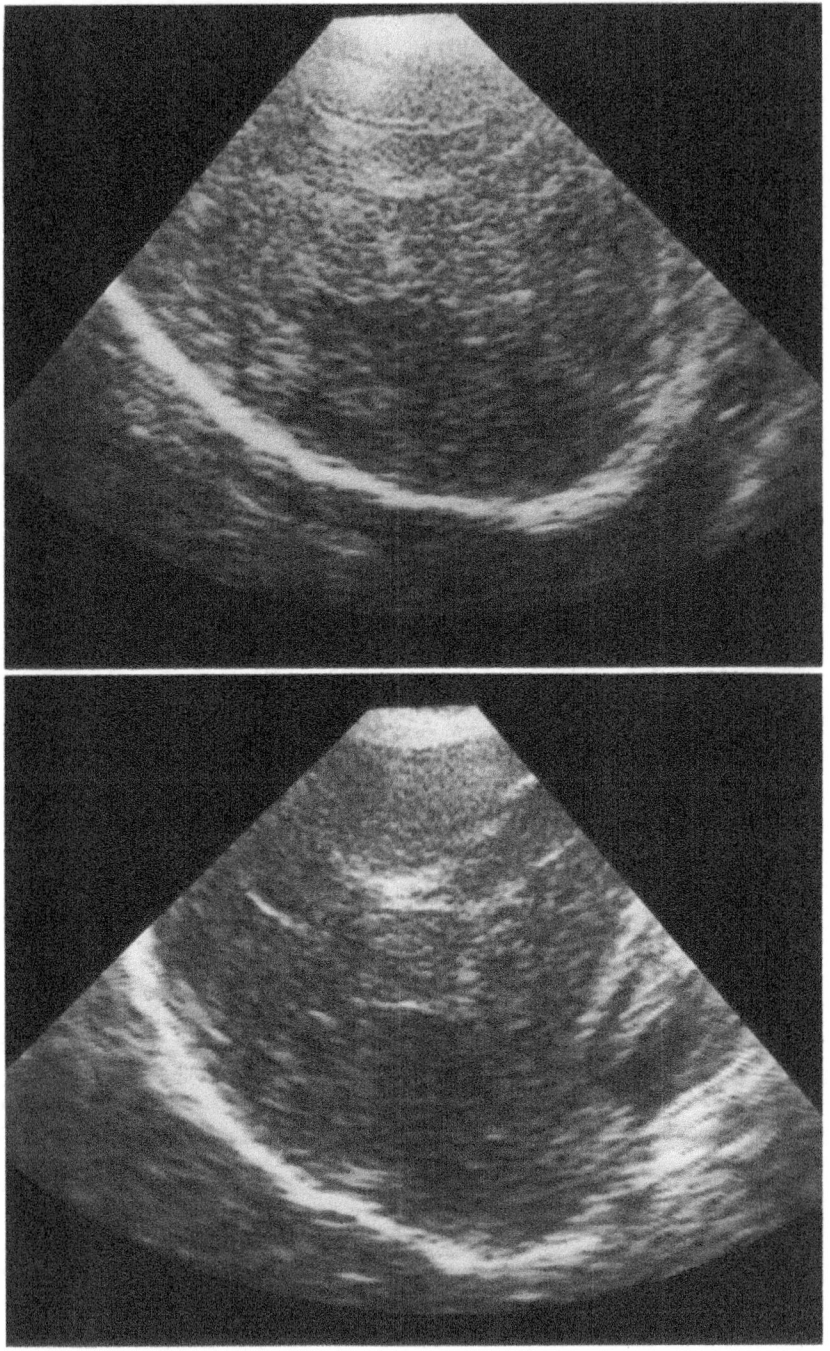

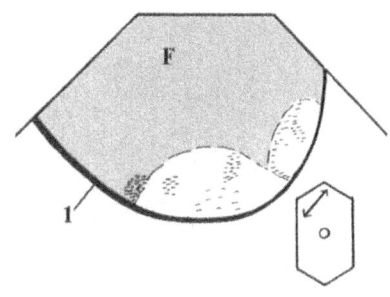

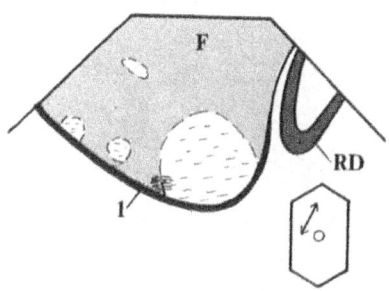

Case 46

Clinical data: A 50-year-old woman suffering from Hodgkin's disease stage II was investigated to monitor her progress.

Description: There is a large hypoechogenic area in segments V and VI with a more echogenic centre. Its borders are ill-defined. The size of the liver is normal. There is no hilar adenopathy. The patient has had splenectomy.

Diagnosis: This is easy since the history is known: hepatic sites in Hodgkin's disease.

Comments: The echo pattern of hepatic lymphomas is nonspecific and variable: decreased echogenicity (Case 45), "target" image: hypoechogenic area with hyperechogenic centre (8.7% of cases), increased echogenicity (13% of cases). Hilar adenopathy and compression of the bile duct may also be detected simultaneously.

At postmortem, 50%−80% of cases show involvement of the liver in Hodgkin's disease, usually as diffuse infiltration, rarely as nodules. This is also the case with non-hodgkinian lymphomas. The results of sonography are unsatisfactory since diffuse lesions are not detected; only the nodules can be visualized. Involvement of the spleen is almost always associated.

Although sonography is not a satisfactory investigation for the diagnosis of liver involvement in lymphomas, it plays a fundamental role in study of the lymph nodes. Moreover, it is indispensable for monitoring the course of the disease.

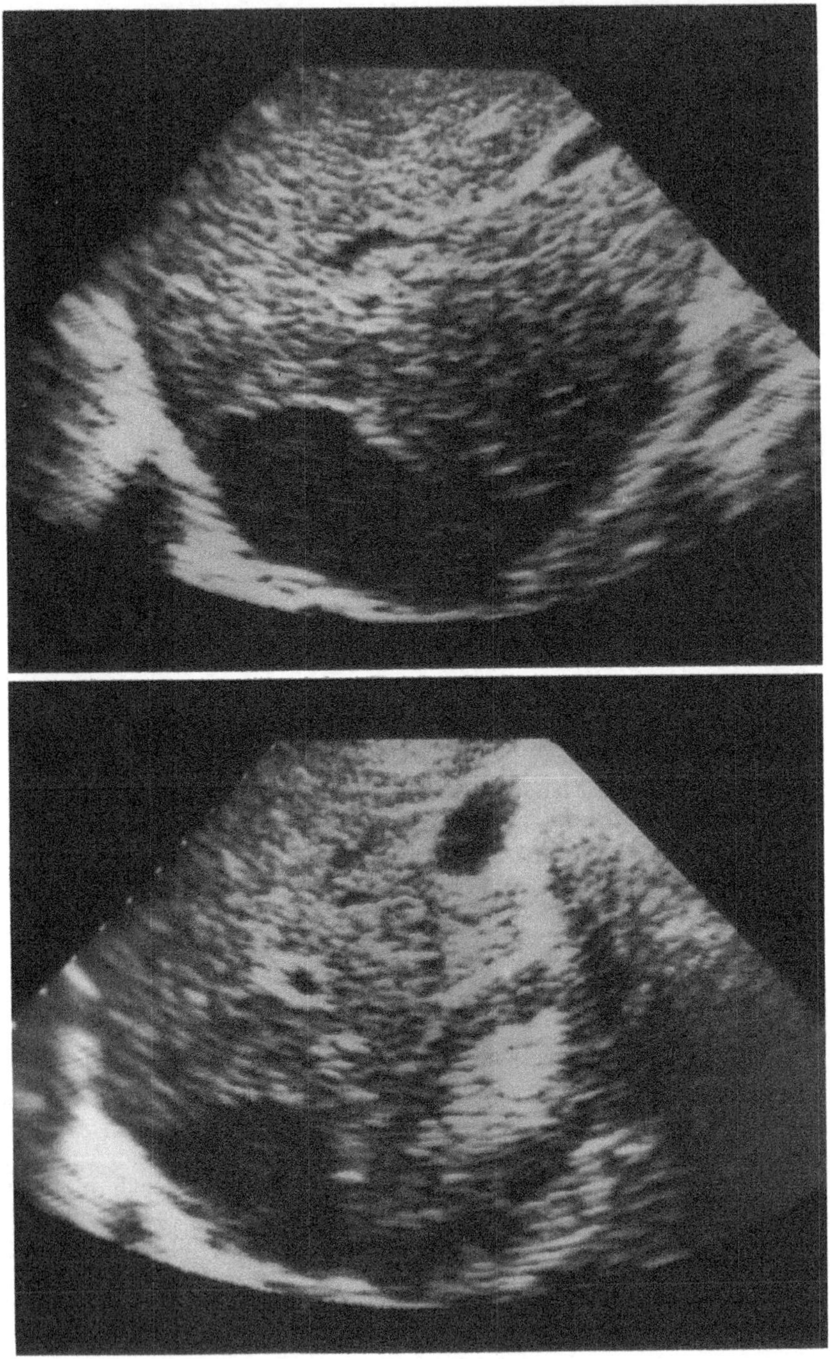

A

B

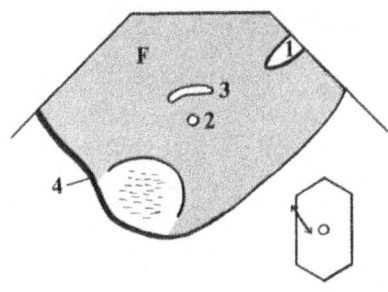

F liver
RD right kidney
1 gallbladder
2 portal vessel
3 hepatic branch
4 diaphragmatic dome

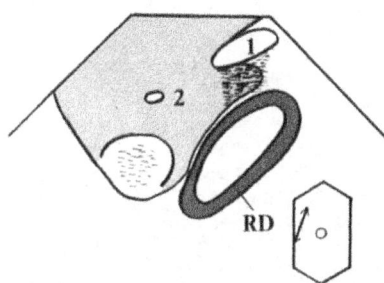

Case 47

Clinical data: A 33-year-old African man has a history of intestinal amoebiases, for which he had been treated 6 years earlier. Presently he complains of pain in the right hypochondrium, fever and diarrhoea.

Description: There is a rounded, pseudo-liquid area of 3 cm diameter, with sharp borders in segment VI. It contains some thin central echoes, which are homogeneously distributed. The presence of a wall cannot be demonstrated. It is located against, and causes deformation of, the diaphragm. There is no pleural effusion.

Diagnosis: The lesion is an amoebic abscess of the liver. This is a classical pattern.

Comments: The thin echoes within the abscess are demonstrated by increasing the gain. The imprint on the diaphragm (Scan A) is an excellent sign. Most amoebic abscesses are located in the right hepatic lobe.

The organism *(Entamoeba histolytica)* invades the colonic mucosa and reaches the liver via the portal system. It settles in the capillaries of the portal vein, which accounts for the peripheral site of the abscesses. Infestation causes necrosis of the hepatocytes with discrete leukocytic infiltration. It is not really a pyogenic abscess, but superinfection may occur. The abscess is usually solitary, especially in Africa, but it can be multiple, as in Asia.

The liver is the second commonest site of amoebiasis, and extension through the diaphragm into the pleural cavity is estimated to occur in 20% of cases. When treated, the course of the disease is variable: the size of the abscess may increase, decrease or remain unchanged. It may become anechogenic with formation of a cyst, or on the contrary show restitution *ad integrum.*

In the absence of a definite history, an amoebic abscess may be confused with a pyogenic abscess or with metastasis.

48

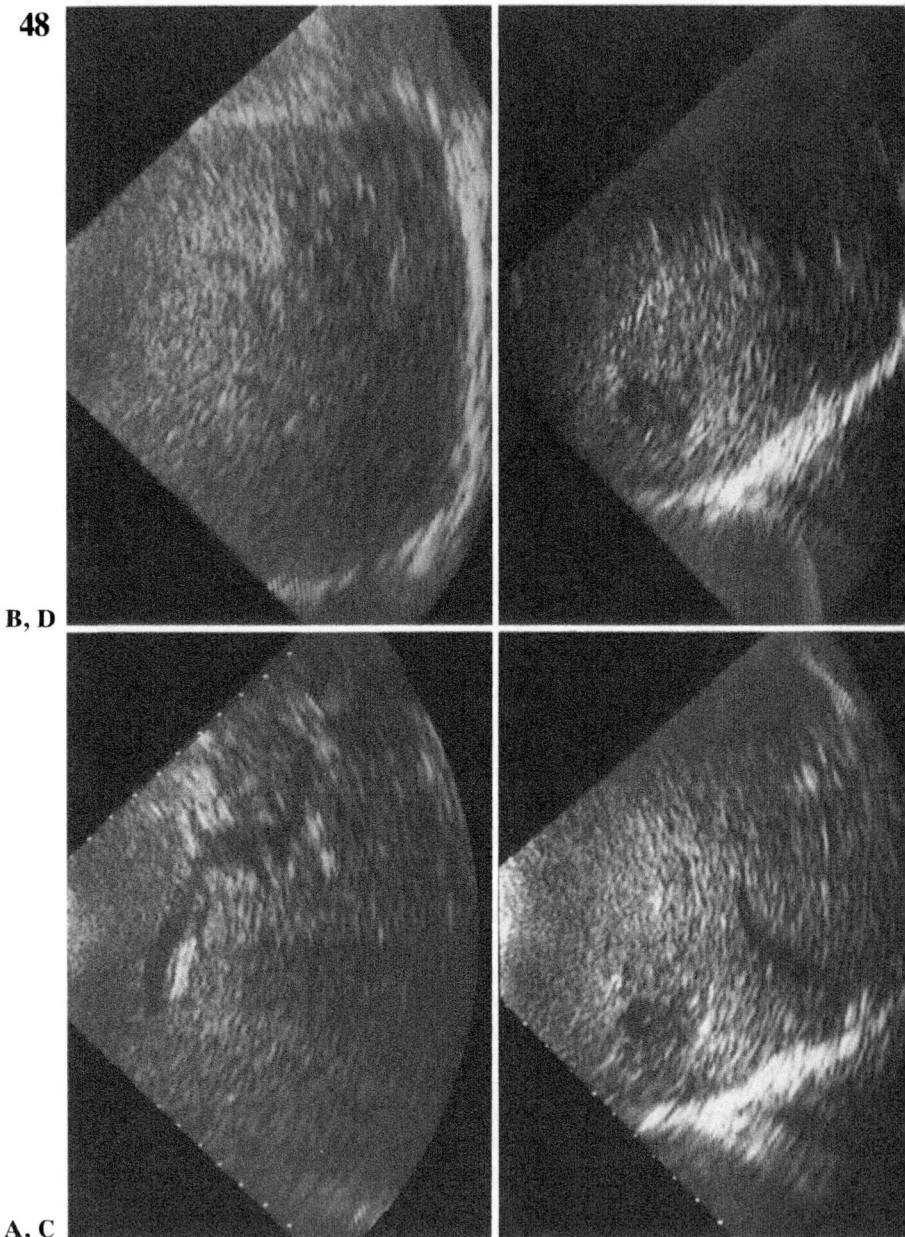

B, D

A, C

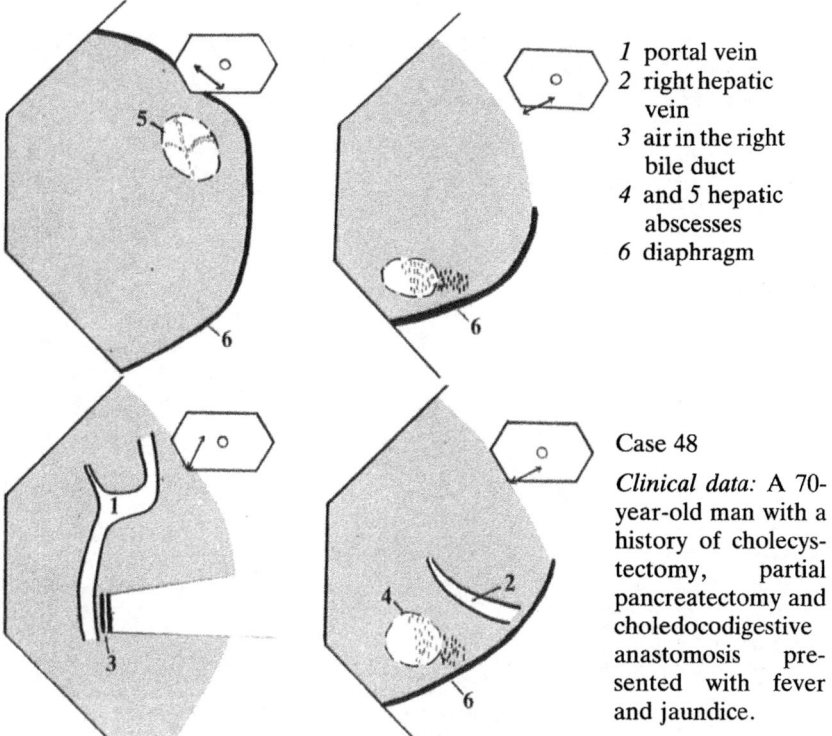

1 portal vein
2 right hepatic vein
3 air in the right bile duct
4 and 5 hepatic abscesses
6 diaphragm

Case 48

Clinical data: A 70-year-old man with a history of cholecystectomy, partial pancreatectomy and choledocodigestive anastomosis presented with fever and jaundice.

Description: The air in the biliary tree is quite obvious (Scan A). In segment VI there is a rounded hypoechogenic area with poorly delineated borders. It contains some central echoes. The same type of area is seen in segment VII. Note the presence of relative echo enhancement. There is also hepatosplenomegaly.

Diagnosis: This is easy: hepatic abscesses secondary to cholangitis. Sonographically guided aspiration yielded several cm^3 of pus.

Comments: Intrahepatic abscess is a severe condition. The mortality is above 50%, despite surgical treatment. Sonography is an excellent diagnostic method. It reveals the abscess in about 90% of cases.

The lesion shown has the classical fluid appearance. This form varies from 3 to 20 cm in size. There are sometimes peculiar appearances – a liquid-liquid interface, numerous internal echoes or septations (Scan B). A hyperechogenic structure stopping the ultrasounds corresponds to gas within the abscess. The most frequent site of an abscess is the right hepatic lobe. There may be an isolated abscess, but they are usually multiple. A peculiar form is seen in immunodepressed patients: micro-abscesses that appear as multiple small hypoechogenic nodules regularly distributed throughout the hepatic parenchyma, sometimes with an echogenic centre.

Without the clinical context it would be impossible to differentiate this from a haemorrhagic cyst, a necrotic tumour, a hydatid cyst, a haematoma or necrotic metastases.

49

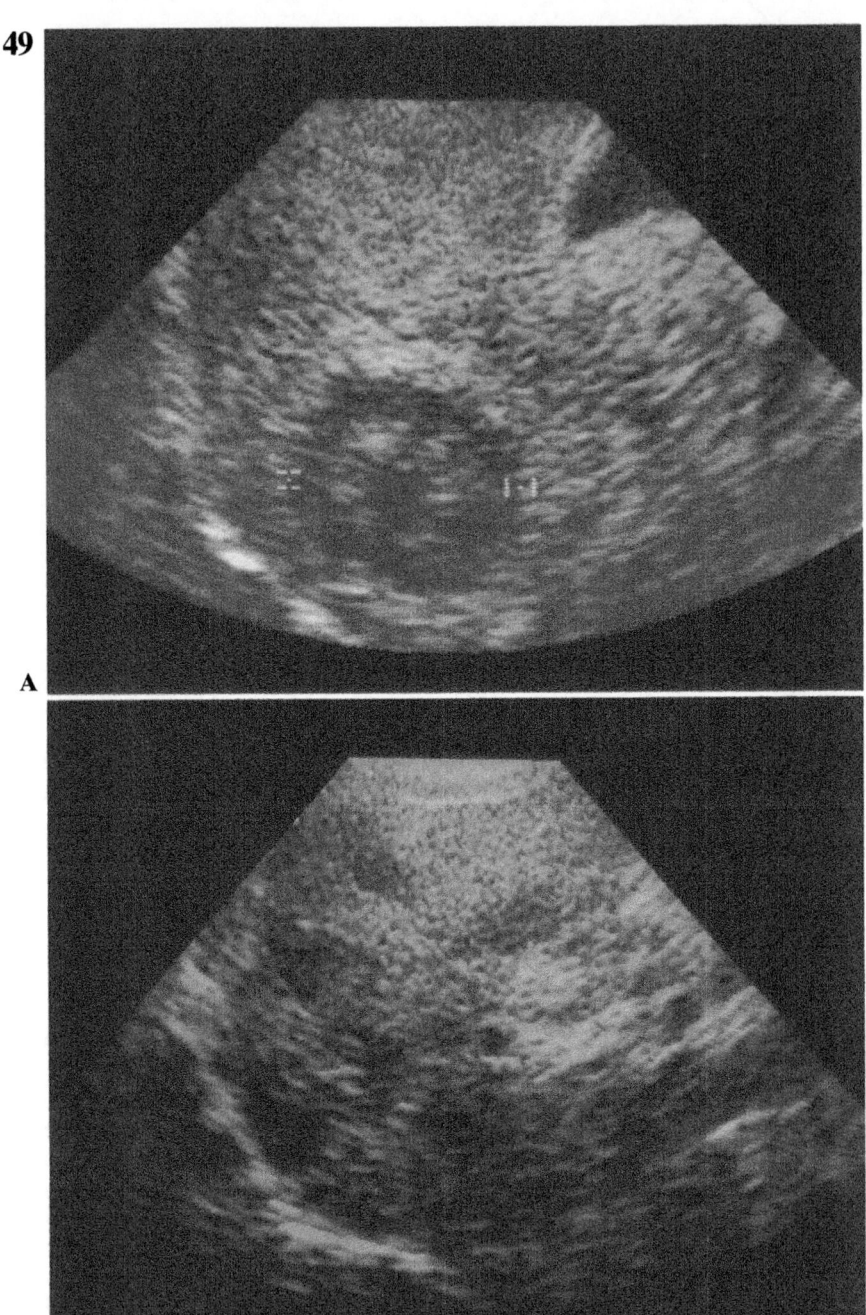

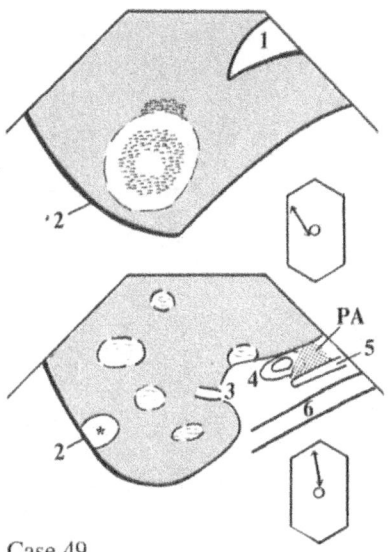

PA hypoechogenic and slightly en- **49**
   larged pancreas (onset of tumoural
   process)
1 gallbladder
2 dome of diaphragm
3 portal vein
4 digestive structure
5 superior mesenteric vein
6 aorta

Case 49

Clinical data: This 60-year-old woman was suffering from non-insulin-dependent diabetes with thoracic pain and alteration of general status.

Description: There is a large (5 cm) rounded mass in segment VII. Its echostructure is mixed – hyperechogenic with a hypoechogenic centre, surrounded by a hypoechogenic area. Its borders are relatively sharp. In the left hepatic lobe (segments II and III) are several rounded, hypoechogenic, homogeneous areas with poorly defined contours. The size of the liver is within normal limits.

Note the rounded anechogenic area, with sharp borders, located against the dome of the diaphragm (Scan B) (*).

Diagnosis: This is easy: hepatic metastases. The ultrasound examination also indicated a neoplasm of the body of the pancreas.

Comments: This classical appearance is also called "bull's eye" lesion; it is found in 20%−35% of all metastases.

Hepatic metastases occur in 50%−70% of pancreatic cancers. The liver is the most frequent secondary site.

An isolated hypoechogenic image may give rise to interpretation problems – is it a simple liver cyst or a secondary site? In fact the same primary cancer can show several echo patterns at the same time.

Regarding additional investigations, computed tomography is sensitive, but there is no specific image; moreover, smaller lesions are difficult to visualize.

Technetium scintigraphy also shows a nonspecific, lacunar image. Arteriography may also be useful, but there are hypovascularized metastases. Although lesions showing any appearance can correspond to hepatic metastases, sonography ultimately takes precedence for this diagnosis. Only the diffuse infiltrative forms, which modify the contours of the liver and cause hepatomegaly catch ultrasounds out.

50

A

B

82

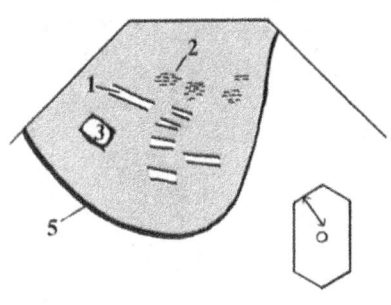

1 dilated intrahepatic bile ducts
2 poorly demarcated hyperechogenic areas
3 biliary cyst
4 hypoechogenic mass
5 diaphragm

50

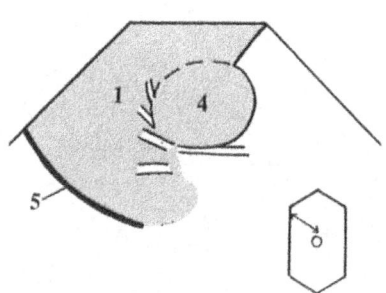

Case 50

Clinical data: A 50-year-old man presented with recent progressive jaundice. There was no remarkable history.

Description: Note the numerous, linear hypoechogenic images in the right hepatic lobe. They correspond to dilated intrahepatic bile ducts. In segments V, VI and VII poorly delimited hyperechogenic areas are visible. In segment V, a rounded mass with a hypoechogenic edge is visible, with no precise limit within the hepatic parenchyma, and a more echogenic centre. Note the well-delineated anechogenic area in segment VII (Scan A). The sonogram is otherwise unremarkable.

Diagnosis: This is easy: there is a hepatoma in segments V, VI and VII.

Comments: The resectability of a hepatocellular carcinoma depends upon its extension to the hepatic parenchyma and upon the absence of venous invasion and of extrahepatic sites. Vascular invasion, especially of the portal vein, is present in 30%−60% of cases, unlike hepatic metastases, in which it is seen in only 5%. Invasion of the portal vein is better detected with ultrasounds and/or angiography than with computed tomography. The latter, however, demonstrates the extrahepatic extension of the lesion better.

The anechogenic area in segment VII corresponds to a biliary cyst.

It is classically said that there is no correlation between cellular type and echostructure. There is therefore no definite criterion for differentiating hepatic metastases from primary carcinoma. A correlation exists, however, between macroscopic appearance and echostructure. A hypoechogenic lesion corresponds to a solid tumour without necrosis. A hyperechogenic pattern can correspond to two different types – either a fatty liver or marked sinusoidal dilatation (producing numerous interfaces). The anechogenic pattern corresponds to extensive liquefaction.

51

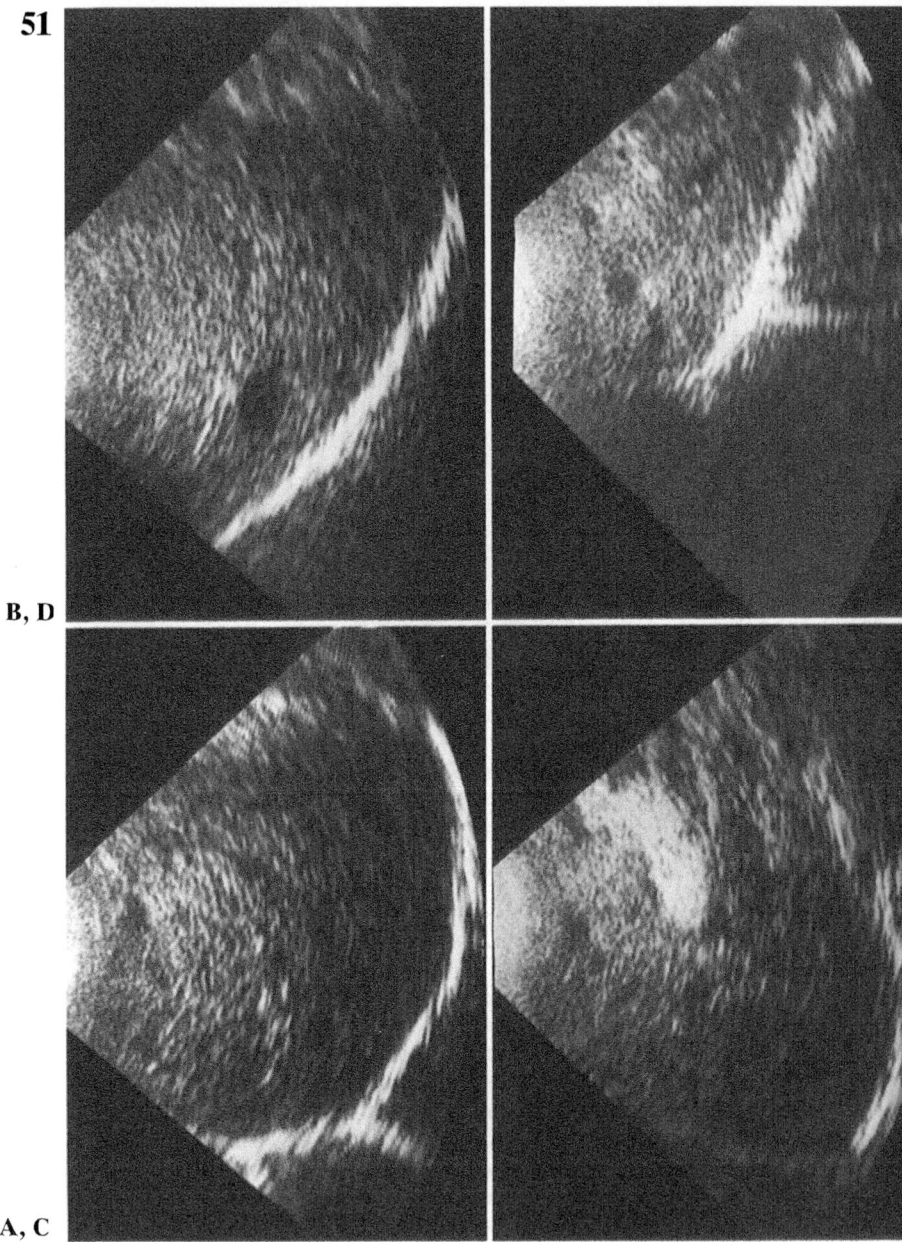

B, D

A, C

84

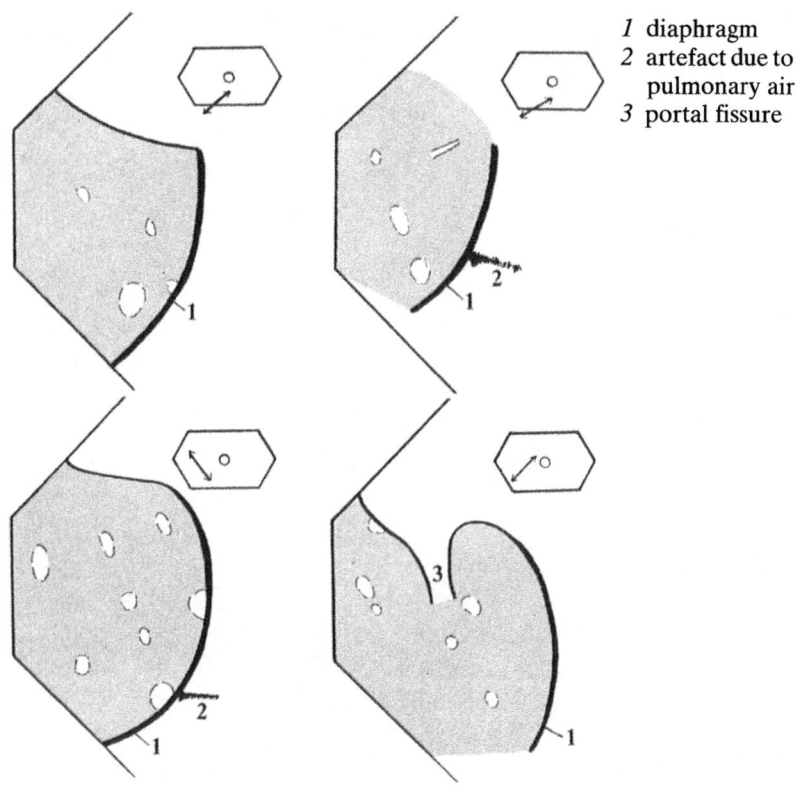

1 diaphragm
2 artefact due to
pulmonary air
3 portal fissure

51

Case 51

Clinical data: A 50-year-old man was hospitalized for investation prior to treatment of a non-hodgkinian lymphoma.

Description: The scan shows multiple hypoechogenic areas that are rounded, well-delimited and small (0.5−1 cm). There is no relative echo enhancement, and the larger lesion presents some fine echoes (Scan B).

The liver has a normal size. The spleen is small and homogenous. The investigation has also shown retroperitoneal adenopathy.

Diagnosis: There is hepatic involvement from non-Hodgkin's lymphoma.

Comments: Only very marked remodelling of the hepatic parenchyma is demonstrated by ultrasounds. Negative investigations do not rule out liver involvement, the more so because patterns, if any exist, are not specific. The hypoechogenic, nodular form is the most frequent (43% of cases). Without clinicobiochemical data it is impossible to differentiate this form from metastases or from micro-abscesses.

Liver enlargement is not a good criterion, since it is nonspecific and also because its absence does not rule out microscopic liver involvement.

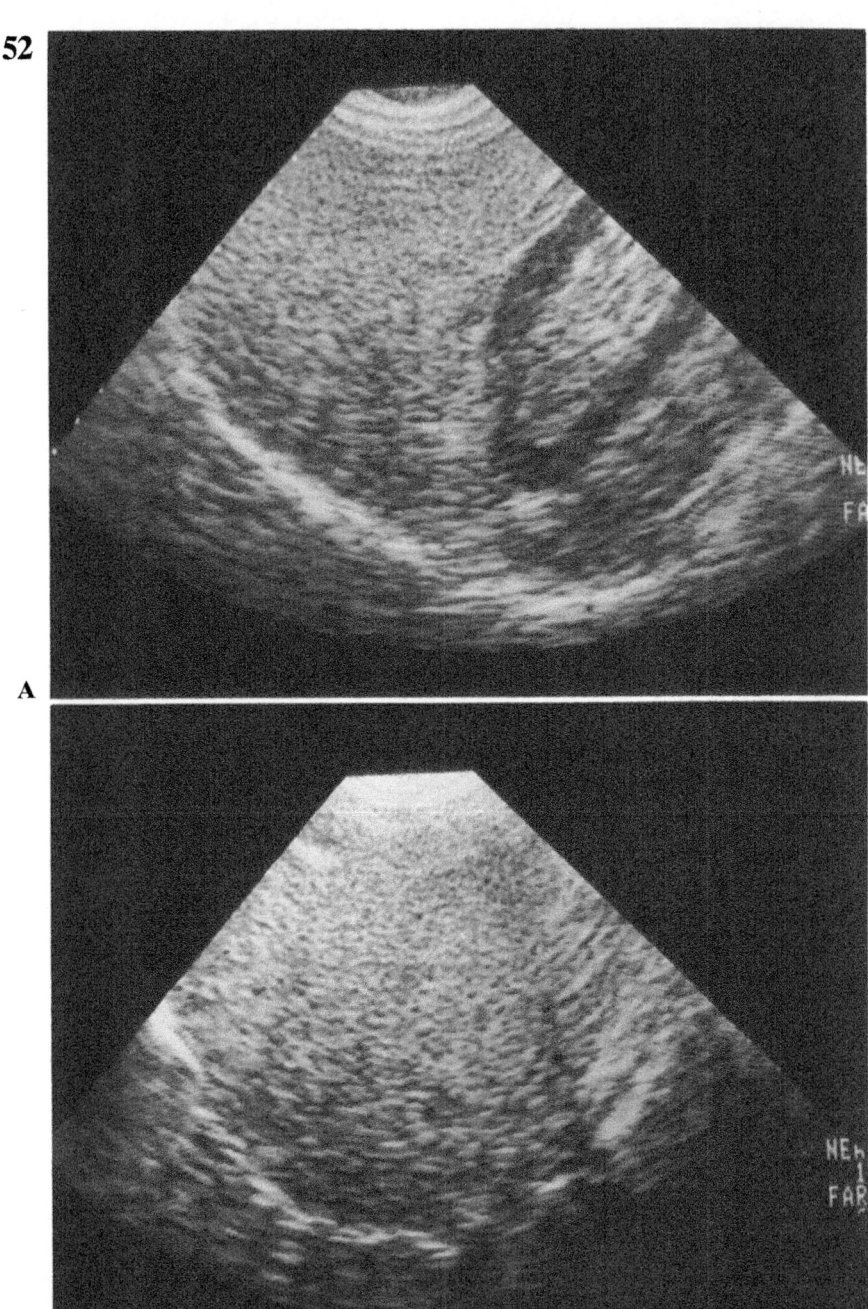

A

B

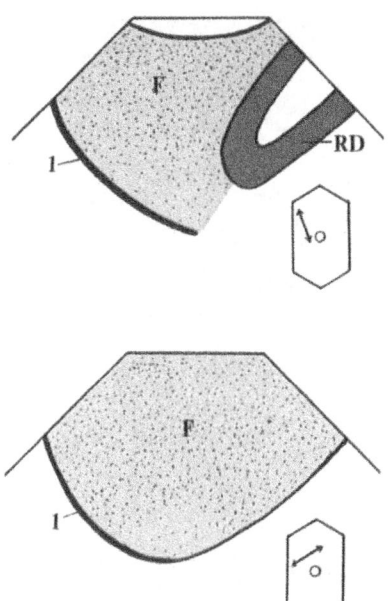

F liver
RD right kidney
1 diaphragm

Case 52

Clinical data: This 36-year-old man has alcoholism.

Description: Analysis of the scans is easy. The liver is globally hyperechogenic and "bright" in a homogeneous way. Its size is normal. Note the hypoechogenic appearance of the renal cortex. The echogenicity of the hepatic parenchyma has become identical to that of the renal sinus. The diaphragmatic dome is well-visualized.

Diagnosis: This is obviously a fatty liver.

Comments: The finding of a hyperechogenic liver is always pathological. This factor is, of course, closely related to the setting of the apparatus; it can thus be produced artificially by increasing the gain. It is very important to carry out correct adjustment with a normal subject.

Involvement of the liver is usually diffuse. Ultrasound assessment of fatty liver is fairly accurate. The accuracy is estimated to be 95%. There are various etiologies of fatty liver: first, alcohol, then prolonged fasting, obesity, diabetes, pregnancy, steroids and hepatotoxic drugs (chemotherapy). Regarding the consequences of alcoholism, one must differentiate between fatty infiltration, hepatitis and cirrhosis. The first of these conditions is reversible, the third is not. Ultrasonography does not have the same diagnostic precision as histologic study after puncture-biopsy of the liver.

"Bright" livers have numerous etiologies – steatosis, cirrhosis, portal fibrosis, severe hepatitis, cardiac failure and haemochromatosis.

53

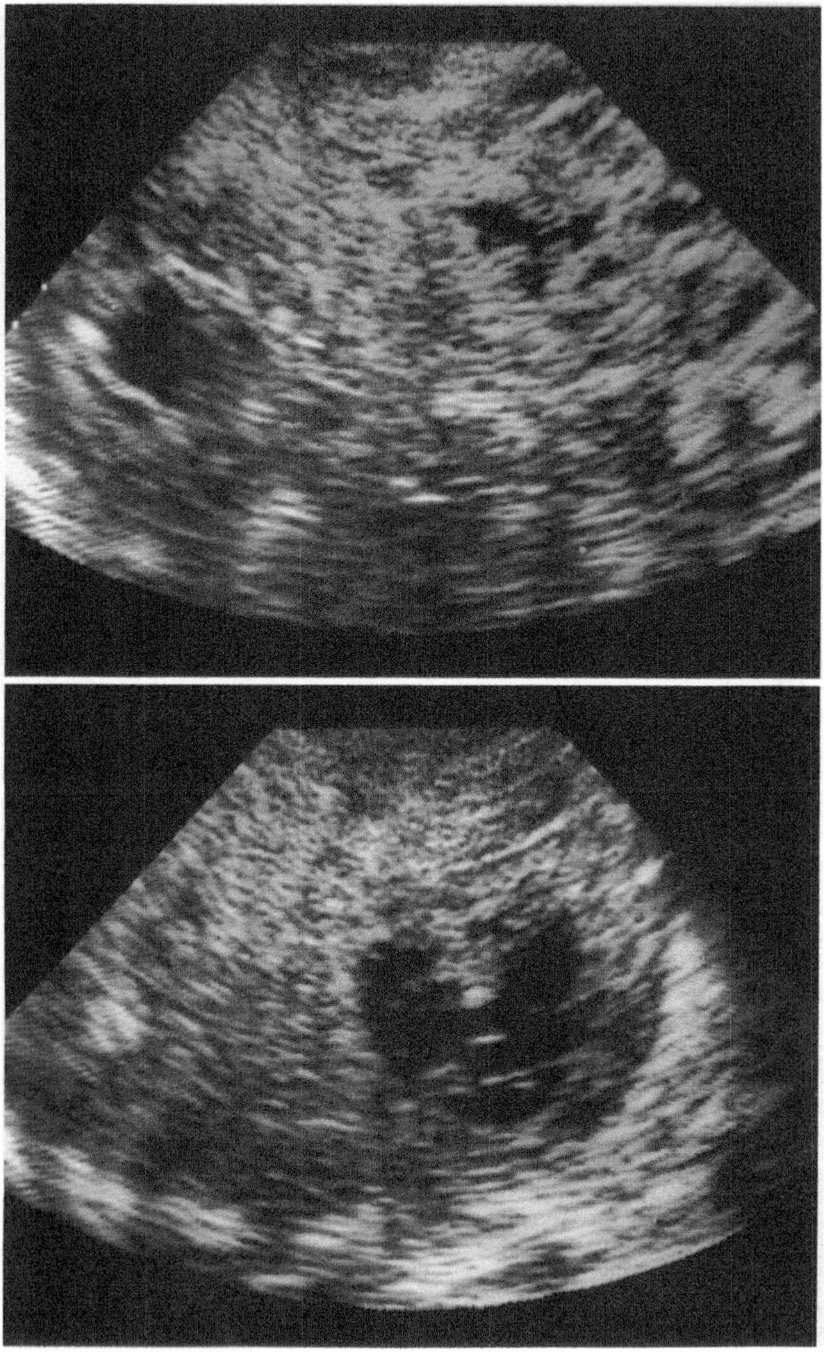

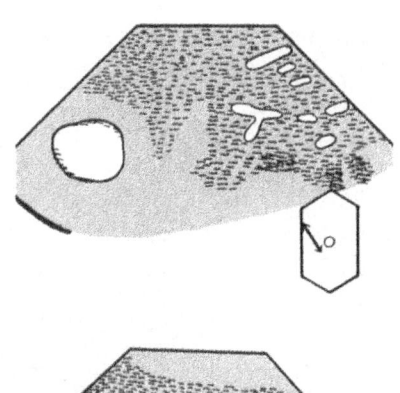

1 large necrotic mass in segment V **53**
2 posterior costal arches

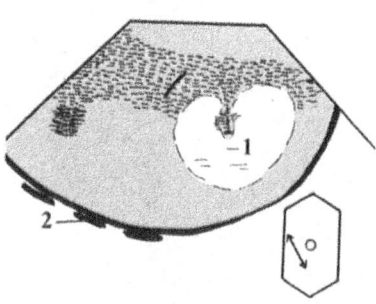

Case 53

Clinical data: The patient is a 50-year-old man with an undifferentiated bronchial neoplasm who is receiving chemotherapy.

Description: The echo-pattern of the liver is entirely remodelled, and both hyperechogenic areas with very blurred contours, and hypoechogenic areas are present. In segment V the scan shows a voluminous mass with an anechogenic centre which is of the fluid type. The mass has irregular internal contours (Scan B).

There is also monstrous hepatomegaly. (In all scans and with the usual field-depth, the liver cannot be entirely visualized on the screen).

Diagnosis: There are obvious diffuse and necrotic metastases of the liver.

Comments: Hepatic metastases occur in 30%−50% of lung cancers. The fluid appearance is uncommon; it indicates central necrosis of the tumour. In such types ultrasonography allows monitoring of chemotherapy. It permits one to assess the number, size and echostructure of the lesions. Increase in number and size is of course pejorative, whereas diminition is a favourable factor. The evolution of the echostructure is variable – a hyperechogenic mass may become hypoechogenic. Conversely, the homogeneous type may become heterogeneous. In such cases it may be difficult to affirm whether the development is favourable or not. The occurrence of central necrosis during chemotherapy is frequent; necrosis is known, however, to be the natural course of larger metastases. In many cases, the response to chemotherapy is difficult to appreciate. Restitutio integrum of the parenchyma is rare.

54

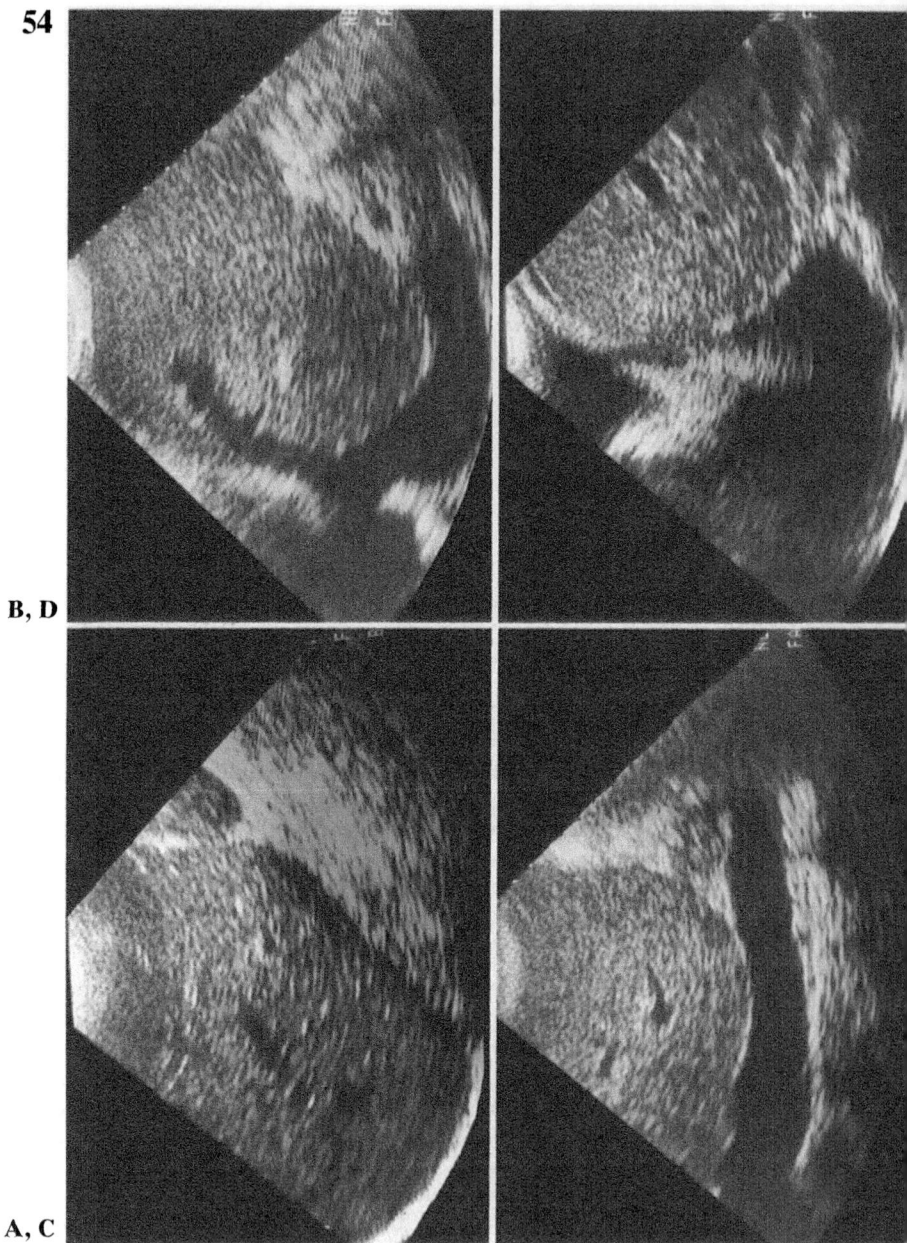

B, D

A, C

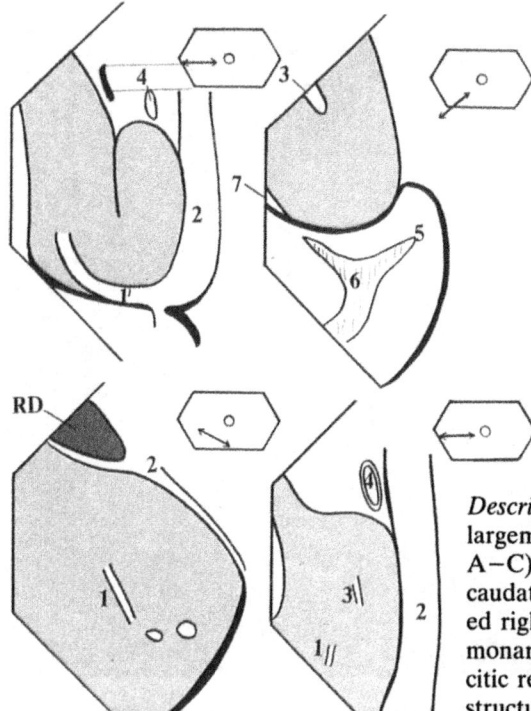

1 right hepatic vessel
1' middle hepatic vein
2 inferior vena cava
3 portal vessel
4 digestive structure
5 pleural effusion
6 pulmonary atelectasis
7 layer of perihepatic ascites

Case 54

Clinical data: A 60-year-old woman with decompensated cardiac insufficiency complained of pain in the abdomen.

Description: There is obvious enlargement of the liver (Scans A−C), involving the right, left and caudate lobes. There is also marked right pleural effusion with pulmonary atelectasis and discrete ascitic reaction (Scan D). The echostructure of the liver is homogeneous.

Note the increased calibre of the inferior vena cava, which measures 2.5 cm, and of the left hepatic vein, which measures 1 cm. Real-time scanning shows the inferior vena cava to have lost its normal respiratory kinetics (especially during the Valsalva manoeuvre).

Diagnosis: This is obvious cardiac cirrhosis.

Comments: Note the hypoechogenic appearance of the caudate lobe (Scan B). This is normal, and due to attenuation of the ultrasound beam by the porta hepatis.

Apart from the nonspecific features − homogeneous hepatomegaly and increased echogenicity (bright liver) there are more suggestive extrahepatic signs − dilatation of the inferior vena cava (wider than 2.5 cm) and of the hepatic veins (wider than 1 cm for the right vein), with unchanged calibre of the inferior vena cava, and of the confluence with the hepatic veins, during respiration. Note that the same phenomenon is seen in thrombosis of the inferior vena cava. One should also search for ascites, pleural effusion, pericardial effusion and cardiac dilatation, especially of the right cardiac chambers.

In this type of disorder sonography plays two roles − on the one hand it allows one to rule out pathology of the liver itself, and on the other hand it permits one to show recovery of the normal respiratory kinetics of the inferior vena cava, which is still an excellent criterion for judging the efficiency of medical treatment.

55

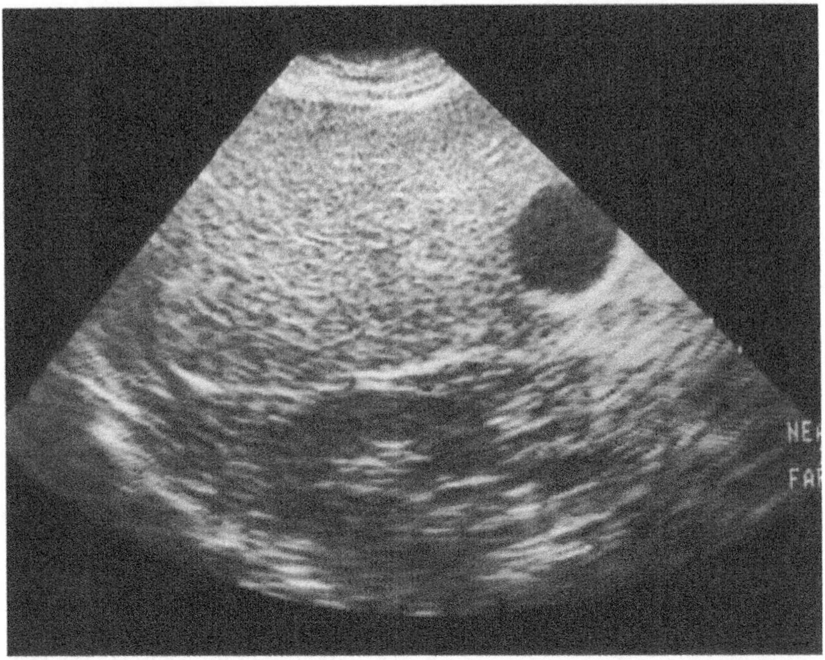

56

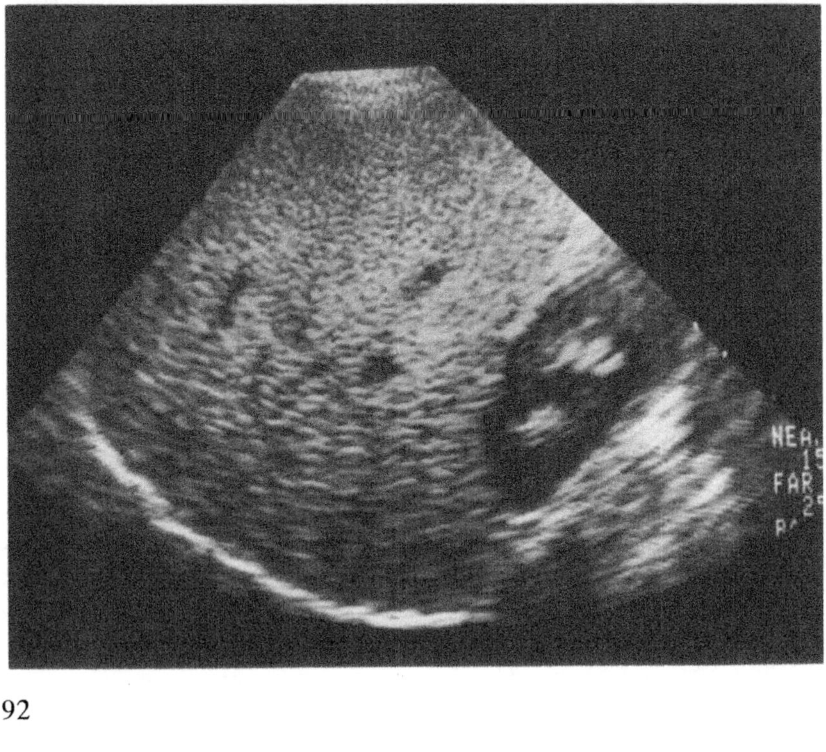

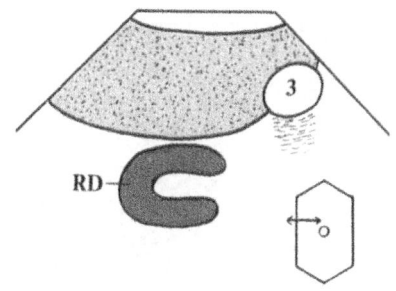

RD right kidney
1 portal branch
2 hepatic branches
3 gallbladder
4 diaphragm

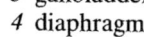

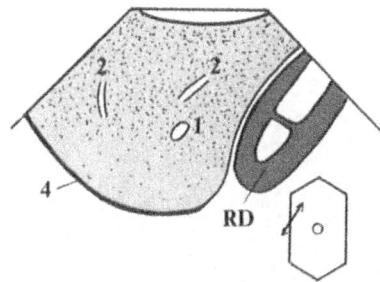

Case 55

Clinical data: A 35-year-old woman, weighing 135 kg, was investigated prior to commencing a weight-loss program.

Description: You have certainly noticed the diffusely increased echogenicity of the liver compared to the renal cortex, and the absence of posterior relative echo-attenuation. These are normal findings in obesity.

Comments: Obesity is a frequent cause of fatty liver. Note the rather thin layer of subcutaneous fat due merely to strong compression of the abdomen by the transducer, indispensable to obtain the scan. Note also that subcutaneous fat without collagen fibres is seen as an area of decreased echogenicity. Experimental studies have shown that the echogenicity is proportional to the volume of fat vacuoles and to the hepatic triglyceride content.

Case 56

Clinical data: A 50-year-old woman underwent surgery 2 years ago for breast cancer, and had chemotherapy.

Description: The size of the liver is within normal limits but its echo pattern is changed and shows diffusely increased echogenicity with slight posterior echo-attenuation. The echostructure is otherwise normal.

Diagnosis: The increased echogenicity of the liver is due to chemotherapy. No secondary deposits are present.

Comments: This appearance is classical but inconstant. The presence of discrete posterior echo-attenuation has been described as existing even in the absence of fibrosis. It is due to marked absorption of the ultrasound beam by the steatosis. The evolution of this steatosis is the same as that of steatoses of other origins. It disappears rapidly as soon as the etiological factor is suppressed.

57

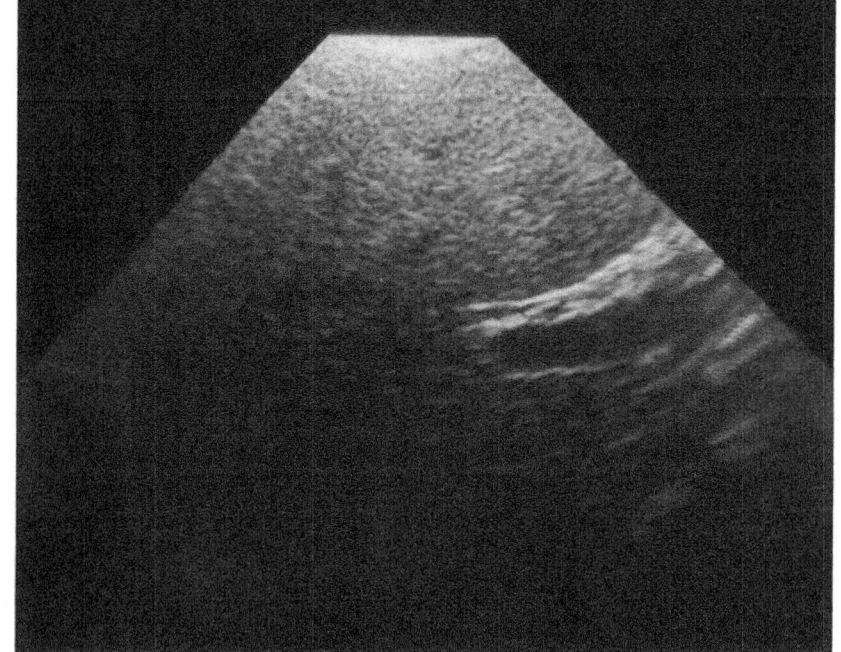

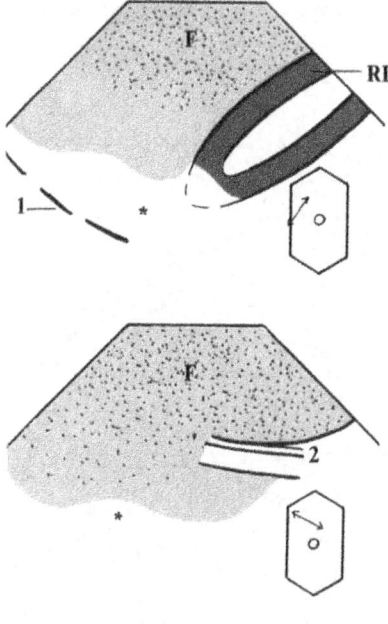

F liver
RD right kidney
1 indistinct diaphragm
2 portal fissure
* pronounced posterior relative
  echo-attenuation

Case 57

Clinical data: A 40-year-old man presented with chronic alcoholism.

Description: There is diffuse enlargement of the liver, with changes in the echo pattern: increased echogenicity in the superficial regions and marked posterior echo-attenuation. The diaphragm is hardly visible (Scan A).

Diagnosis: This is easy: fibrosis of the liver.

Comments: Hepatic fibrosis, already an advanced stage in cirrhosis, causes pronounced posterior echo-attenuation. The diagnosis of an intrahepatic tumoural process therefore becomes difficult. Although steatoses and fibroses usually have a different echo pattern, there is no good correlation with the liver-biopsy data, so that it is not possible to differentiate these two conditions on the basis of sonographic criteria. The diagnostic accuracy is 70%. Moreover, fibrosis does not imply atrophic cirrhosis; other signs are necessary to assess the diagnosis (Case 65). This stage of hepatic fibrosis is irreversible.

Note also that fibrosis resulting from primary biliary cirrhosis or from chronic active hepatitis is detected at an advanced stage, whereas fibrosis secondary to alcoholism is more easily detected on account of the pre-existent steatosis.

Although the most frequent cause of cirrhosis in France is alcoholism, the signs of hepatic fibrosis are neither specific nor sensitive. The criteria are moreover strongly subjective and the sonographer's experience plays a significant role.

58

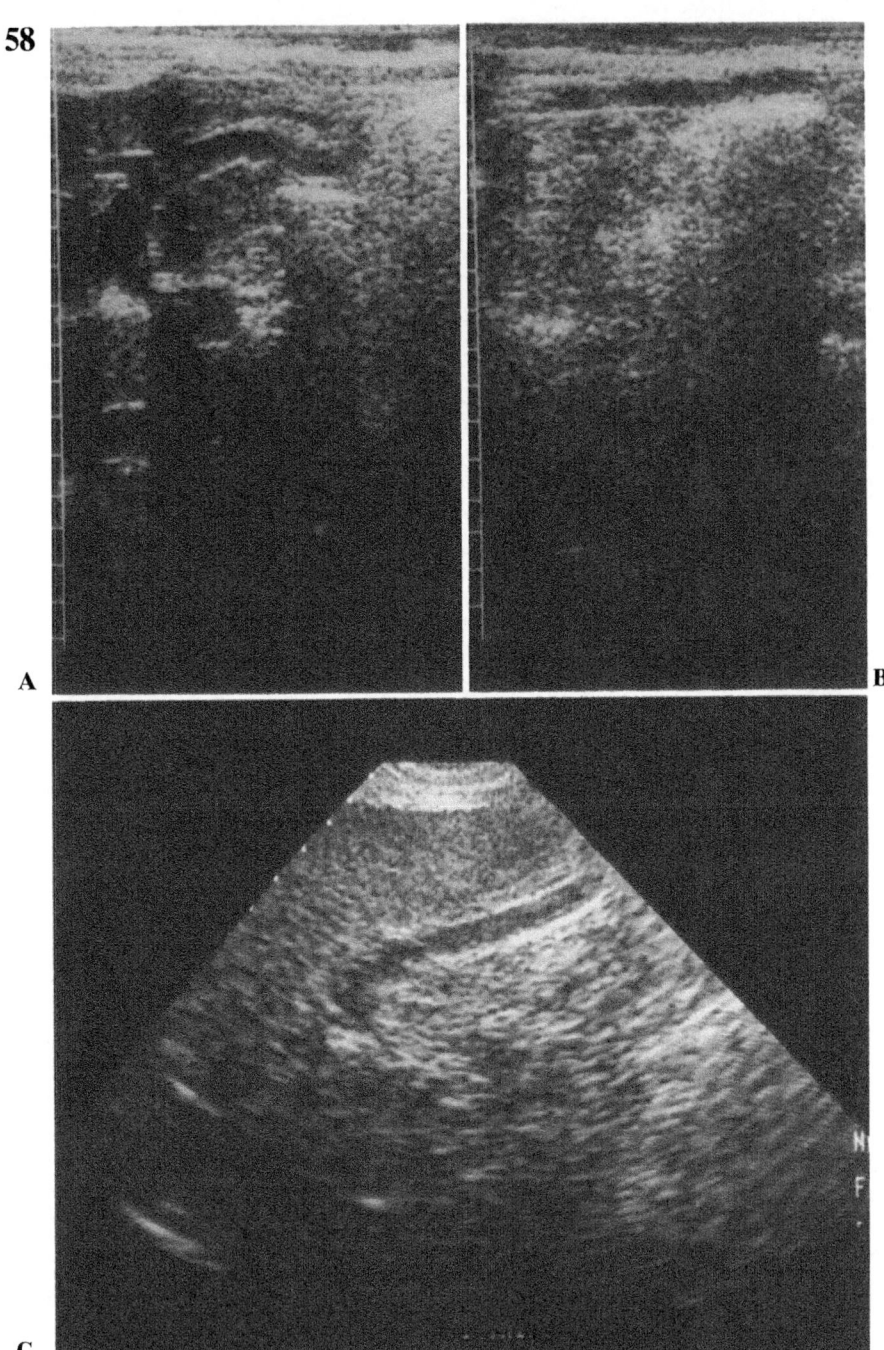

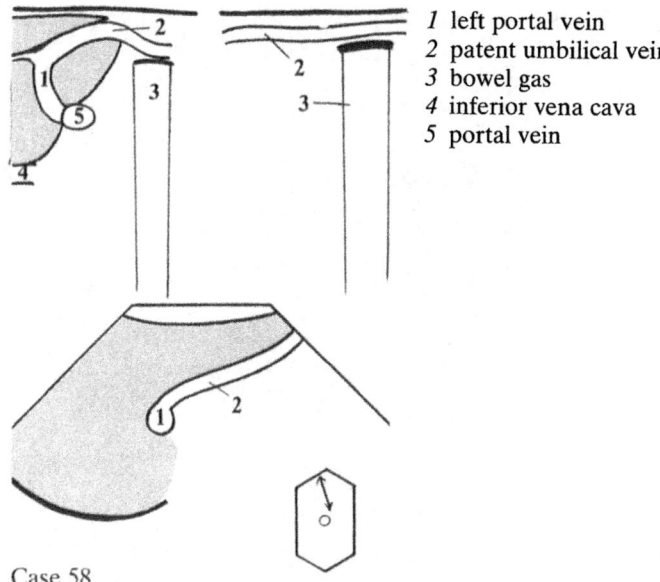

1 left portal vein
2 patent umbilical vein
3 bowel gas
4 inferior vena cava
5 portal vein

Case 58

Clinical data: A 55-year-old alcoholic man with hepatomegaly was hospitalized because of myeloma.

Description: The scan shows a tubular image that commences at the left portal tributary and runs towards the anterior abdominal wall, continuing up to the umbilicus. Note, on scan A, the width of the portal vein (1.5 cm) and of the left portal tributary (1 cm).

Diagnosis: This is easy: reperfusion of the umbilical vein, a sign of portal hypertension. The umbilical vein is located in the falciform ligament.

Comments: There are several types of venous deviations resulting from obstruction of the portal circulation: portocaval or hepatofugal, and portoportal or hepatopetal anastomoses (Case 67). Besides the superficial systems, which are of minor importance since they are of less functional significance, there are two types of portocaval anastomosis: with the superior or with the inferior vena cava. There is also a third hepatofugal shunt, namely reperfusion of the umbilical vein. This is considered to be pathological when the vein is more than 3 mm in diameter. Its detection is of prominent importance since it may be the only ultrasonographic sign of portal hypertension. Sonography is very accurate, since it permits detection in 90% of cases. There is no correlation between the degree of umbilical vein dilatation and the presence ot other signs indicating portal hypertension.

Increased diameter of the portal vein, above 13 mm, is a very reliable sign of portal hypertension. Some authors consider this to be a debatable point; they set more value upon the size of the splenic vein (diameter of more than 15 mm). This is far from being specific, since the splenic vein is widened in splenomegaly due to any cause.

59

B, D

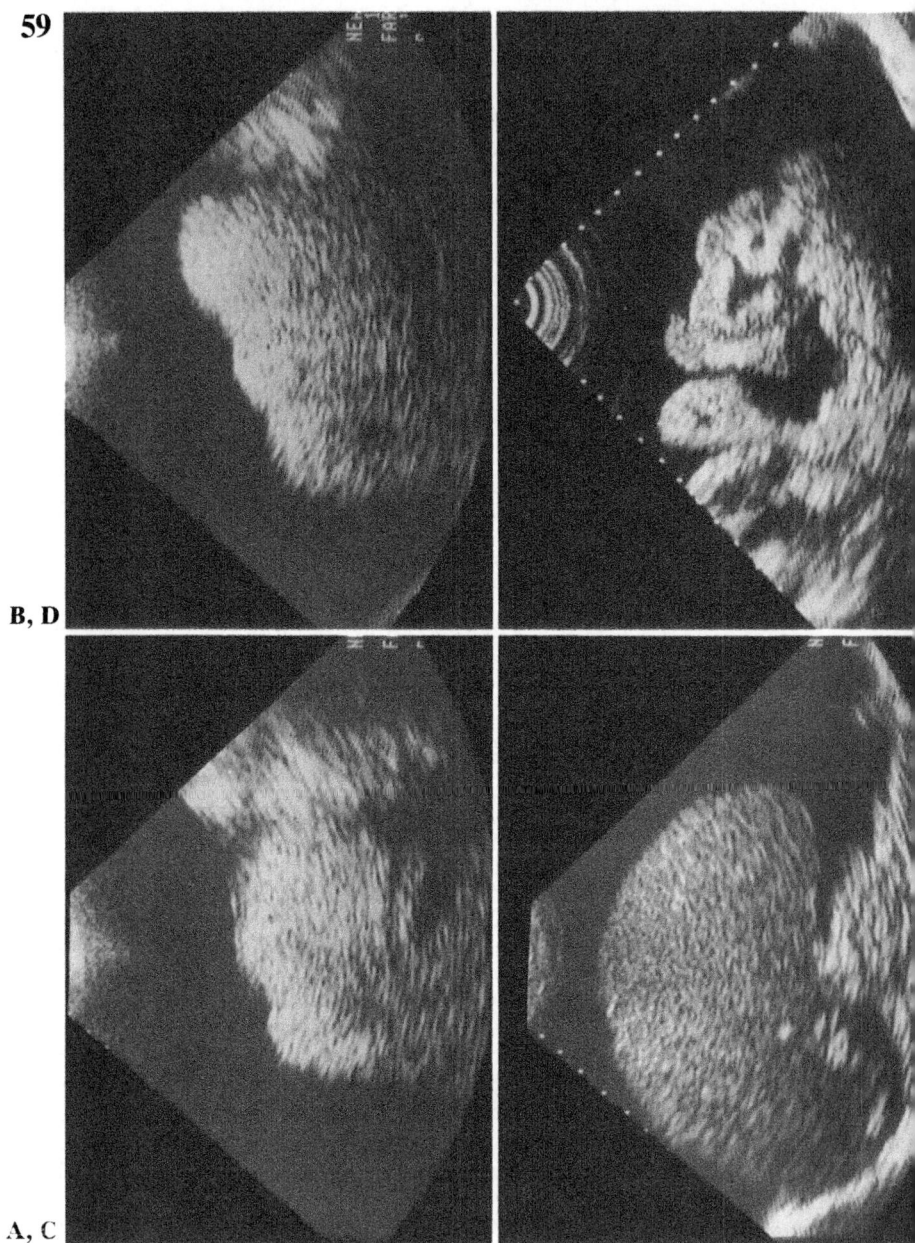

A, C

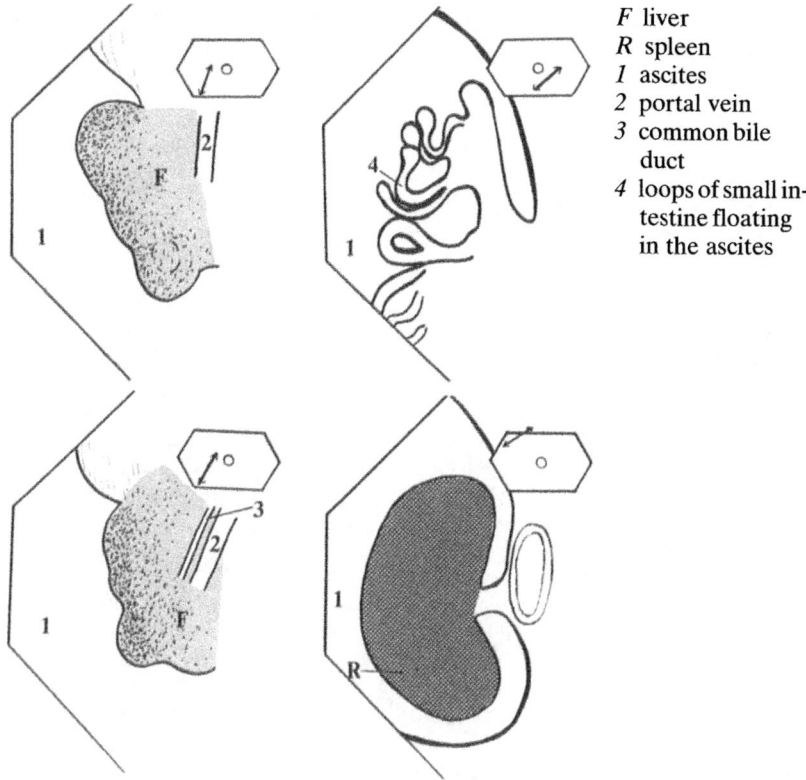

F liver **59**
R spleen
1 ascites
2 portal vein
3 common bile
  duct
4 loops of small in-
  testine floating
  in the ascites

Case 59

Clinical data: This 35-year-old man has chronic active hepatitis.

Description: There is abundant ascites evenly distributed throughout the peritoneal cavity. Note, in Scan D, the bowel loops floating in the ascitic fluid. The liver is very small. It is atrophic and has bosselated contours, which are visible because of the ascites. The echogenicity is increased but you must take account of the enhancement due to the ascites. Note the hypertrophic portal vein with a width jof 1.5 cm (Scan A). Scan C shows uniform splenomegaly.

Diagnosis: Atrophic cirrhosis with portal hypertension.

Comments: The portocaval venous circulation has not been visualized in this case. Sonographic investigations are sometimes unusually difficult (in obese patients, for instance) especially when abundant ascites prevents visualization of the pancreas. The difficultly is increased when there is excessive intestinal gas. Computed tomography and angiographic study of venous backflow may be useful in such cases.

Portoportal, hepatopetal anastomoses are usually due to obstruction of the splenic or portal vein.

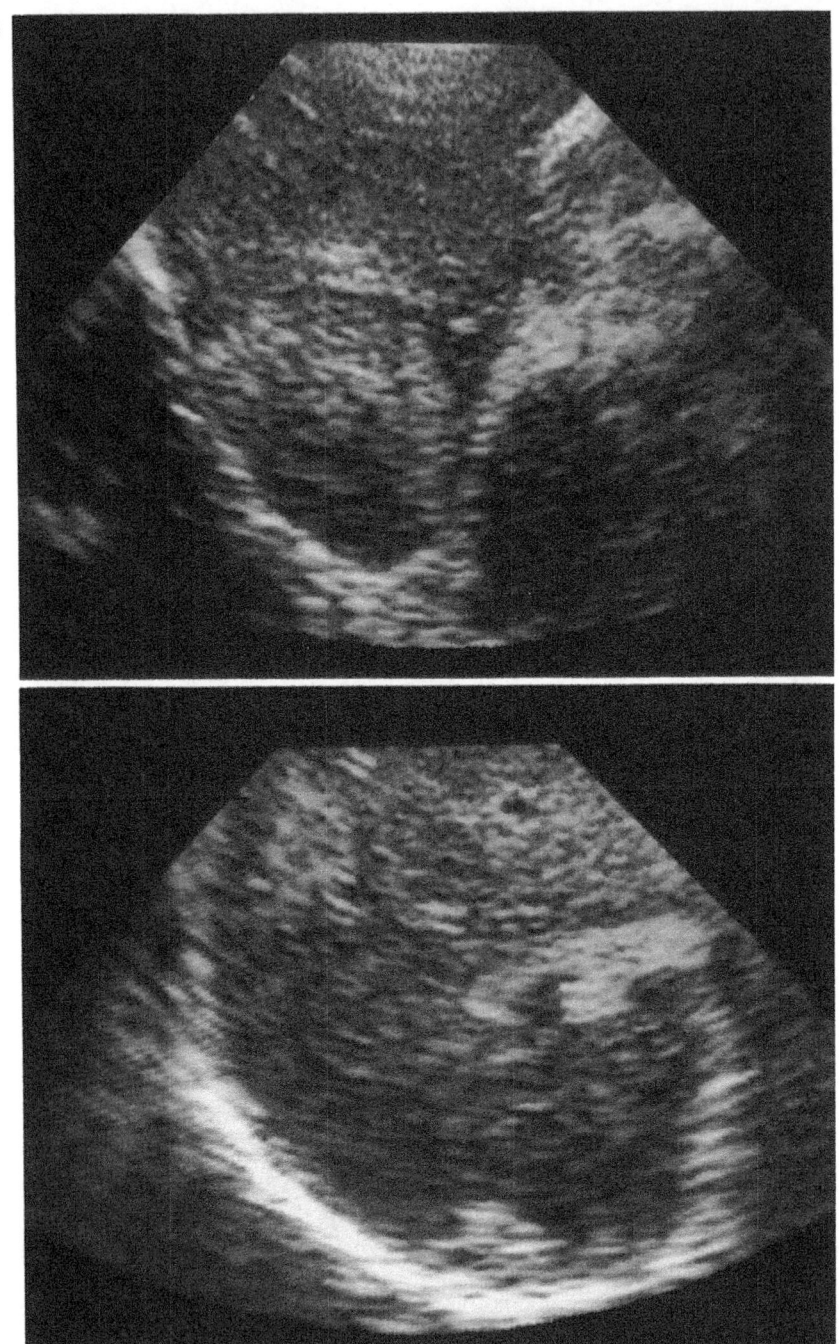

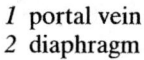
1 portal vein
2 diaphragm

60

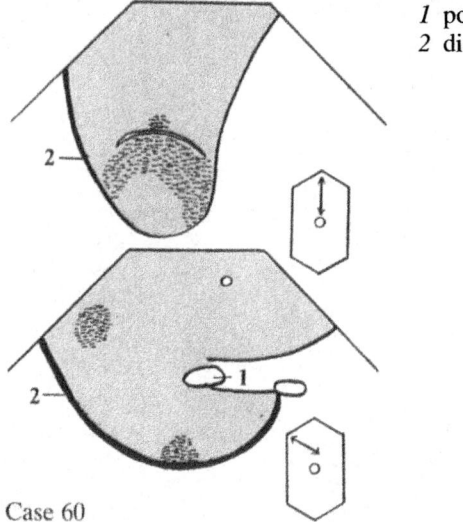

Case 60

Clinical data: A 55-year-old man presented with alternating diarrhoea and constipation, and general ill-health.

Description: The scan shows a rounded, heterogeneous area of increased echogenicity, bordered by a hypoechogenic ring, occupying segment IV. It measures 4 cm in diameter. There are also two smaller areas of increased echogenicity with irregular heterogeneous contours, located in segments VI and VII. Compare these findings with those of Case 38.

Diagnosis: There are metastases in the liver. The primary lesion is a carcinoma of the sigmoid colon.

Comments: Detection of a colonic carcinoma through hepatic metastases is uncommon (1% of cases) and associated with a poor prognosis. Age and sex have no appreciable correlation with the incidence of metastases, which do, however, occur more frequently with longer survival, despite chemotherapy.

Although it is difficult to relate the primary tumour to the appearance and site of a secondary lesion, it is classically suggested that hyperechogenic metastases are of colonic origin (in fact, 57% of hyperechogenic forms are colonic). This is a common sonographic pattern occurring in 27%–30% of all liver metastases. The hyperechogenicity is due to the rich vascularization of the lesions.

Purely hypoechogenic forms are rare and are due to lymphomas (case 51). Mixed forms are common.

It is mainly cancers depending on the portal system which give rise to hepatic metastases (stomach, colon, pancreas, biliary system), in contrast to tumours depending on the systemic arterial system (choroidal melanomas, neuroblastomas, carcinomas of the breast and of the testis).

For small tumours (up to 2 cm) sonography and arteriography are more accurate than computed tomography.

61

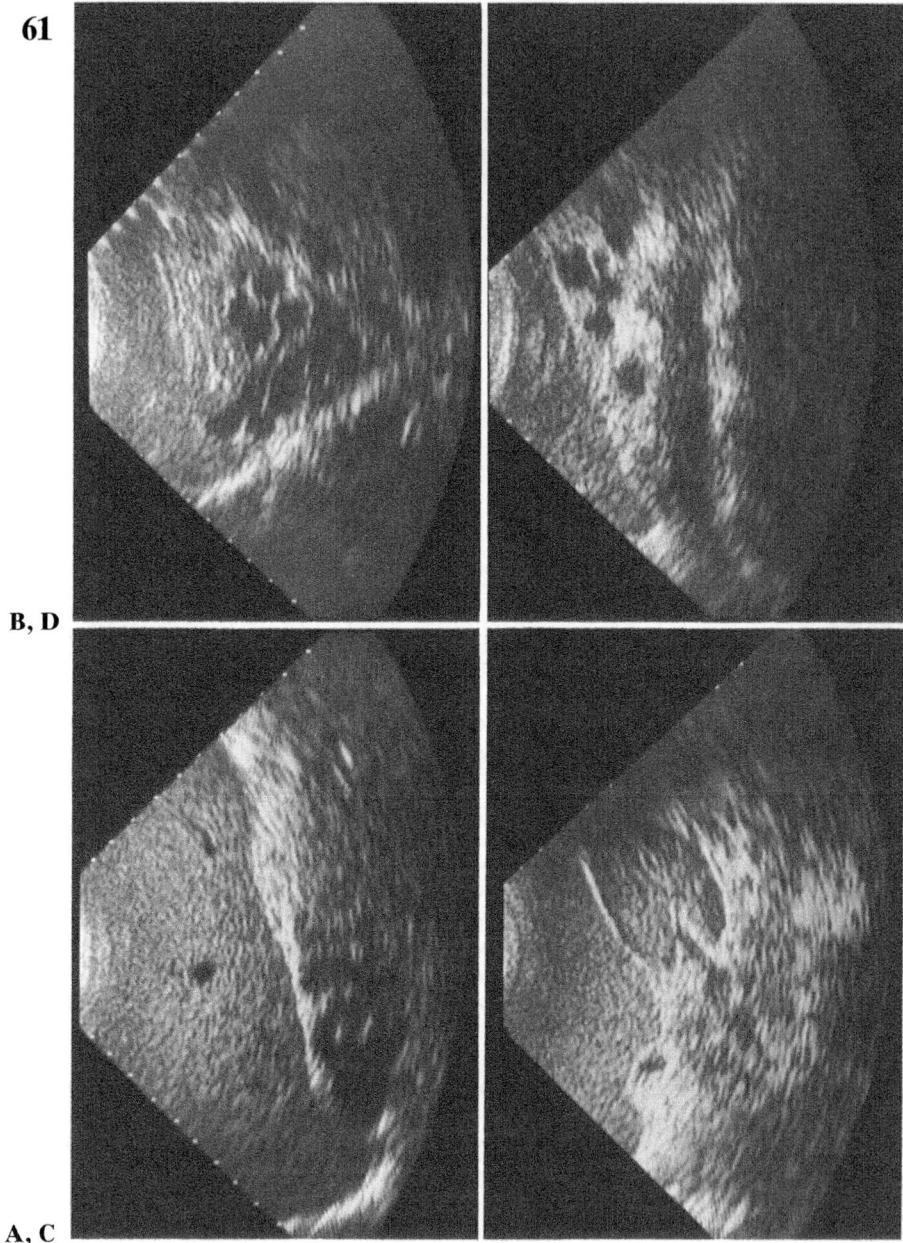

B, D

A, C

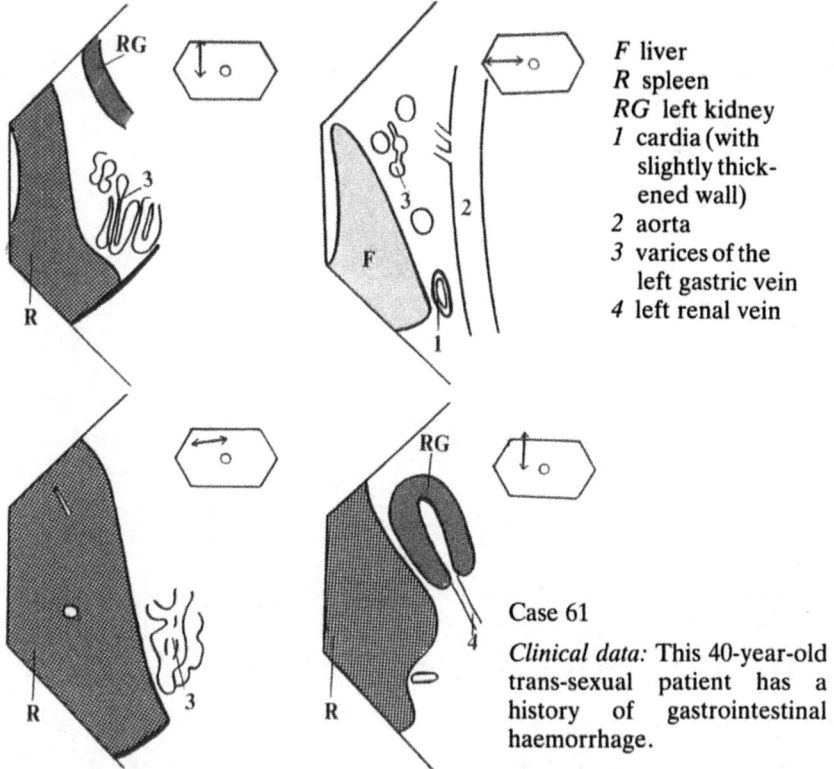

F liver
R spleen
RG left kidney
1 cardia (with slightly thick-ened wall)
2 aorta
3 varices of the left gastric vein
4 left renal vein

Case 61

Clinical data: This 40-year-old trans-sexual patient has a history of gastrointestinal haemorrhage.

Description: In scan B, you have certainly noted the vascular network between the spleen and the diaphragm. A sagittal scan (Scan D) passing between the aorta and the left hepatic lobe shows numerous rounded echo-free areas, which are of liquid type and confluent. Scan A also shows splenomegaly: the spleen measures 17 cm in its long axis and shows a homogeneous echostructure.

Note that the left renal vein has normal dimensions.

Diagnosis: There are obvious gastro-oesophageal varices with a dilated gastric vein, reflecting portal hypertension.

Comments: Hepatofugal portocaval anastomoses with the superior vena cava at the level of the cardia are of prominent importance. Dilatation of the gastric vein is the most frequent and the most specific feature. It is normally not visualized. When it becomes pathological because of portal hypertension, the gastric vein is dilated and can be recognized by ultrasounds as soon as it measures 5 mm in diameter. Moreover, its course becomes tortuous, and it is usually serpiginous. It arises in the cardiotuberous region, runs along the lesser curvature of the stomach and empties into the portal vein or, more rarely, into the splenic vein. It is visualized by ultrasounds in 80% of cases. Its size is directly proportional to that of the cardio-oesophageal varices and thus to the *bleeding potential of the patient.* This criterion is much more significant than the size of the portal vein or the splenic vein for the evaluation of portal hypertension.

62

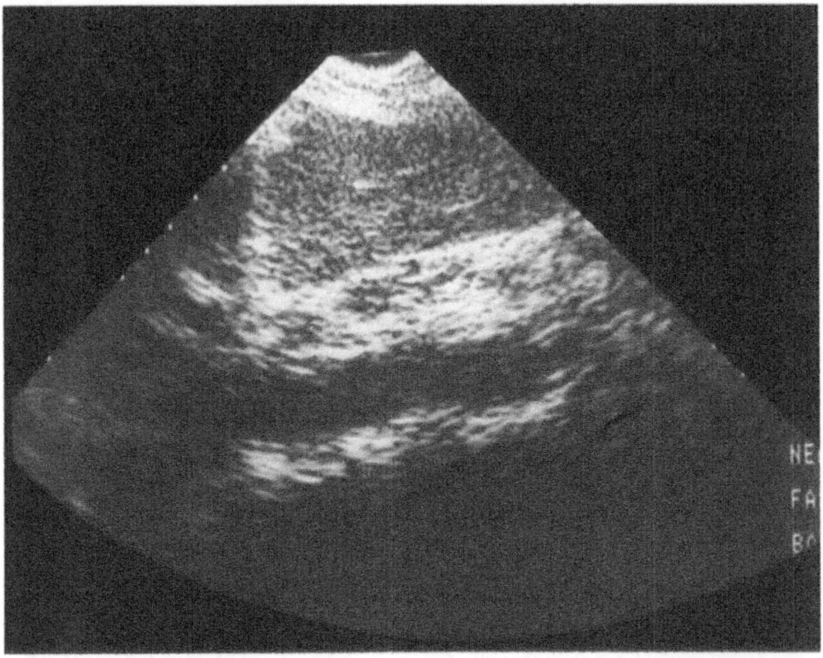

63

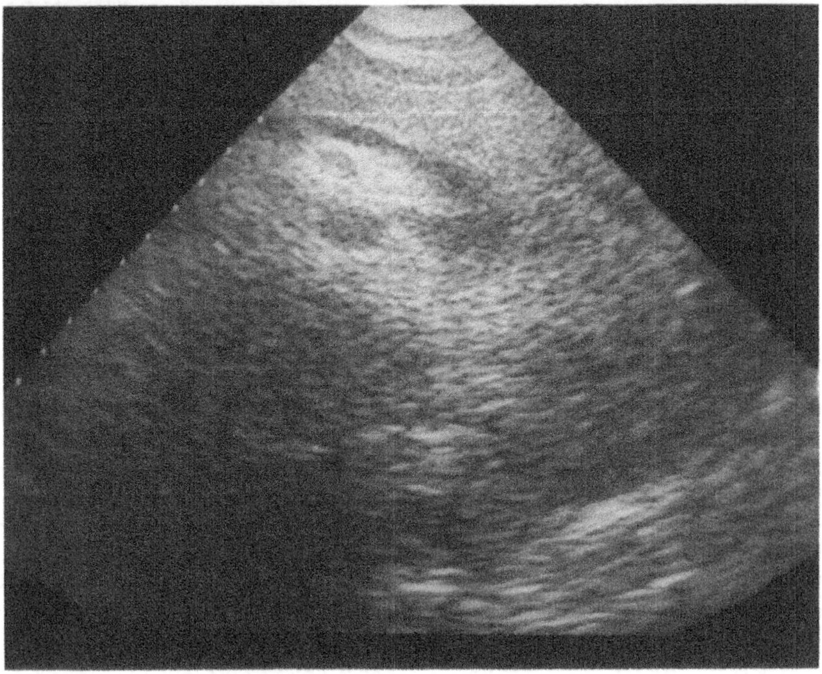

F liver
PA pancreas
1 aorta
2 infradiaphragmatic portion of the oesophagus (note the thickening of its wall due to variceal dilatations)
3 varices
4 superior mesenteric artery
5 splenic vein
6 dilated left renal vein
7 body of vertebra

Case 62
Clinical data: A 60-year-old woman requires assessment of alcoholism.

Description: The midsagittal scan passing anterior to the abdominal aorta shows confluent, oval or rounded echofree structures.

Diagnosis: There are moderate dilatations of the gastric vein, reflecting portal hypertension.

Comments: Varices in the lower portion of the oesophagus are detected by paramedian sagittal scans passing through the abdominal aorta inferiorly, the left lobe of the liver superiorly and (the annular digestive structure) the lower oesophagus (Cases 62 and 63). Sonography is less accurate when the dilatations are discrete. When the stomach is filled with air or with liquid, the cardio-oesophageal varices are compressed and therefore less easily seen. Another sign has been described and seems reliable: absence of a decrease in the calibre of the splenic vein and of the superior mesenteric vein during expiration.

Sonography has brought about a change in the investigation of portal hypertension. Angiography is carried out when portocaval anastomosis is being considered.

Case 63
Clinical data: This is the same patient as in Case 61, after splenectomy and portocaval anastomosis.

Description: Direct anastomosis between the proximal part of the splenic vein and the left renal vein is seen. Note the increased calibre of the left renal vein and the disappearance of the gastric-vein varices.

Comments: Ultrasonography allows postoperative assessment of portal hypertension. Function is assessed by visualization of the anastomosis itself when this is trunkular. Radicular or submesocolic anastomoses are more difficult to depict. The disappearance of oesophageal varices also demonstrates patency of the anastomosis. An increase in calibre of the inferior vena cava and, especially, absence of respiratory movements of this vessel are valuable but inconstant signs.

64

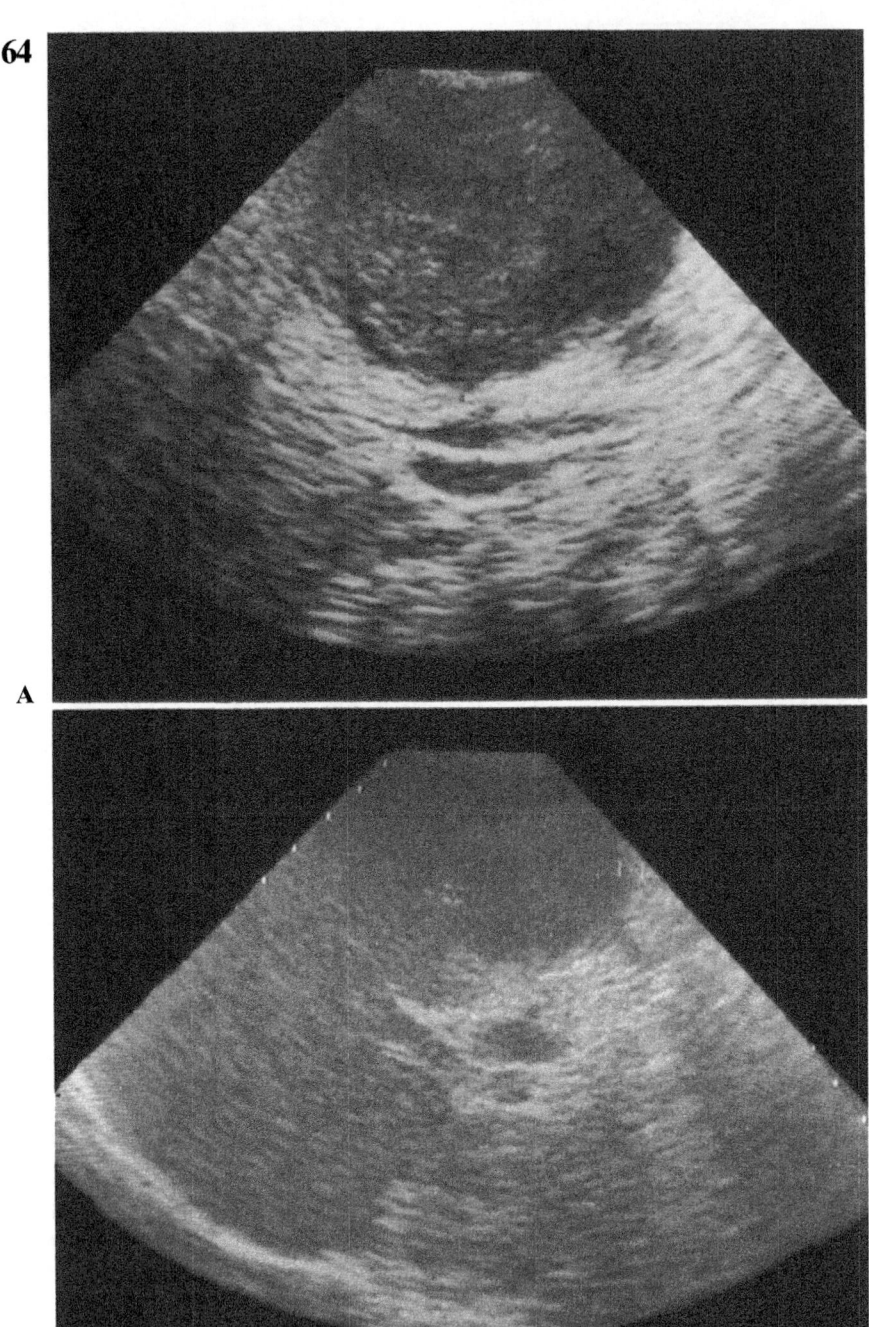

A

B

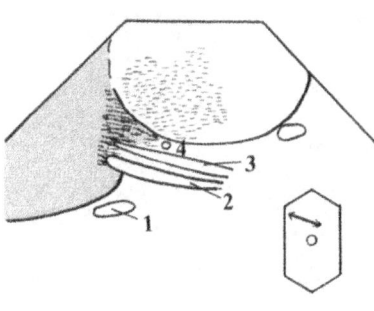

1 inferior vena cava
2 portal vein
3 common bile duct
4 right hepatic artery

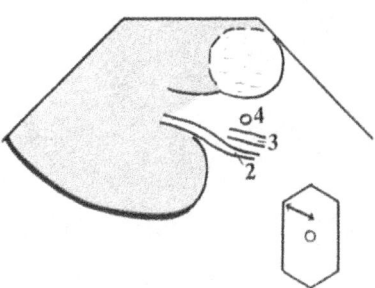

Case 64

Clinical data: This 70-year-old man with an unremarkable history was hospitalized with E. coli septicaemia. Scan A corresponds to the initial investigation. Scan B was taken 3 weeks later.

Description: A voluminous oval mass is detected in segment IV. It measures 9 cm in diameter. It is heterogeneous, with alternating hypo- and hyperechogenic areas, slight posterior enhancement, and vague demarcation from the hepatic parenchyma. Fine-needle apiration obtained pus containing colibacilli.

Diagnosis: There is an intrahepatic abscess.

Comments: A liver abscess may present as a solid mass, but this is rare (9% of cases). This appearance is due to the presence of cholesterol crystals, protein debris, or microbubbles within the abscess. Suggestive elements are posterior echo-enhancement and a fine peripheral halo. This is the appearance of the subacute stage. In the acute stage, poorly demarcated focal areas that are more echogenic than normal parenchyma are seen. There may be difficulties in differential diagnosis from metastases (which do not show posterior relative echo-enhancement).

In fact, there are many appearances, depending on the time of detection, and none is specific. Anything can be seen, from an echo-free lesion to a hyperechogenic solid mass.

Ultrasonography permits fine-needle guided biopsy and installation of drainage.

65

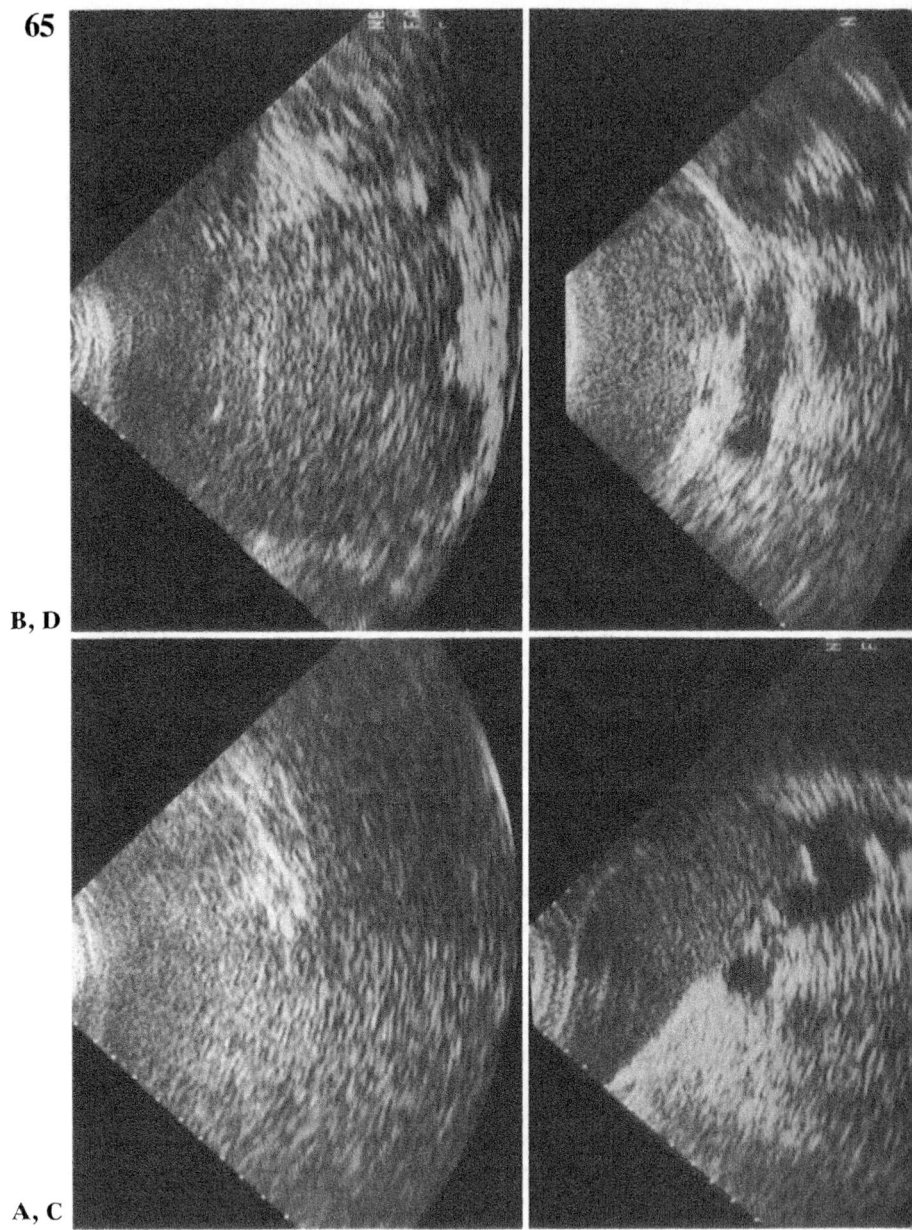

B, D

A, C

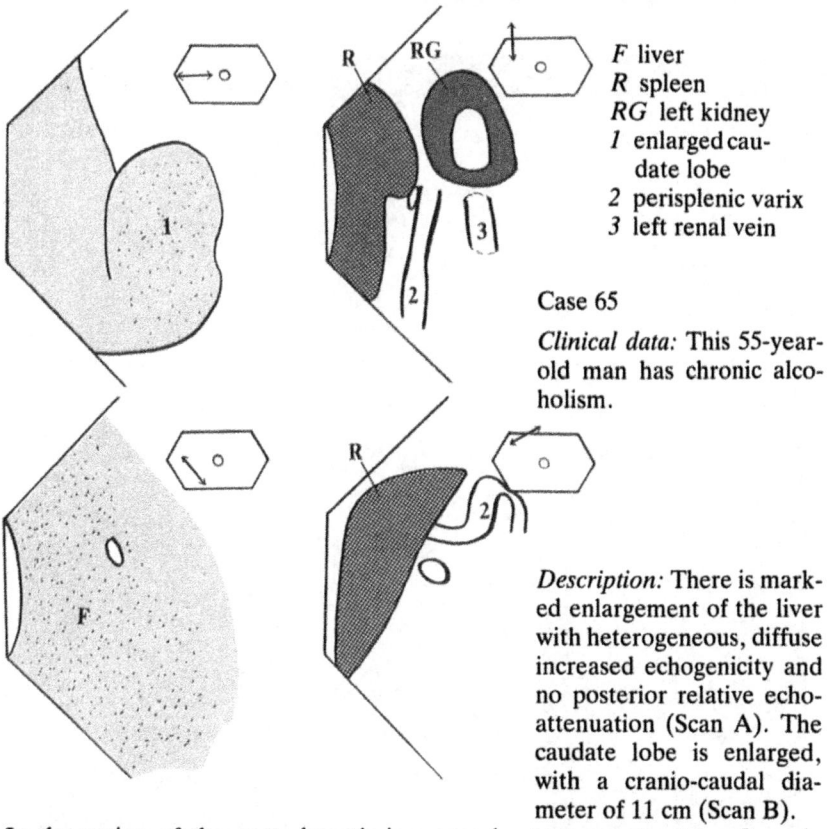

F liver
R spleen
RG left kidney
1 enlarged caudate lobe
2 perisplenic varix
3 left renal vein

Case 65

Clinical data: This 55-year-old man has chronic alcoholism.

Description: There is marked enlargement of the liver with heterogeneous, diffuse increased echogenicity and no posterior relative echo-attenuation (Scan A). The caudate lobe is enlarged, with a cranio-caudal diameter of 11 cm (Scan B). In the region of the porta hepatis is a vascular tortuous structure, 2 cm in diameter (Scan C). The left renal vein is dilated (Scan D). The size of the spleen is within normal limits. There is also a small amount of perihepatic ascites.

Diagnosis: There is exogenic hepatopathy with spontaneous splenorenal anastomosis, reflecting portal hypertension.

Comments: Centrifugal portocaval anastomoses towards the inferior vena cava have two pathways – spleno-renal or mesenterico-haemorrhoidal. The first is more easily visualized by ultrasounds and more frequent. The anastomoses originate from the distal part of the splenic vein, from the veins of the gastric wall and/or from the left suprarenal vein. The left renal vein and the inferior vena cava become dilated because of the increased blood-flow. They may develop in isolation or along with gastro-oesophageal varices.

Enlargement of the caudate lobe (normal value 5 cm) has been described as a sign of cirrhosis. This sign is not specific, since it is also seen in the Budd-Chiari syndrome.

On the whole, ultrasonography is a very good investigation for this type of pathology. It has three roles – in positive diagnosis (detection of collateral circulation, ascites, splenomegaly and abnormal echostructure of the liver), etiologic diagnosis and prognosis (haemorrhage potential).

66

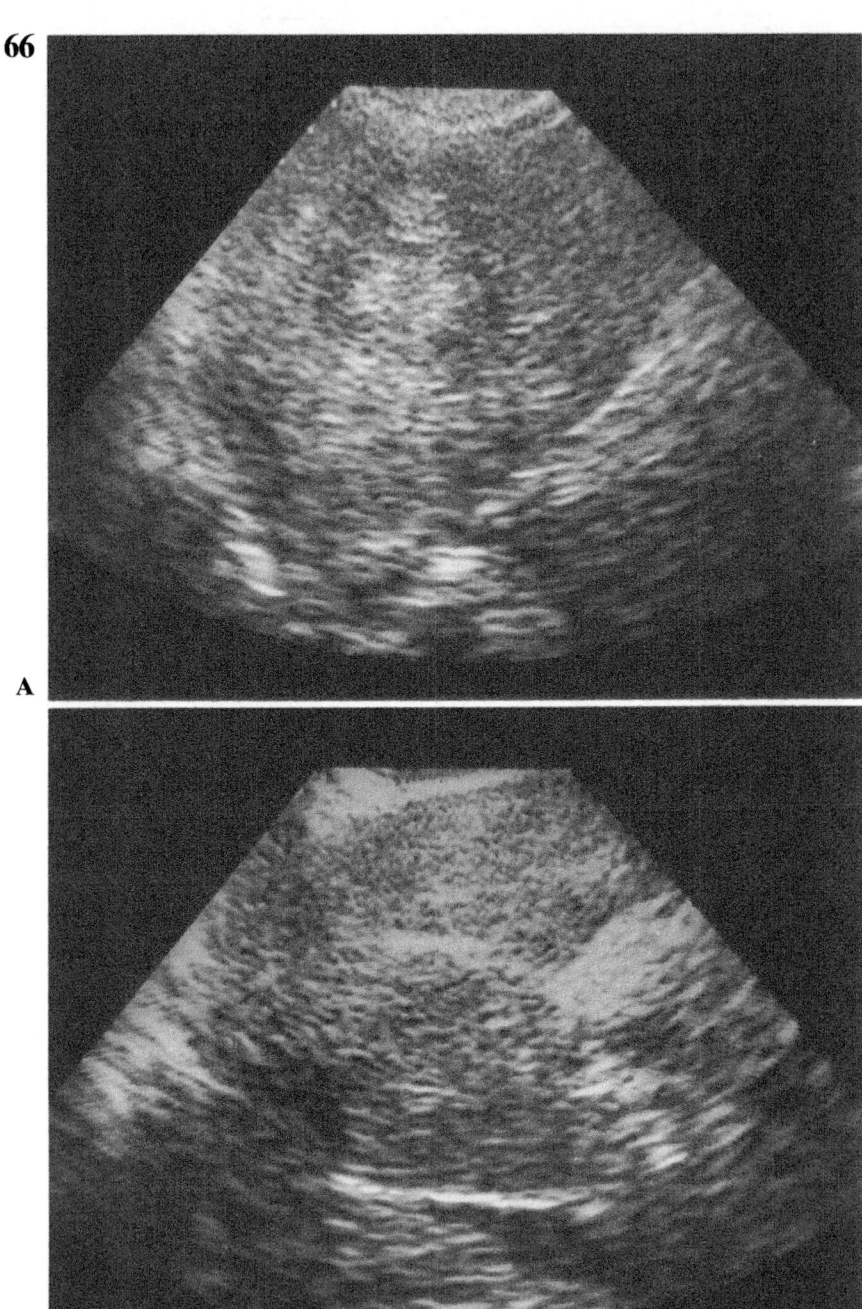

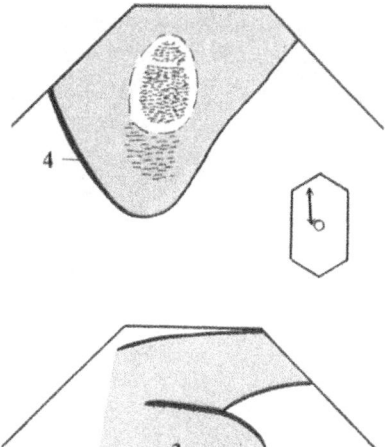

1 portal vein
2 inferior vena cava
3 enlarged caudate lobe
4 diaphragm

Case 66

Clinical data: A 55-year-old patient with alcoholism and nicotinism presented with progressive jaundice.

Description: A rounded mass, 5 cm in diameter, is seen in segment VII. It has a hyperechogenic centre, surrounded by a hypoechogenic area with irregular borders. Note the discrete posterior relative echo-enhancement. On a midsagittal scan (Scan A) note the enlarged caudate lobe, reflecting cirrhotic involvement.

Diagnosis: This was initially thought to be hepatoma on cirrhosis. Eventually, it was histologically proved to be a cholangiocarcinoma.

Comments: There are two histological forms of primary hepatic carcinoma – hepatocellular carcinoma or hepatoma derived from the parenchymal cells of the liver (Case 45), and cholangocellular carcinoma or cholangiocarcinoma developing in the intrahepatic bile ducts. The latter type is much more rare. There are also mixed forms and sarcomas, which are even more rare.

Three forms of cholangiocarcinoma can be distinguished:
– Peripheral or distal (Case 66) developing in the intrahepatic biliary canalicules
– Proximal, revealed by isolated dilatation of the intrahepatic bile ducts proximal to the obstruction
– Extrahepatic, involving the main bile duct (Case 32)

Macroscopically and histologically, the peripheral form may be difficult to differentiate from adenocarcinoma.
   This lesion occurs in 25% of cases in cirrhotic livers. The hypoechogenic ring corresponds to a fibrous capsule. Its progression is slower than that of classical adenocarcinoma, so that surgery is possible.
   In this case too, sonography is a morphological investigation. It participates especially in the assessment of extension.

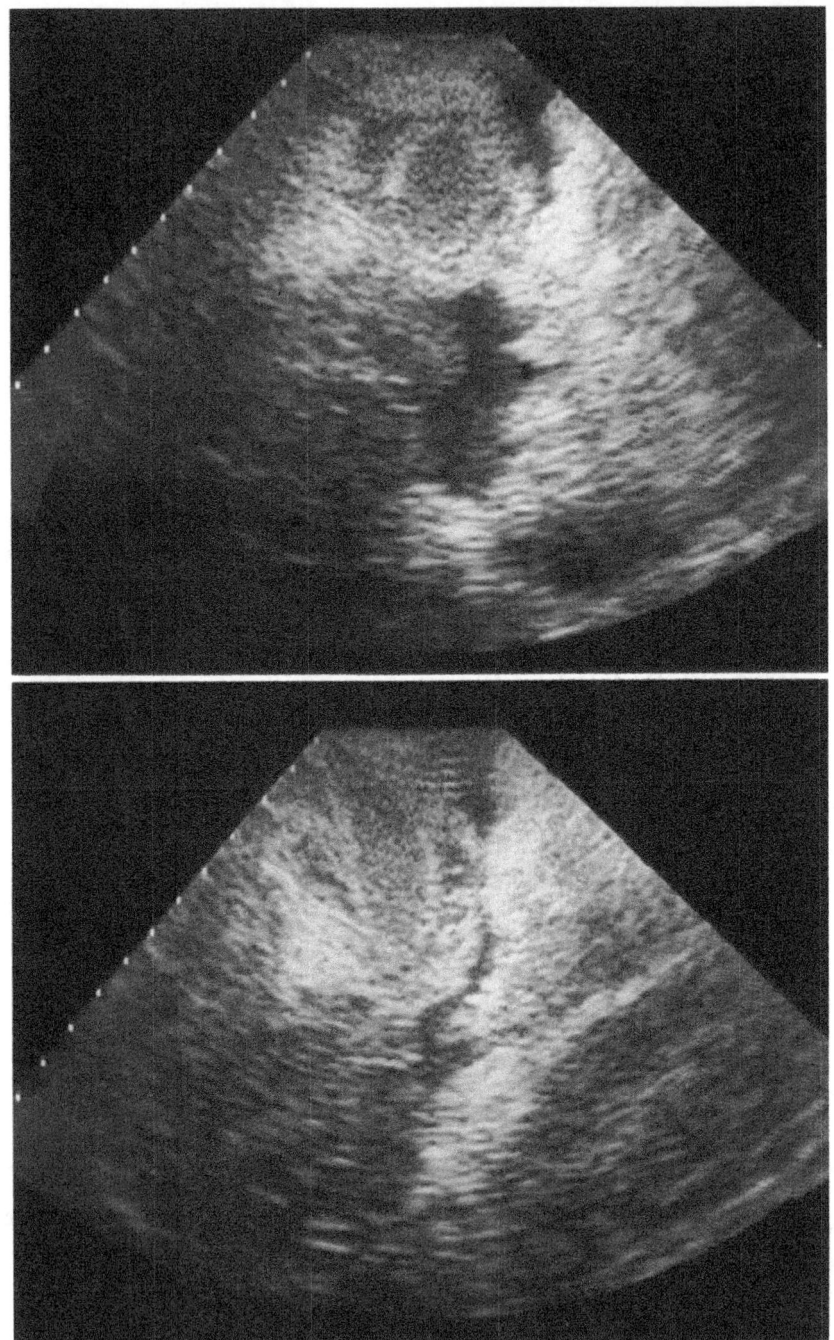

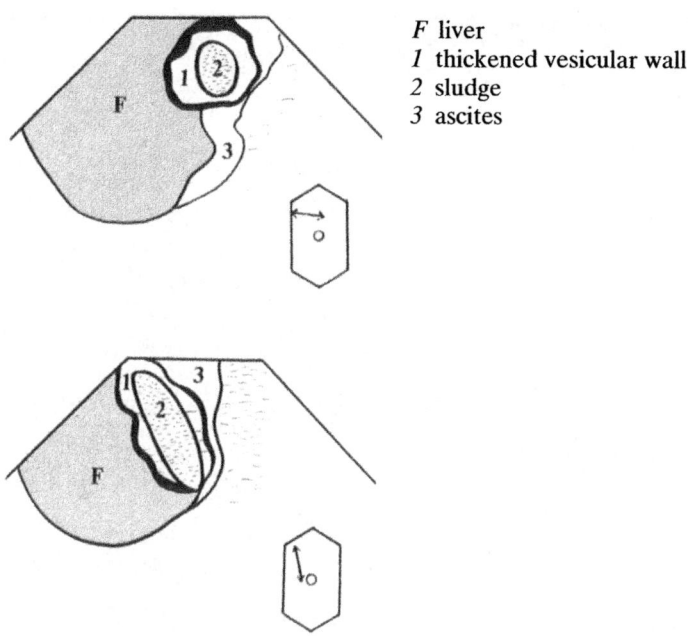

F liver

67

1 thickened vesicular wall
2 sludge
3 ascites

Case 67

Clinical data: This 50-year-old man has decompensated alcoholic cirrhosis.

Description: The gallbladder is abnormal. Regularly distributed intravesicular echoes correspond to sludge. The considerable thickening of the gallbladder wall consists of several echo-free structures, which are irregular and tortuous, and located in the middle of the wall. You have certainly noted the presence of ascites.

Diagnosis: There is dilatation of the perivesicular veins, a sign of portal hypertension.

Comments: Portal hypertension is defined on purely clinical grounds by associating collateral circulation, splenomegaly, ascites, gastrointestinal haemorrhage from ruptured varices, and manometrical alterations.

Dilatation of the perivesicular veins – also termed Sappey's veins by some authors, has seldom been described in the literature. It is seen in cirrhoses and, more particularly, in portal vein thrombosis. Dilatations are usually located outside the muscular tissue and are associated with thickening of the walls. Their size varies from 1–5 cm. Continuity of the varices with the portal system is hardly ever demonstrated using ultrasonography. When they are normal, these veins correspond to an accessory portal system; it is not an anastomosis. Their dimensions are not proportional to the degree of portal hypertension.

68

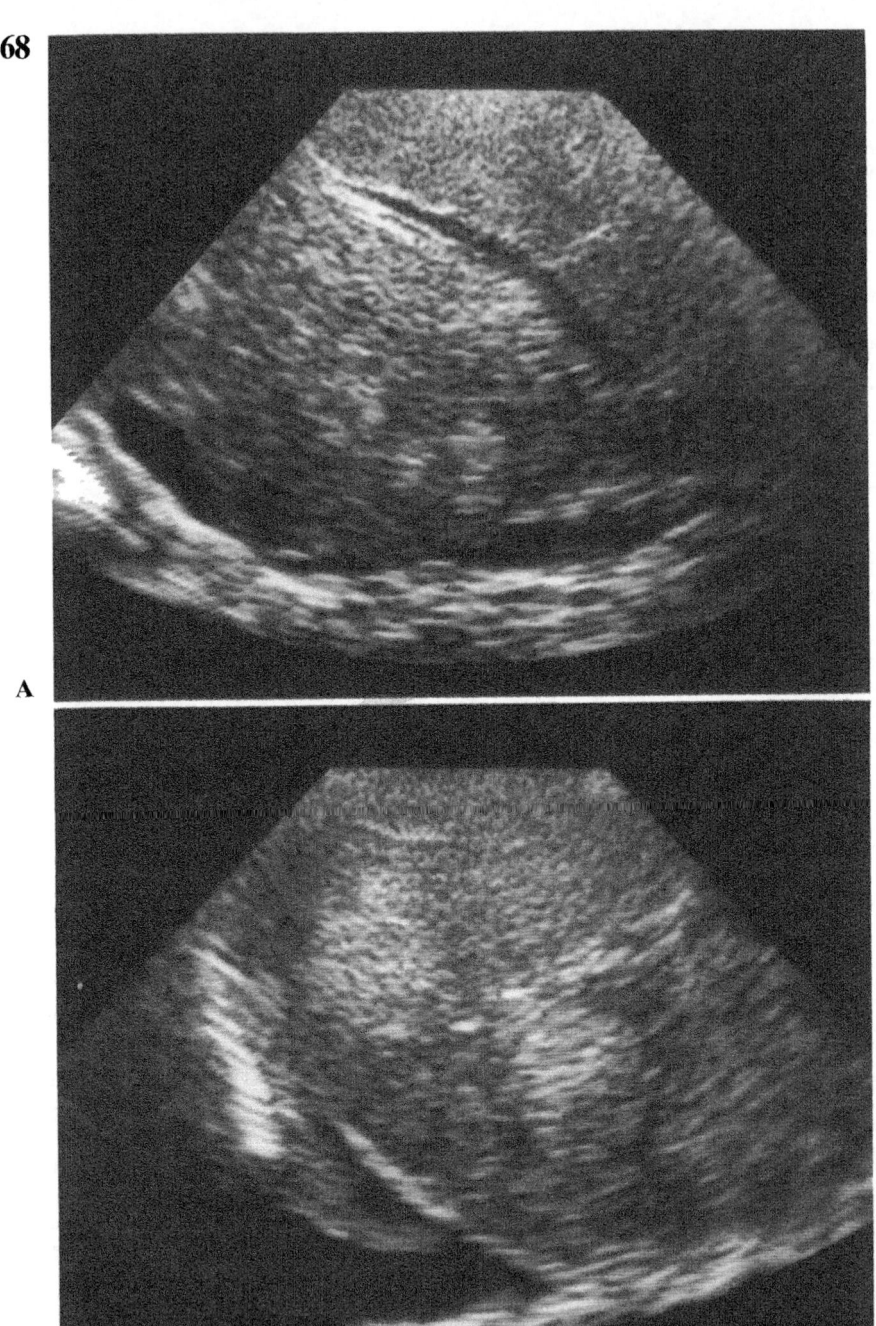

A

B

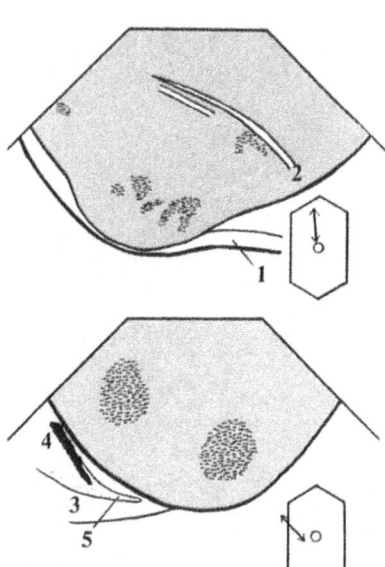

1 inferior vena cava **68**
2 right portal vein with biliary tributary
3 right pleural effusion
4 pulmonary air
5 segmental atelectasis

Case 68

Clinical data: A 50-year-old woman with carcinoma of the colon was operated 1 year ago, and received chemotherapy. She is being investigated for reassessment.

Description: There is a voluminous mass, 7 cm in diameter, situated in segments I and IV; it is heterogeneous and contains some structures of increased echogenicity causing compression of the inferior vena cava and displacement of the left portal vein. In segments VII and VIII, two hyperechogenic structures with irregular borders are seen. Note the right pleural effusion and partial atelectasis of the lower part of the right lobe, which is floating in the pleural fluid. The hyperechogenic band corresponds to pleural air (Scan B).

Diagnosis: This is easy: hepatic metastases from a colonic carcinoma.

Comments: Some metastases are associated with a poor prognosis – those from hepatoma and oesophageal, gastric and pancreatic lesions. Others, however, permit more prolonged survival: oto-rhino-laryngeal tumours and non-colonic carcinomas. In 20%–35% of colonic carcinomas there are metastases to the liver.

Sonography alone has a sensitivity of 90% and a specificity of 75%. Although it does not allow one to diagnose the nature of the lesion, it provides precise information about the primary site, the lymph nodes, vascular thrombosis, ascites and involvement of the spleen. When it is combined with biochemical tests of hepatic function, the specificity of sonography increases. It also permits guided puncture. Some teams have pointed out the advantage of peroperative sonography for determination of the exact number and size of lesions as well as of their topography with regard to surgical landmarks.

The accuracy of computed tomography is no better.

69

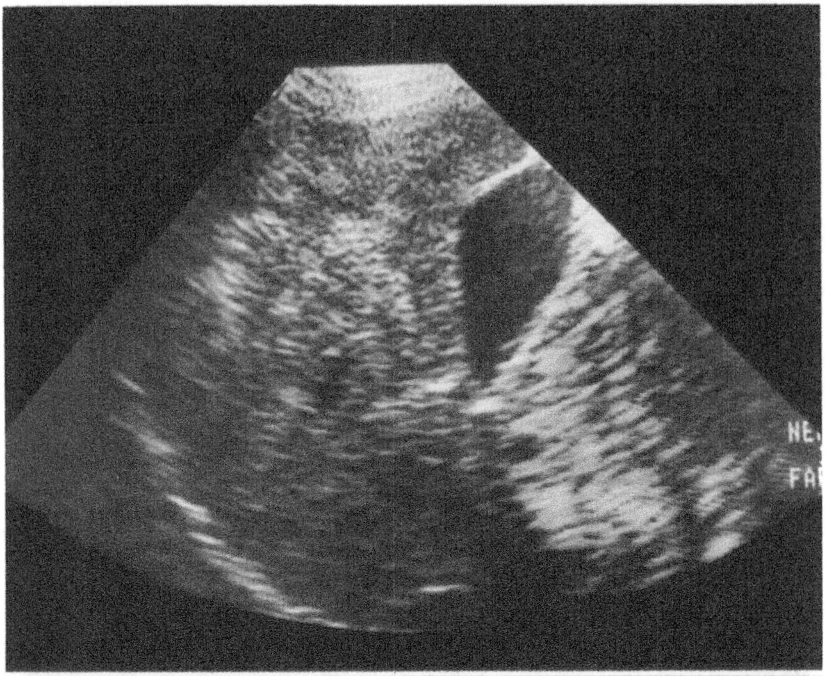

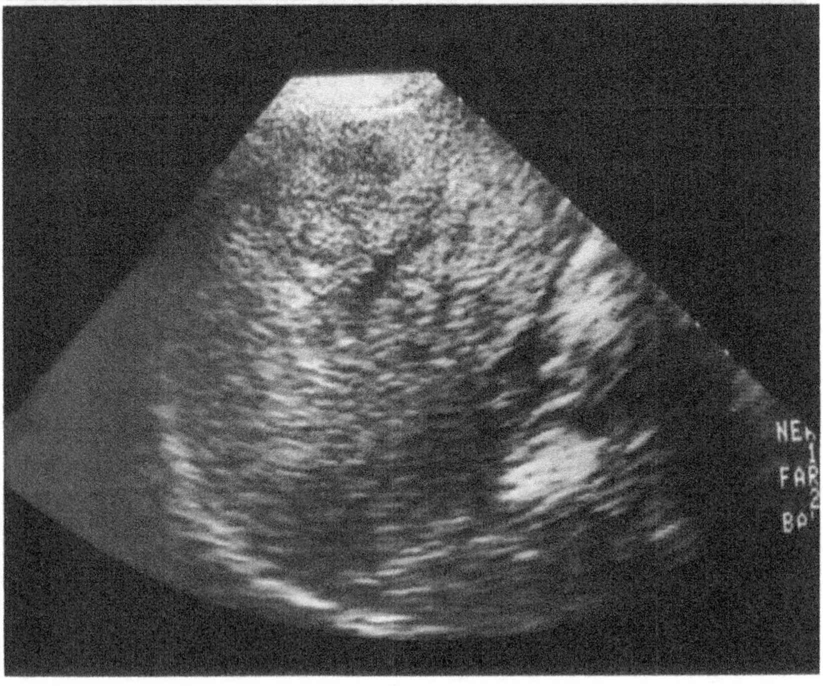

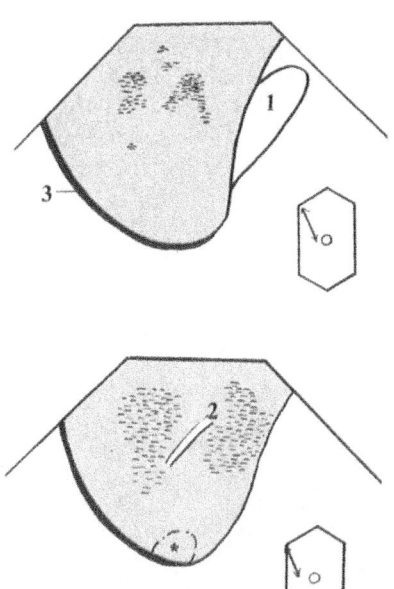

1 gallbladder
2 branch of right hepatic vein
3 diaphragm

Case 69

Clinical data: This 50-year-old man has diabetes and hypertriglyceridaemia.

Description: Note the poorly demarcated hyperechogenic areas, distributed throughout the whole right hepatic lobe. Their echostructure is homogeneous. There is no compression of the vascular structures and no "mass effect". The size of the liver is normal.

Diagnosis: You are wrong, this is not a primary or secondary tumoural process, but localized steatosis. The diagnosis is difficult, because the lesions are usually more circumscribed. Computed tomography and puncture-biopsy of the liver confirmed the diagnosis.

Comments: Steatosis of the liver is usually considered to be diffuse. Localized fatty infiltrations have been seen however. The sonographic appearance always leads one to suspect a neoplastic process. There are, however, some semiologic criteria – the image is not spherical, *there is no mass effect on the hepatic borders or vessels,* the borders of the steatosic area are sharp. The etiology of this form is the same as that of diffuse involvement, but the reason for the heterogeneous distribution remains unknown. Computed tomography shows localized hypodense areas, which are not spherical and have no mass effect. Diagnosis is based on measurement of the density, which is negative or near zero. When doubt remains, puncture-biopsy of the liver will provide the definite diagnosis.

The roughly rounded hypoechogenic area in segment VI (Scan B) (*) corresponds to normal parenchyma. Here again, there is a risk that a false diagnosis of a hypoechogenic mass will be made.

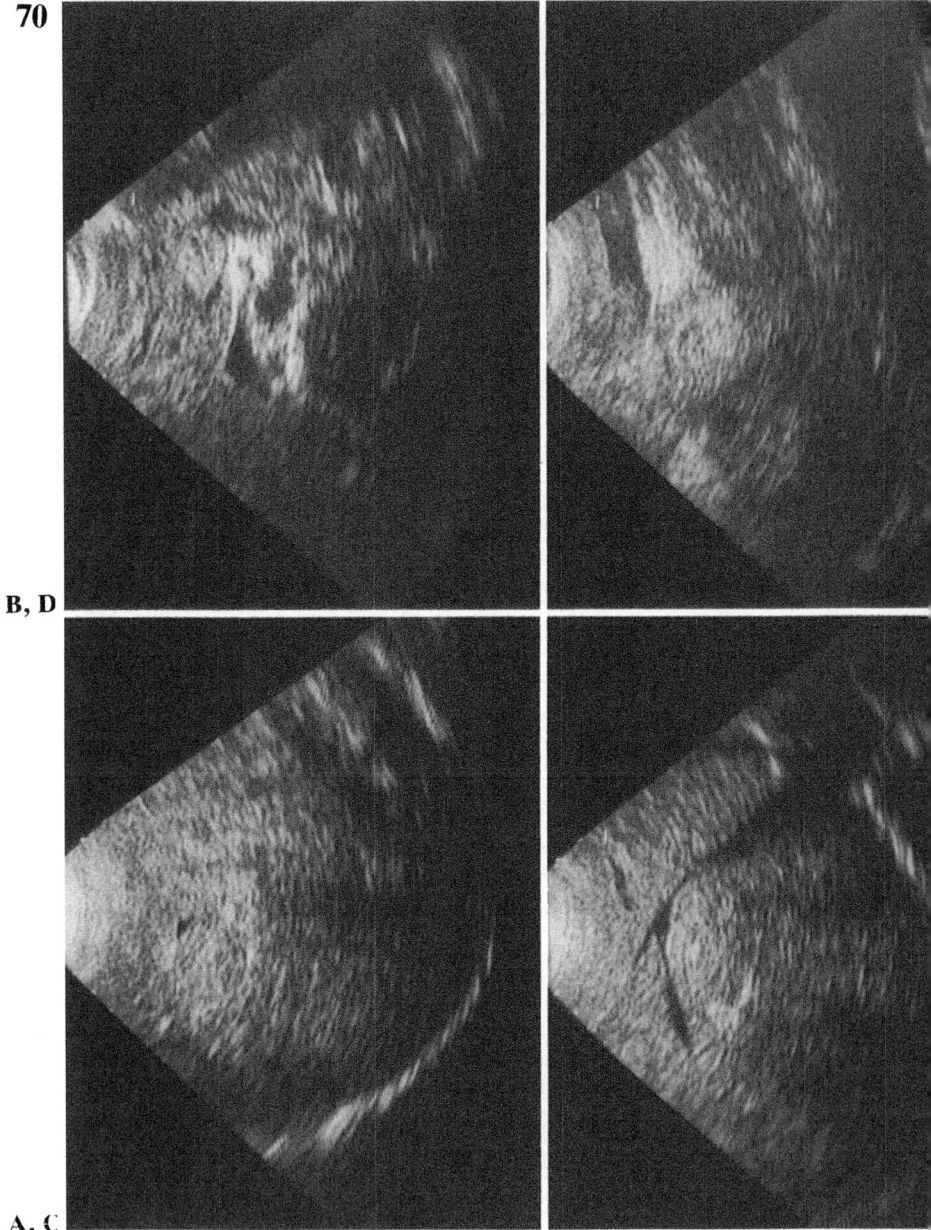

B, D

A, C

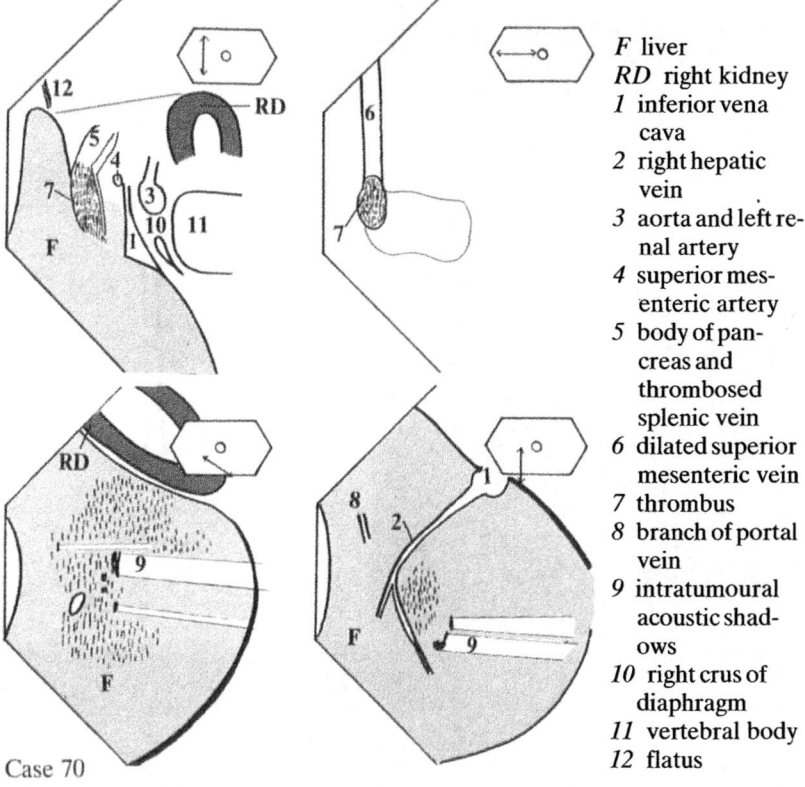

F liver
RD right kidney
1 inferior vena cava
2 right hepatic vein
3 aorta and left renal artery
4 superior mesenteric artery
5 body of pancreas and thrombosed splenic vein
6 dilated superior mesenteric vein
7 thrombus
8 branch of portal vein
9 intratumoural acoustic shadows
10 right crus of diaphragm
11 vertebral body
12 flatus

Case 70

Clinical data: This 35-year-old Senegalese man has alteration of general status and pain in the right hypochondrium.

Description: You should have noted the following features:
a) A heterogeneous mass with indistinct limits in the right hepatic lobe has shifted the right hepatic vein (Scan C) and compressed the right side of the inferior vena cave (Scan B).
b) The portal vein is replaced by an elongated echogenic structure, 1 cm thick, corresponding to a thrombus in the portal vein. This extends from the splenic vein to the superior mesenteric vein (Scans B–D).
Note also the dilatation of the superior mesenteric vein.

Diagnosis: Hepatoma of the right liver lobe with extensive venous thrombosis.

Comments: Hepatoma is very frequent in Asia and in Southern Africa, and occurs in men and women. It represents 10%–40% of all cancers. The HbS antigen in present in one case out of two. Thrombosis of the portal trunk is responsible for presinusoidal portal hypertension and sometimes for arterioportal shunt. Note the intratumoural acoustic shadows (Scan A). They do not correspond to intratumoural calcifications, but are artefacts due to reflection of the ultrasound beam on a curved surface in two structures with different acoustic impedances – normal liver and tumoural tissue.

71

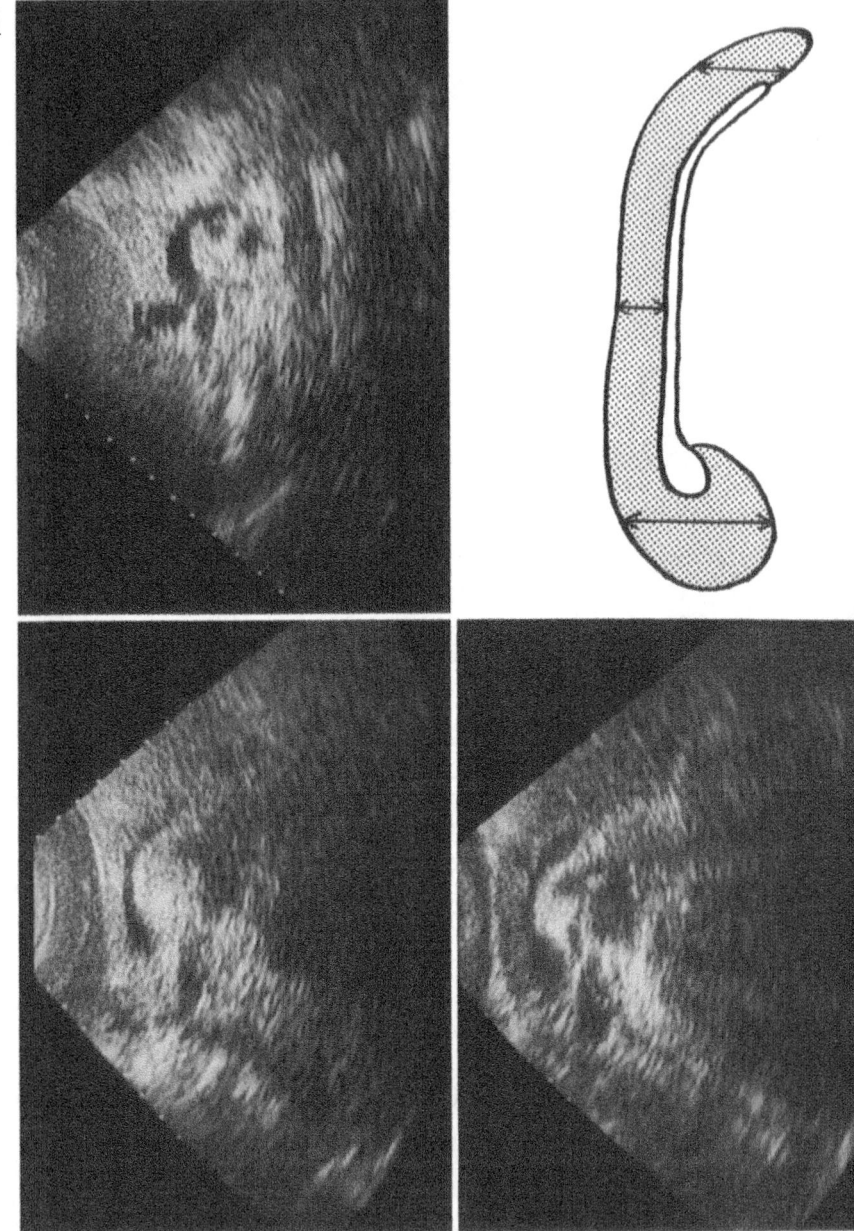

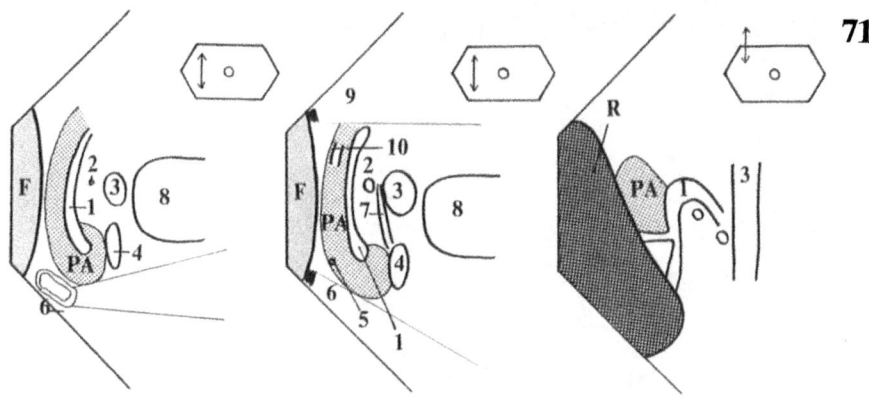

F liver	*2* superior mesenteric artery	*6* duodenum
PA pancreas	*3* aorta	*7* left renal vein
R spleen	*4* inferior vena cava	*8* vertebral body
1 splenic vein	*5* gastroduodenal artery	*9* gas in the stomach
		10 splenic artery

Case 71

Visualization of the pancreas is usually easy, but it may require compression of the epigastric region to eliminate bowel gas, or placement of the patient in the erect position. Limitations in visualization may also be overcome by asking the patient to drink several glasses of water to create a fluid-filled ultrasound window.

The pancreas is visualized by means of its vascular landmarks: the splenic vein (1); superior mesenteric artery (2); aorta (3); inferior vena cava (4); gastroduodenal artery (5). The size and shape of the pancreas are variable. Its dimensions measured in the transverse plane are 2.5−3 cm for the head, 0.4− 2 cm for the neck and 0.7−3 cm for the corporeo-caudal region. Values below or equal to 3.5 cm in the head region are considered normal.

Sonography does not always permit satisfactory visualization of the pancreatic tail, even with the transrenal approach. The previously described manoeuvres, as well as placement of the patient in the prone position, may be helpful.

The echogenicity of the pancreas is similar or superior to that of the liver. It actually depends on the patient's age and on the subcutaneous fat layer. These two factors are independent and cause increased echogenicity of the pancreatic parenchyma. Histopathological studies have shown that after the age of 60 years there is moderate or significant accumulation of fat in the acinar cells. Analysis of the parenchyma in acute or chronic pancreatis in old patients is therefore difficult.

The accuracy of ultrasonography for the detection of pancreatic diseases is 70%; its specificity is 80%.

72

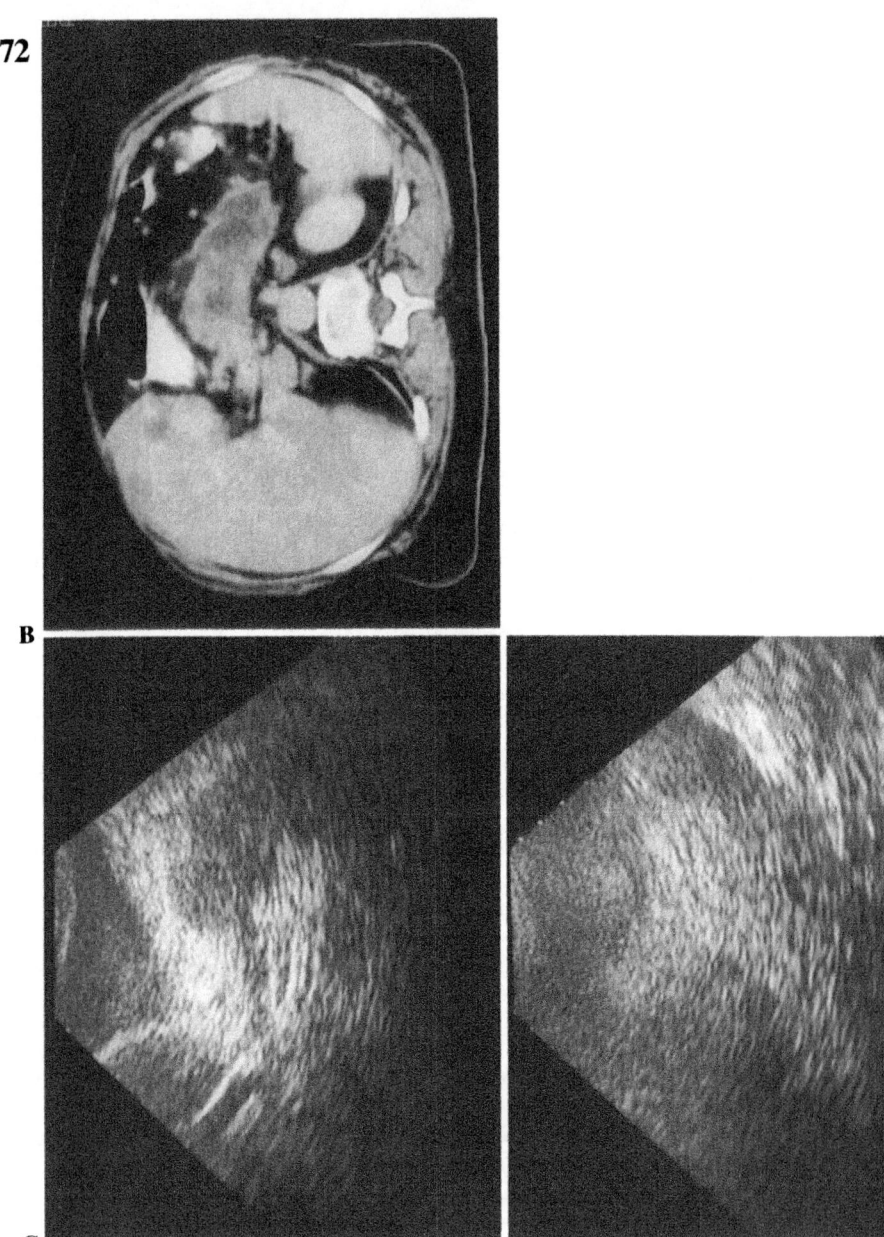

B

A, C

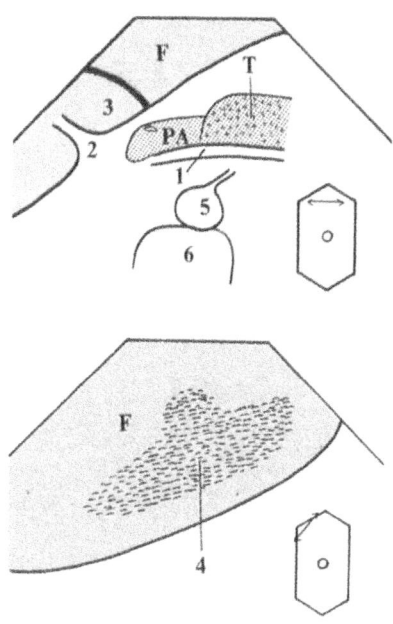

F liver
PA pancreas
T tumour
1 splenic vein
2 portal vein
3 round ligament
4 hepatic metastases
5 aorta
6 body of vertebra

72

Case 72

Clinical data: A 60-year-old woman had been complaining of heaviness in the epigastric region.

Description: There is a hypoechogenic, homogeneous mass with indistinct borders in the body of the pancreas; it commences roughly at the level of the superior mesenteric artery and is responsible for enlargement of the pancreas. Note that the tail of the pancreas is not visualized. There are also hyperechogenic, homogeneous and poorly demarcated areas in the right hepatic lobe.

Diagnosis: There is a tumour of the body and tail of the pancreas with metastases to the liver. Note the very clear visualization of the tail of the pancreas, which had not been seen with ultrasonography. Note also the hypertrophy of the left adrenal gland, also not shown sonographically (Scan B).

Comments: Most primary tumours of the pancreas are adenocarcinomas of the glandular epithelium with various degrees of differentiation. In about two-thirds of cases, the site involved is the head of the pancreas. Tumours involving the entire pancreas are very rare. According to some authors, diabetes is a predisposing factor.

The sensitivity of sonography is about 70%. Lesions below 2 cm are difficult to detect, especially when the echostructure is not greatly modified. In such cases ingestion of a large volume of water will help by creating an acoustic window. The accuracy of computed tomography is better with tumours of the pancreatic tail. Remember, however, that at the time when the tumour is detected, 90% of the patients are incurable.

73

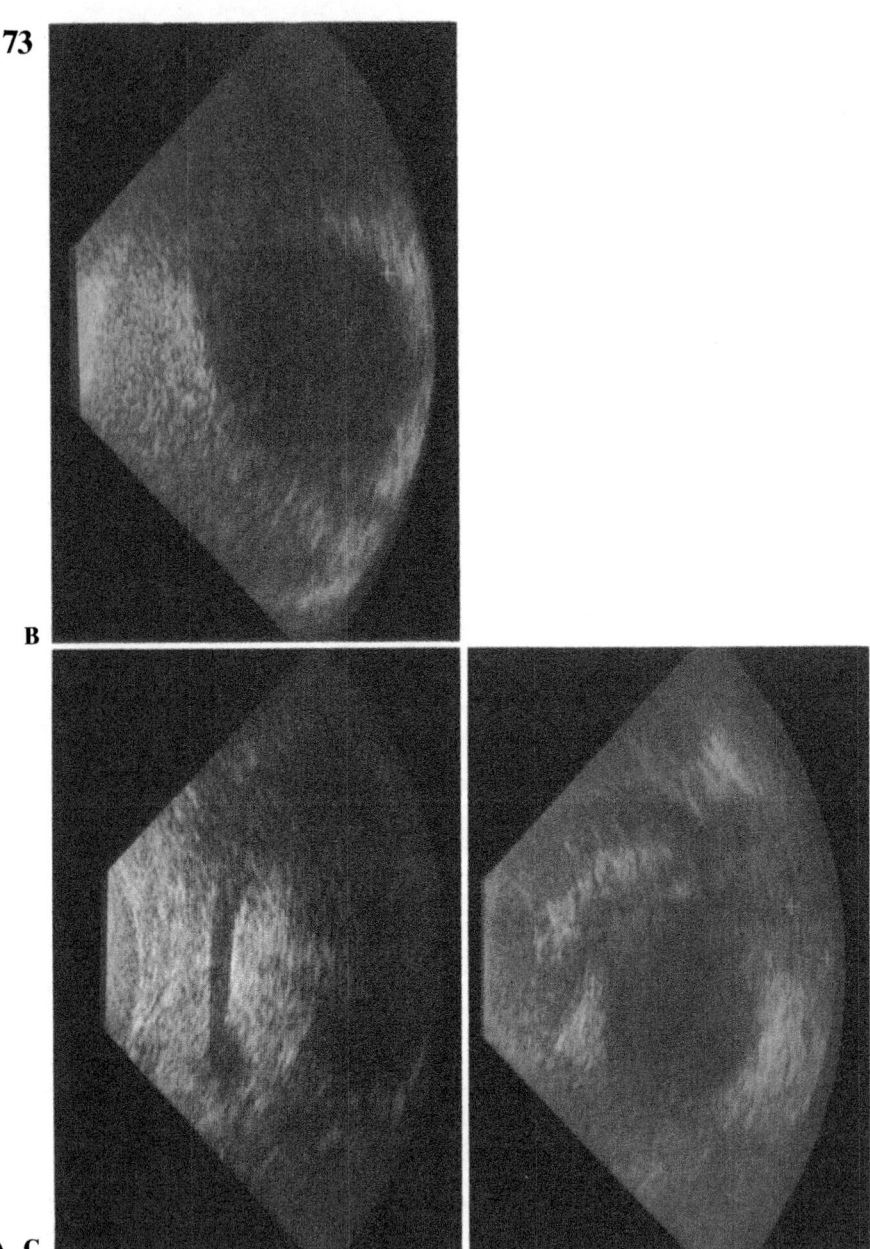

B

A, C

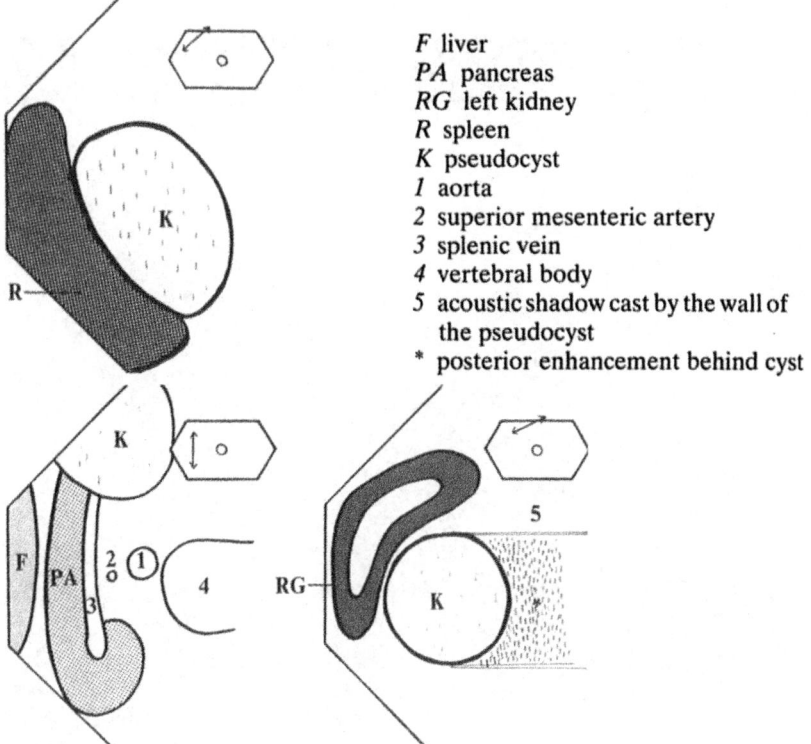

F liver
PA pancreas
RG left kidney
R spleen
K pseudocyst
1 aorta
2 superior mesenteric artery
3 splenic vein
4 vertebral body
5 acoustic shadow cast by the wall of
  the pseudocyst
* posterior enhancement behind cyst

Case 73

Clinical data: A 60-year-old man had complained about pain in the epigastric region for 3 months.

Description: There is a hypoechogenic structure in the left hypochondrium. It is very large – 7 cm in diameter – with smooth walls and contains some fine echos. It causes displacement of the left kidney (Scan C). At the level of the head and of the body the pancreatic parenchyma appears discretely heterogeneous but has normal echogenicity with regard to the patient's age. It has normal dimensions. Note the presence of posterior relative echo enhancement (Scan C) (*) reflecting the presence of a liquid mass.

Diagnosis: There is a pseudocyst in the tail of the pancreas.

Comments: It is not always easy to affirm that a lesion involves the pancreas, especially when it concerns the tail. One must rule out renal, adrenal and mesenteric cysts, a cystic pancreatic tumour and finally a hypoechogenic structure in lymphomatosis.

Pseudocysts are secondary to segmental liquefaction of the adrenal, associated with exudative reactions. They are evolutive. About 10 days after the onset of clinical manifestations of acute pancreatitis, a poorly demarcated echo-free area appears within the pancreatic parenchyma. Its volume is variable. Some – usually 3 – weeks later, a fibrous capsule or wall appears. The term

73

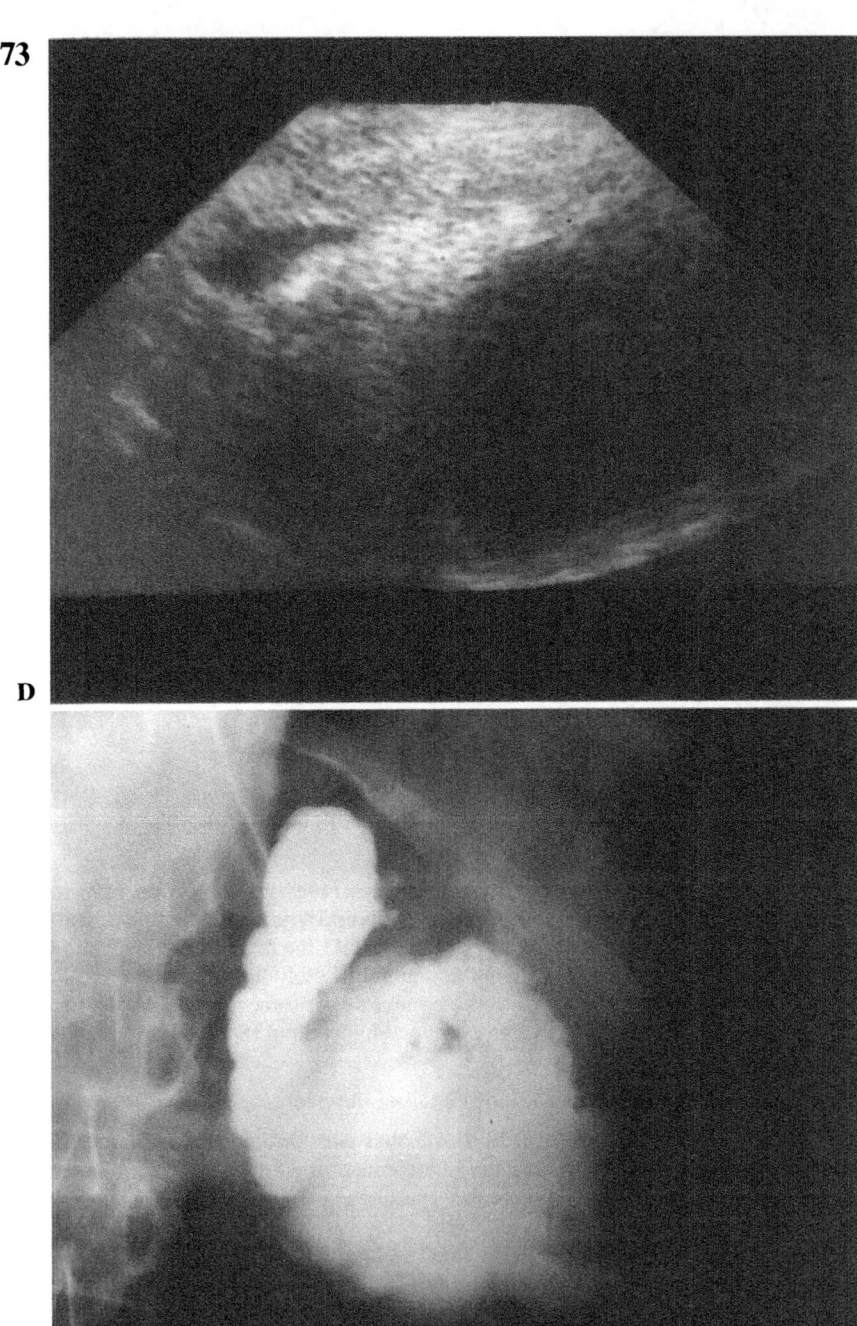

D

E

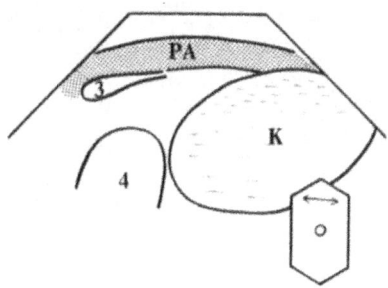

pseudocyst is then appropriate; until then it was only a fluid collection. The wall thickens progressively and may even calcify. The echo-pattern described here corresponds to an advanced stage. The heterogeneity of the mass is due to the presence of necrotic debris or of blood clots. These may be located in the most downward-sloping parts or be regularly scattered throughout the mass.

Pseudocysts may be solitary or multiple; they may be located in the pancreas or outside the liver (in the omenta, left anterior pararenal space, posterior pararenal space, mesentery, mediastinum or pelvis). Pseudocysts are found in 10% of acute pancreatitis cases, but they can also be a complication of an acute exacerbation of chronic pancreatitis. They seem to occur more commonly in acute pancreatitis of alcoholic origin.

Ultrasonography permits detection of masses above 2 cm in size. In fact, the rate of detection also depends on the site and on the equipment which is utilized. Anyhow, computed tomography is more accurate.

The course of the disease is variable – spontaneous regression by fistulization in a hollow viscera, or, most commonly, aggravation may occur. Increase in size is a sign of communication with the pancreatic secretory system. Some small cysts of the pancreas may remain asymptomatic for a long time. Sometimes the complications require surgery – incomplete fistulization in a hollow viscera, intracystic haemorrhage, secondary infection and intraperitoneal rupture.

Ultrasound detection of the pseudocystic stage is fundamental for monitoring progress and treatment. After a certain delay – 6 weeks, according to certain authors – drainage with sonographically guided puncture of a pseudocyst with capsule is advisable (Scan E). Ultrasound assessment of the presence and thickness of a wall is fundamental, since premature drainage of a poorly delimited collection is a source of complications. Some authors recommend immediate recourse to surgery in order to avoid any risk of infection.

74

B, D

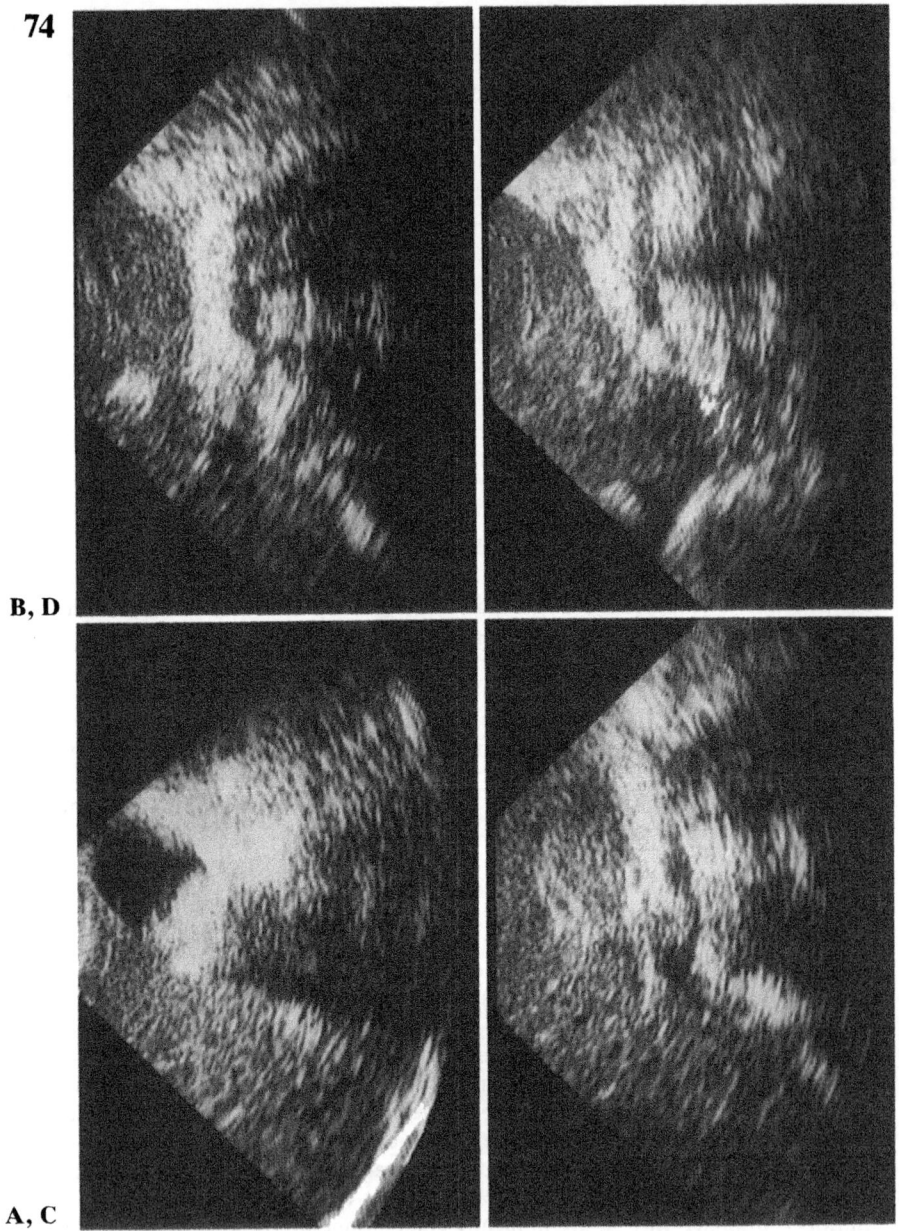

A, C

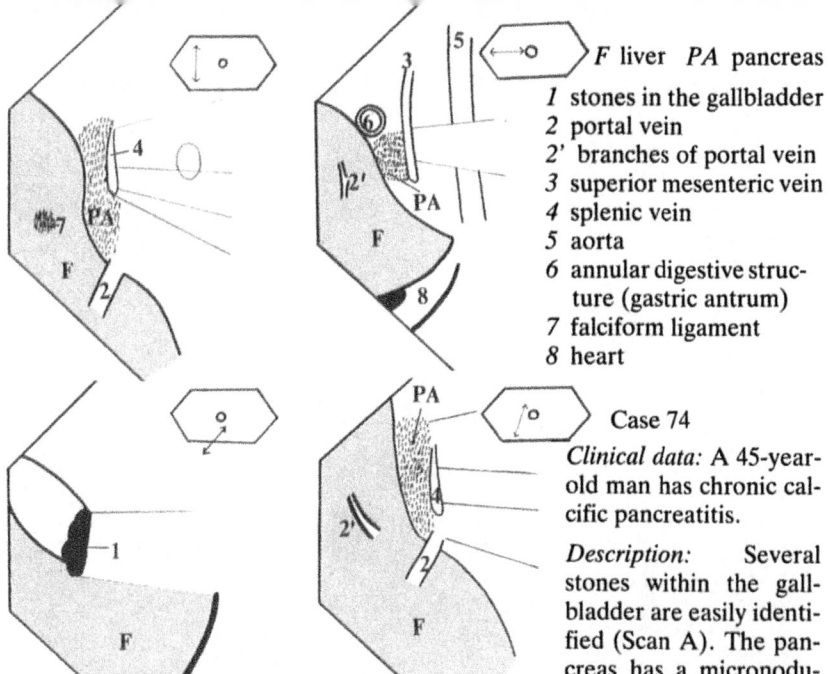

1 stones in the gallbladder
2 portal vein
2' branches of portal vein
3 superior mesenteric vein
4 splenic vein
5 aorta
6 annular digestive structure (gastric antrum)
7 falciform ligament
8 heart

Case 74

Clinical data: A 45-year-old man has chronic calcific pancreatitis.

Description: Several stones within the gallbladder are easily identified (Scan A). The pancreas has a micronodular, intensely echogenic structure. Its size is normal. Acoustic shadows reflect the presence of calcifications throughout the gland. Note also the poor visualization of the distal part of the splenic vein (Scans B and D). The hyperechogenic structure in the hepatic parenchyma corresponds to the falciform ligament (Scan B).

Diagnosis: This is calcifying chronic pancreatitis. The presence of calcification is pathognomonic, but the echostructure of the pancreas shown here is atypical; it is usually of the heterogeneous type. In fact the sonographic appearance of chronic pancreatitis varies greatly.

Comments: Pancreatic calcification is seen mainly in alcoholic chronic pancreatitis and more rarely in reccurent chronic pancreatitis with gallstones. The calcifications always correspond to intraductal or intracanalicular calculi. Parenchymatous calcifications occur in a different context after traumatic of iatrogenic intraparenchymatous haemorrhage.

The sonographic findings in calcifying chronic pancreatitis are: normal size, localized enlargement, diffuse enlargement or atrophy; and a localized reflective echo-pattern with or without acoustic shadow, reflecting the presence of lithiasis or of fibrosis. Signs of compression must be sought systematically: dilatation of the main bile duct; disappearance of the splenic vein with splenomegaly (a sign of its thrombosis, either global or segmental regular or irregular dilatation of the main pancreatic (Wirsung's) duct; signs of disease progression, such as an attack of acute pancreatitis (a hypoechogenic area associated with sometimes localized enlargement); pseudocyst formation.

You should also search for the cause. Changes in the echo-pattern of the liver may be consistent with exogenous intoxication. Gallbladder lithiasis may be present.

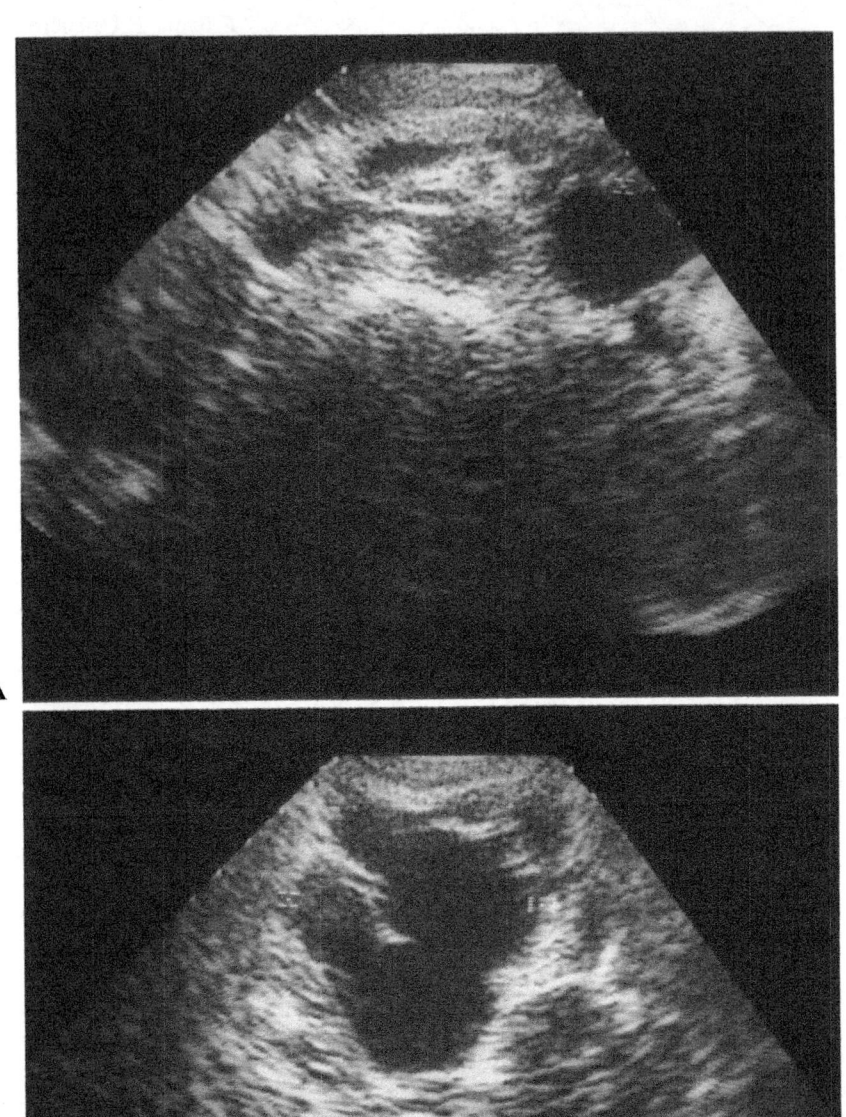

A

B

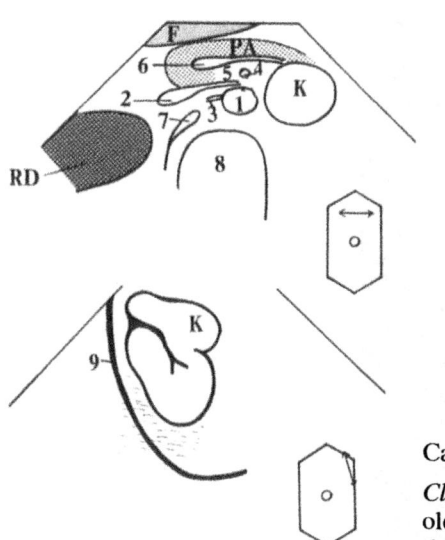

F liver
RD right kidney
PA pancreas
K cyst
1 aorta
2 inferior vena cava
3 right renal artery
4 superior mesenteric artery
5 left renal vein
6 splenic vein
7 right crus of the diaphragm
8 vertebra
9 diaphragm

Case 75

Clinical data: This patient is a 60-year-old diabetic man in poor physical condition.

Description: Scan B shows a roughly rounded, echo-free left hypochondrial mass, with septations and posterior relative echo-enhancement. Its borders are smooth, and its long axis is 6.5 cm. The most difficult part of the investigation is localization of the mass in the tail of the pancreas and exclusion of an adrenal, or even renal tumour. This requires several scans and eventually having the patient drink several glasses of water.

Diagnosis: This is a macrocystic cystadenoma of the tail of the pancreas.

Comments: The most frequent cystic lesions in the pancreas are, of course, pseudocysts (85%). Real cysts are rare and of two types, micro- and macrocysts. The macrocystic adenoma is more frequent in women. Its favoured site is the tail of the pancreas. It is lined by muciparous glandular cells. Its wall may show localized thickening, or even true vegetations. It is rather large, usually above 2 cm in size. This form is to be considered malignant; differentiation from cystadenocarcinoma is often difficult, even histologically. The description given here is typical; there may also be calcification. Mucinous adenocarcinoma is even more rare; it consists of a solid and a cystic part. The prognosis is good when surgery has resulted in complete removal.

The main problem remains the differential diagnosis from pseudocyst. This is easy when the latter has a typical appearance: a unilocular, purely liquid rounded mass with a thin, smooth wall, that is intra- or extrapancreatic. The differential diagnosis is difficult with atypical pseudocysts: these have heterogeneous contents due to haemorrhage or to necrotic debris, and demonstrate the presence of septations. In some rare cases differentiation from a malignant tumour with a necrotic centre, a metastasis arising from a primary mucin-secreting tumour (carcinoma of the ovary) or a cyst in echinococcosis should also be considered. Also, do not forget that a tumour can be associated with pseudocysts.

76

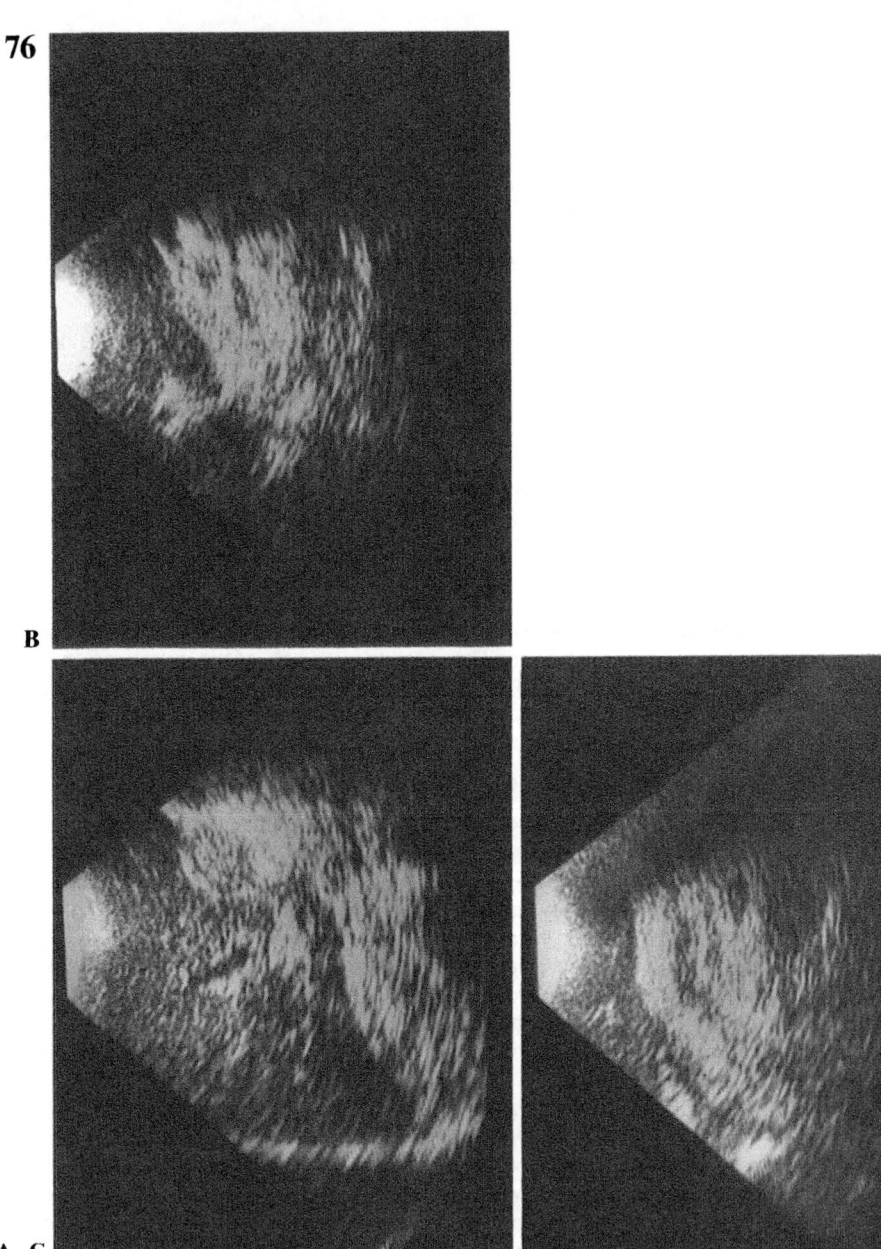

B

A, C

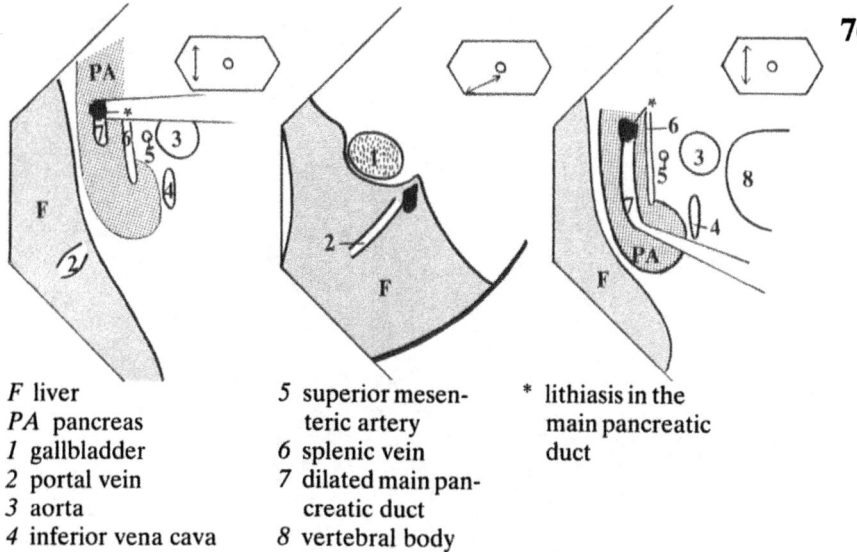

F liver	*5* superior mesen-	* lithiasis in the
PA pancreas	teric artery	main pancreatic
1 gallbladder	*6* splenic vein	duct
2 portal vein	*7* dilated main pan-	
3 aorta	creatic duct	
4 inferior vena cava	*8* vertebral body	

Case 76

Clinical data: A 70-year-old man presented with abdominal pain and signs of an inflammatory process.

Description: The scan shows the increased volume of the body of the pancreas, which is 2.5 cm in thickness. Above all, it shows increased echogenicity, taking into account the patient's age. In the centre of the body of the pancreas, a canalar structure of 1 cm diameter is seen parallel to the splenic vein, with an intraluminal hyperechogenic structure that casts an acoustic shadow. Note the atrophic gallbladder, with a lumen occupied by sludge.

Diagnosis: This is chronic pancreatitis with dilatation of the main pancreatic duct and intracanalar lithiasis.

Comments: The main pancreas duct (Wirsung's duct) is visualized in 55% of normal cases, usually in the corporeal region. It is more difficult to identify in the head of the pancreas because of its anteroposterior course. The same is true for the tail. The pancreatic duct usually appears as two echogenic bands delimiting a sonolucent line, the diameter of which is below or equal to 2 mm. Exceptionally, it may appear as a linear echogenic structure without a lumen. These variations in its appearance are due to physiological variations in pancreatic secretion. Be careful not to confuse the main pancreatic duct with the posterior aspect of the gastric wall, the hepatic artery or the splenic artery (Case 71 C).

Dilatation of the pancreatic duct can be seen in all pancreatic diseases. In chronic pancreatitis, the dilatation is irregular, whereas it is regular and smooth in carcinoma. The presence of calcifications strongly suggests chronic pancreatitis. As a rule, the main pancreatic duct is more dilated in tumours of the pancreas than in chronic pancreatitis.

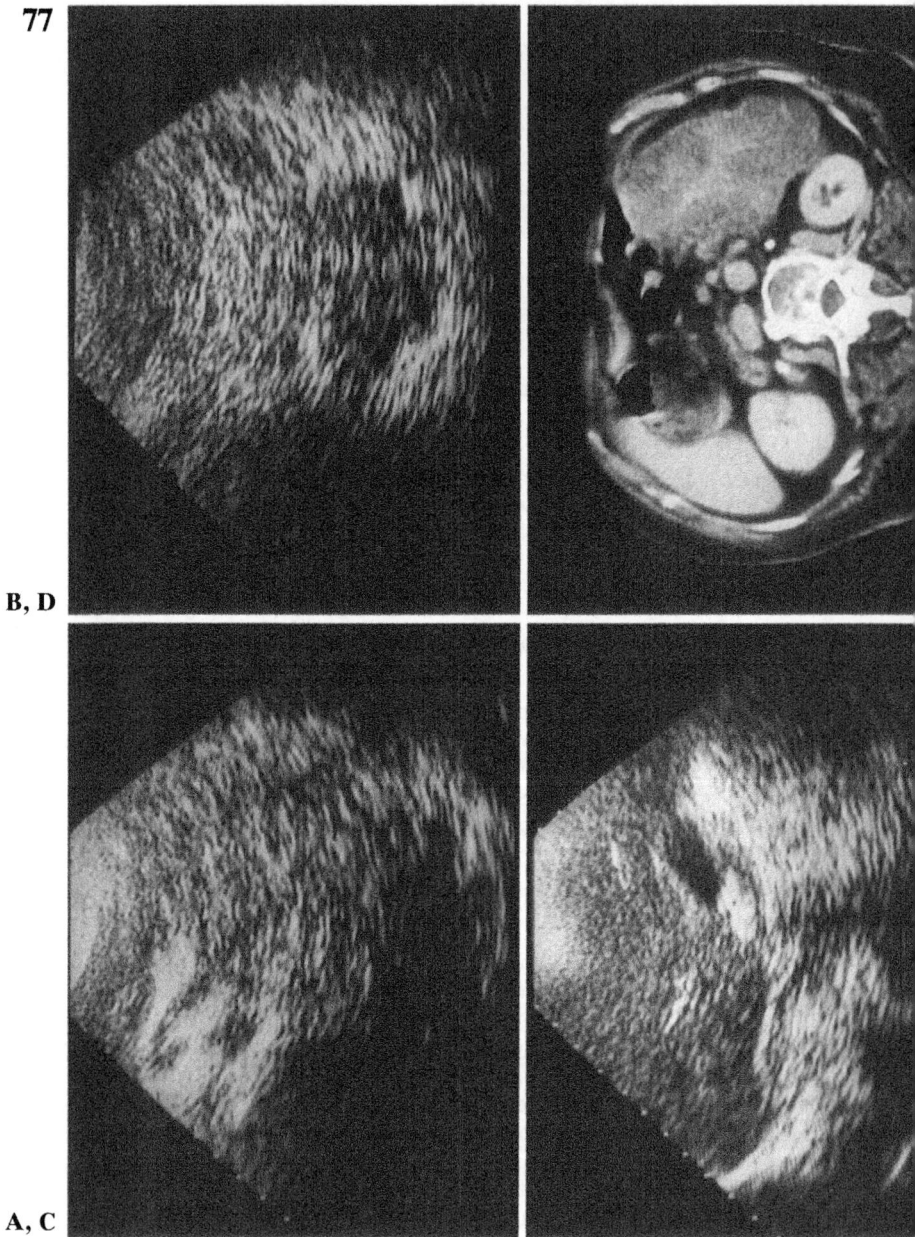

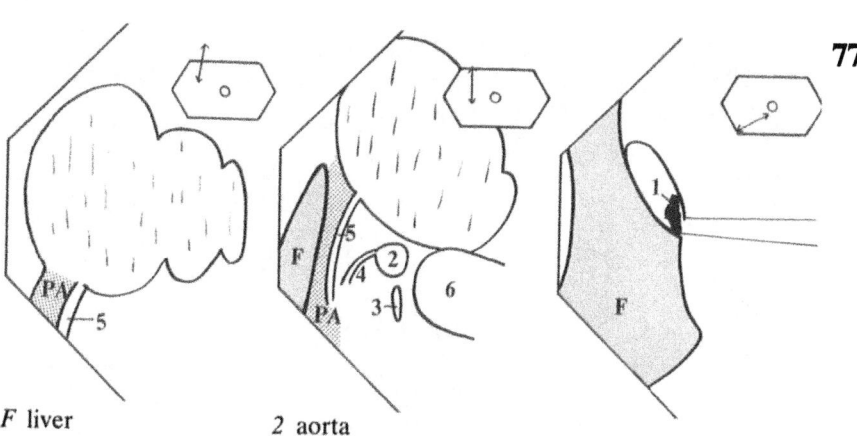

F liver
PA pancreas
1 gallbladder lithiasis

2 aorta
3 inferior vena cava
4 superior mesenteric artery

5 splenic vein
6 vertebral body

Case 77

Clinical data: An 80-year-old woman has a palpable mass in the left flank.

Description: There is a voluminous mass, 9 cm in diameter, arising from the tail of the pancreas. It is very heterogeneous and contains small hypoechogenic areas (less than 1 cm in diameter), separated by dense echoes corresponding to septations. There is no calcification. The remainder of the pancreas is unremarkable.

It is very difficult to differentiate this mass from the gastrointestinal structures. Two criteria are helpful – there is no brownian movement and no modification in this area after a 2-day interval.

You have certainly noted the presence of calculi in the gallbladder.

Diagnosis: This is very difficult. It was a microcystic adenoma of the pancreas. Computed tomography showed a voluminous tumour composed of cystic areas separated by septations. The radiate arrangement of these septations is characteristic (Scan D).

Comments: The microcystic adenoma is of the serous type and is lined with squamous or flattened cuboidal cells. It is formed of numerous cysts of less than 2 cm, with clear contents, rich in glycogen. This type is always benign. It is more frequent in women but has no peculiar affinity for the tail of the pancreas.

The small size of the cysts, their multiplicity and the fact that they are superposed may be responsible for the solid-type appearance, and thus render diagnosis with ultrasounds difficult. In 20% of the cases there are also calcifications.

True pancreatic cysts of the microcystic adenoma type are found in 72% of patients with Von Hippel-Lindau disease (which may include angioma of the retina, haemangioblastoma, tumour of the kidney and pheochromocytoma).

78

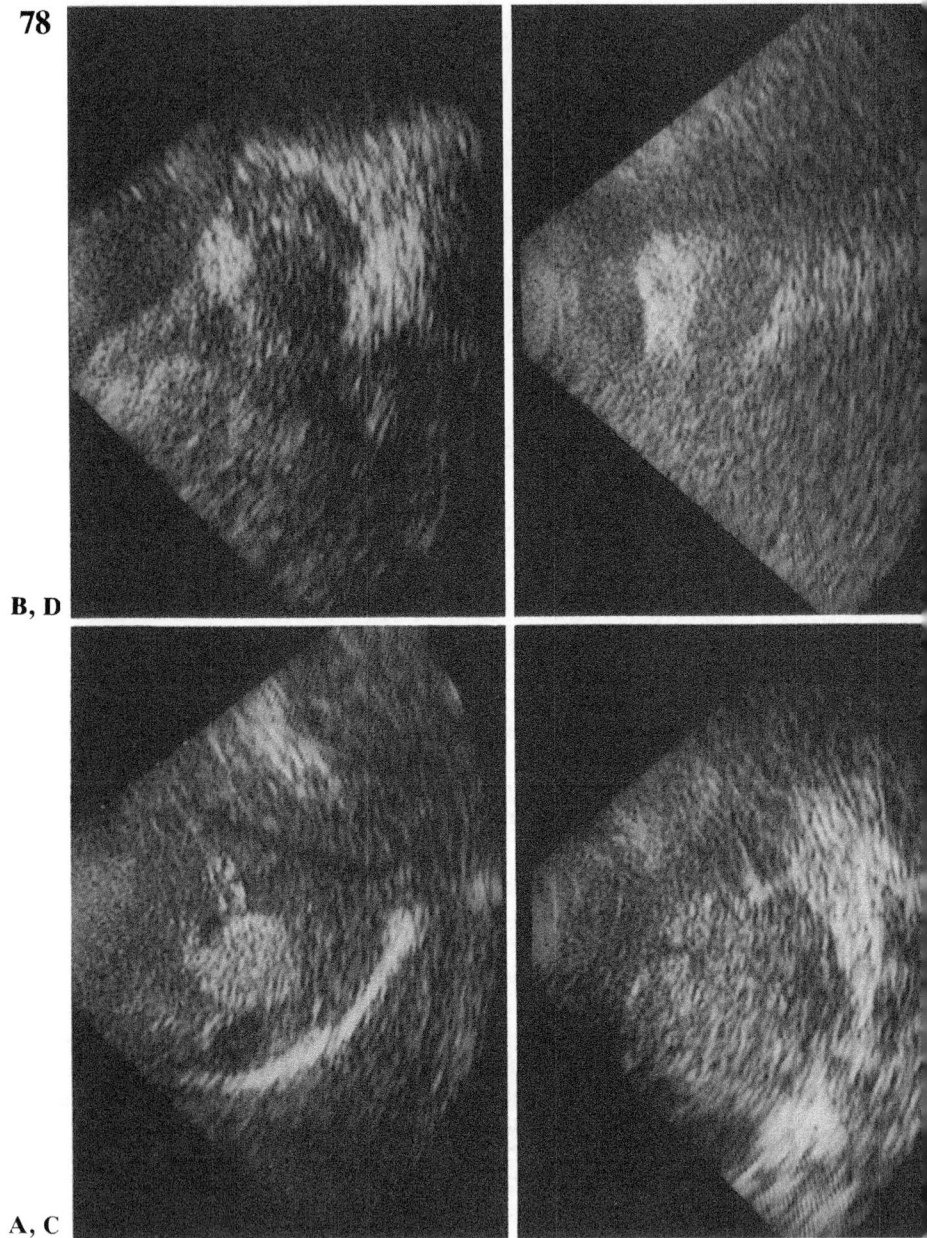

B, D

A, C

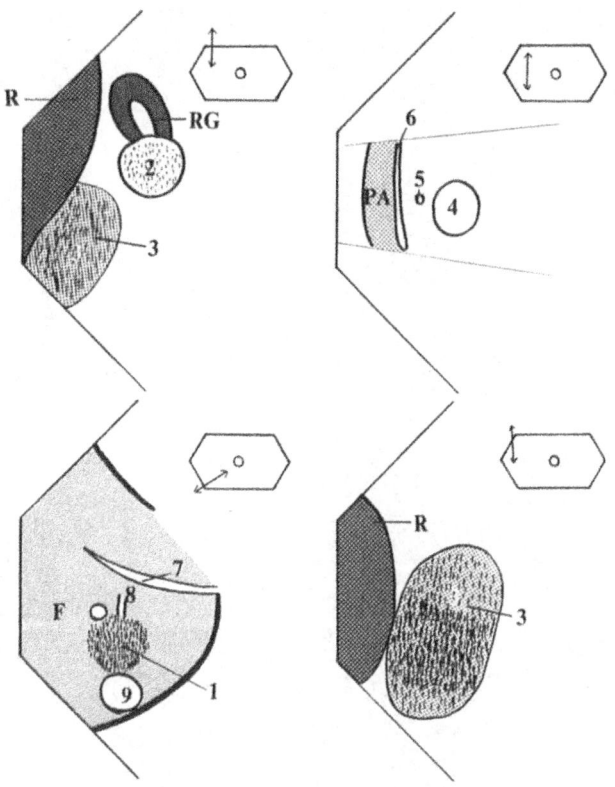

F liver
PA pancreas
R spleen
RG left kidney
1 hepatic metas-
   tases
2 left adrenal me-
   tastasis
3 carcinoma of the
   pancreatic tail
4 aorta
5 superior mesen-
   teric artery
6 splenic vein
7 right hepatic
   vein
8 branch of the
   right portal vein
9 cystic formation
   in the liver

Case 78

Clinical data: A 70-year-old woman complains of pain in the thoracic region.

Description: There is a voluminous mass at the level of the tail of the pancreas, i. e. within the region occupied by the spleen and kidney. It has a thickness of 6 cm, irregular borders and a hyperechogenic, heterogeneous structure (Scans B and C). The body of the pancreas is enlarged, and homogeneously hypoechogenic, showing an oedematous reaction (Scan D).

Note the presence of metastases in the liver (Scan A) and left adrenal (Scan B).

Diagnosis: This is carcinoma of the tail of the pancreas with hepatic and left adrenal metastases.

Comments: This tumour has an atypical echostructure, a hypoechogenic or anechogenic appearance being the rule. The metastases, however, have the typical appearance of pancreatic carcinoma. Ultrasound-guided fine-needle biopsy provides histological proof.

Note that dilatation of the main pancreatic duct is an inconstant finding, found mainly in carcinomas of the pancreatic head.

79

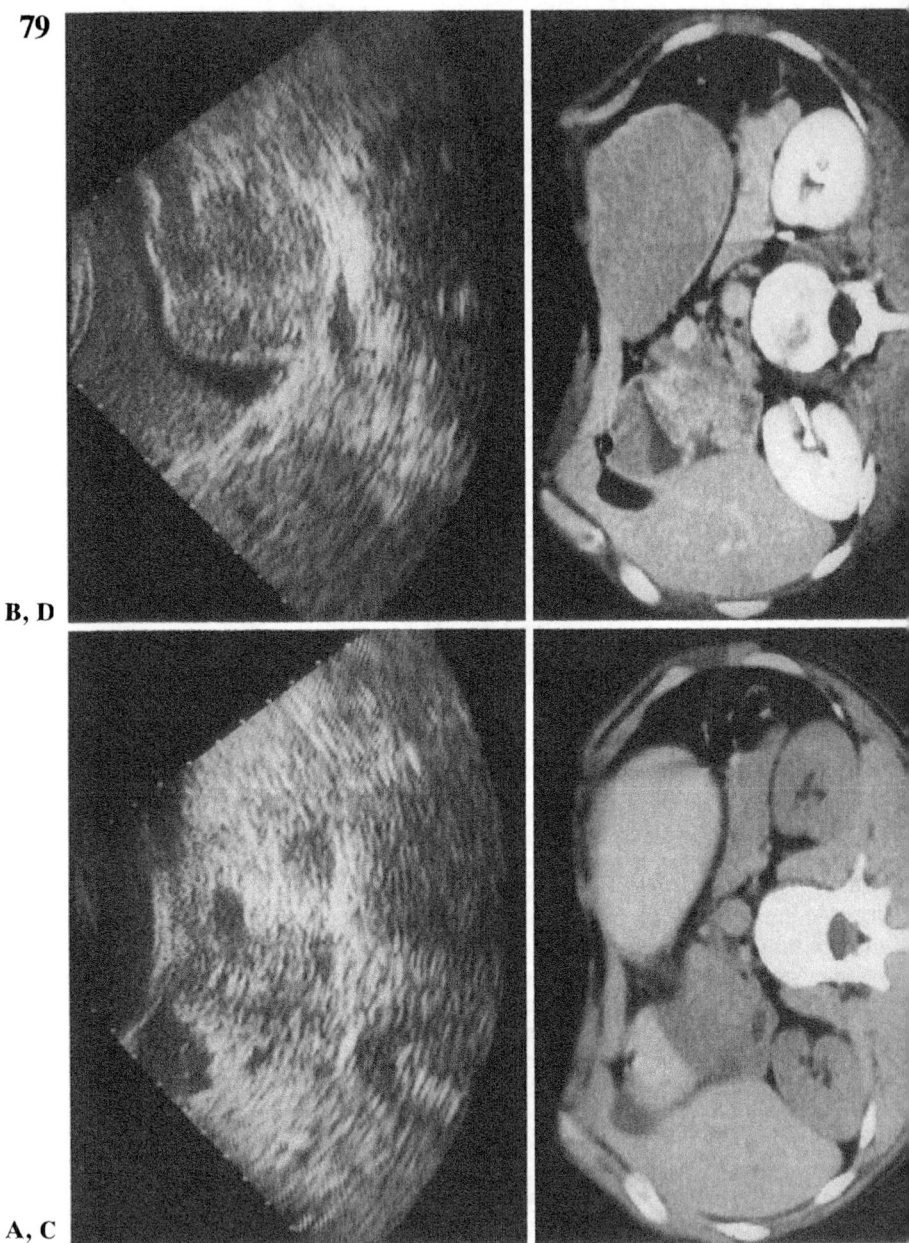

B, D

A, C

138

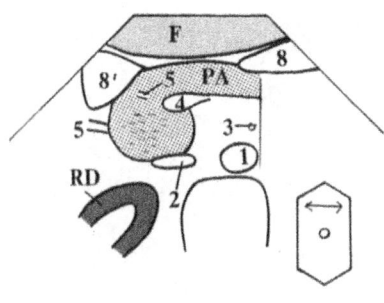

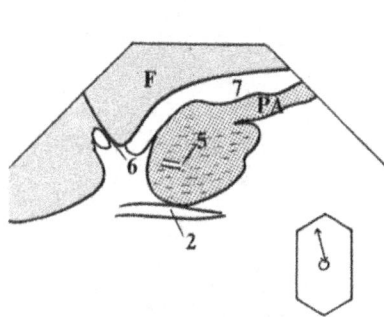

F liver **79**
PA pancreas
1 aorta
2 inferior vena cava
3 superior mesenteric artery
4 splenic vein
5 bile duct
6 portal vein
7 gallbladder
8 gastric antrum
8' first part of duodenum

Case 79

Clinical data: This 50-year-old man was complaining of vomiting and weight loss of 15 kg within 3 months. There was no jaundice.

Description: A mass of 5 cm in diameter, heterogeneous and predominantly hypoechogenic is seen in the head of the pancreas. The borders are irregular (Scans A and B). The lower part of the gallbladder is compressed, but the remainder is not dilated (Scan B). The bile duct is clearly visible (Scan A) and displaced by the mass, but not dilated. In contrast, the first part of the duodenum and the pyloric antrum are dilated (Scan A).

Diagnosis: This is not a tumour of the pancreatic head. The histological diagnosis was chronic pancreatitis with marked fibrosis involving the head of the pancreas.

Comments: This is a difficult diagnosis. The absence of biliary duct dilatation hints at a benign condition. In chronic pancreatitis, dilatation of the biliary ducts is moderate or absent. In chronic pancreatitis, the sonographic changes seen are variable and diversely combined; moreover, in 15% of cases the pancreas is unremarkable. The specific diagnosis is only made one time out of two. At best ultrasound findings permit one to speak of "pancreatopathy". When combined with a plain radiograph of the abdomen and computed tomography, sonography is much more informative. Also, it should be kept in mind that the incidence of pancreatic carcinoma is higher in patients with chronic pancreatitis.

A tumour of the pancreatic head is always associated with marked dilatation of the main bile duct and of the intrahepatic bile ducts.

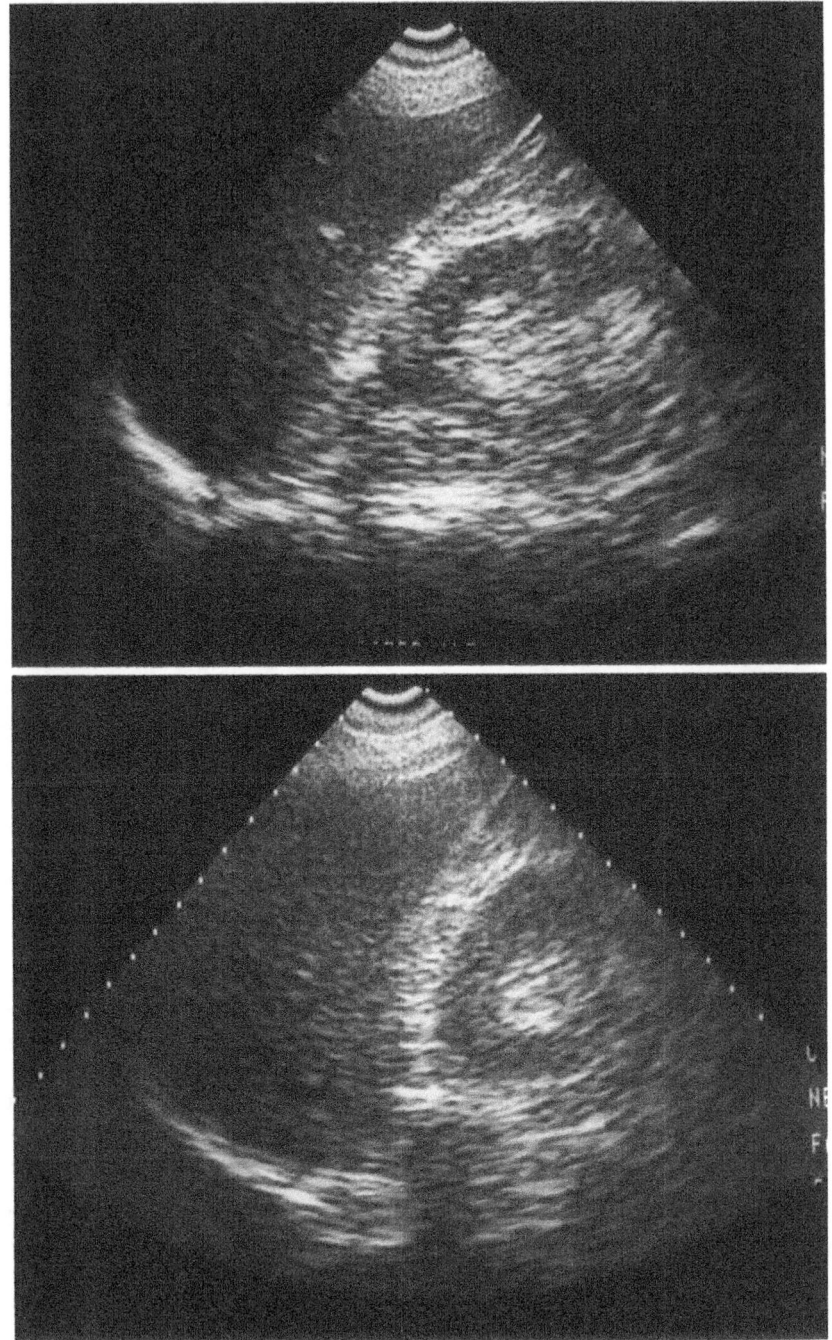

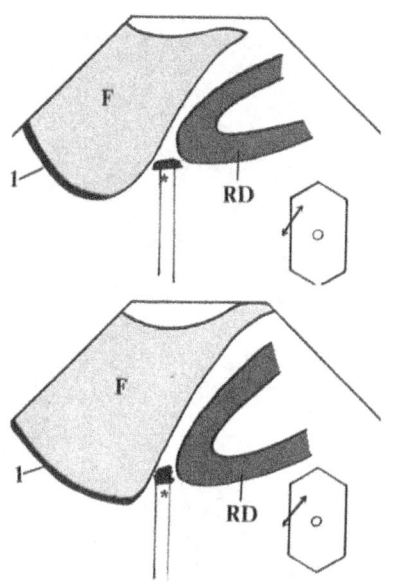

F liver
RD right kidney
1 diaphragm
* right adrenal calcification with
acoustic shadow

Case 80

Clinical data: A 50-year-old man presented with phlebitis of the left lower limb.

Description: A 1.5 cm-long hyperechogenic area with an acoustic shadow is seen above the upper pole of the right kidney. There is, however, no evidence of an abnormal mass.

Diagnosis: This is easy: calcification of the right adrenal gland.

Comments: Addison's disease is a rare cause of bilateral adrenal calcification. Much more frequent are asymptomatic adrenal-gland calcifications without symptoms, secondary to remote haemorrhage or, more rarely, to histoplasmosis, haemochromatosis or amyloidosis. Adrenal tumours, for instance carcinoma of the adrenal cortex, certain cysts, pheochromocytomas and adenomas, can also calcify.

The technique of examining the adrenals is simple: scanning is mainly perpendicular, and then parallel to the long axis of the kidney, one scan visualizing the superior pole of the kidney, the liver and the inferior vena cava. The examination is carried out in deep inspiration. On the right, the adrenal bed is visualized between the superior pole of the kidney and the inferior vena cava as an echogenic structure that is roughly V-shaped. It is more difficult to visualize the left adrenal bed. In current practice it is useless to persist in trying to visualize normal adrenals. Moreover, variability in the (hyper- or hypo-)echogenicity of the perirenal fat sometimes renders the diagnosis of adrenal-gland lesions difficult. The fat of the perirenal fascia may be poorly echogenic, whereas the fat in the anterior and posterior pararenal spaces is markedly echogenic. Moreover, localized areas of fat within the perirenal fascia can be echogenic, thus mimicking an adrenal tumour.

On the right, it is possible to detect adrenal lesions with dimensions greater than 1.5 to 2 cm; on the left, lesions above 2−3 cm in size are detectable. A definite diagnosis is provided by computed tomography.

81

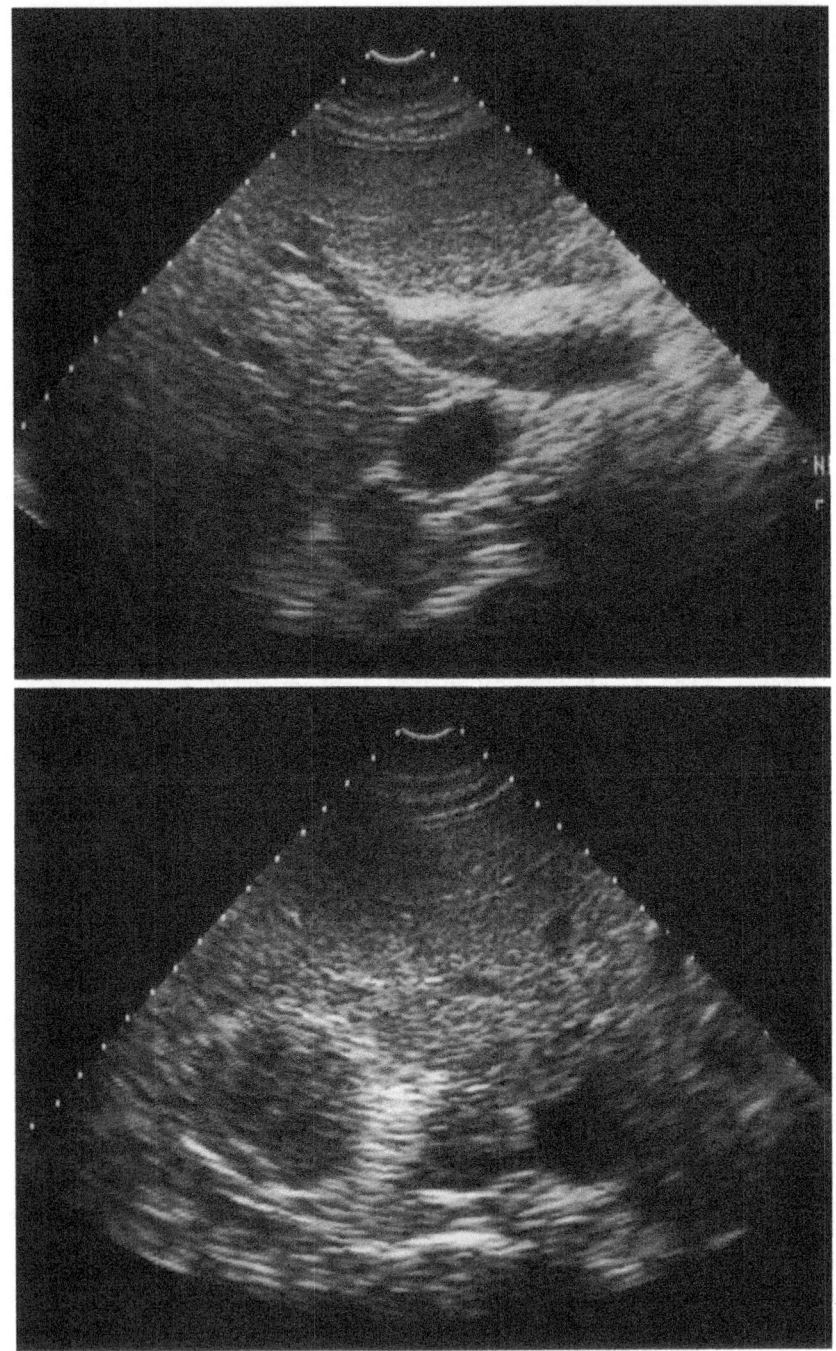

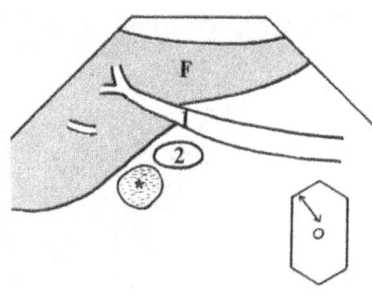

F liver
RD superior pole of the right kidney
1 portal vein
2 inferior vena cava
3 hepatic vein tributaries
* right adrenal tumour

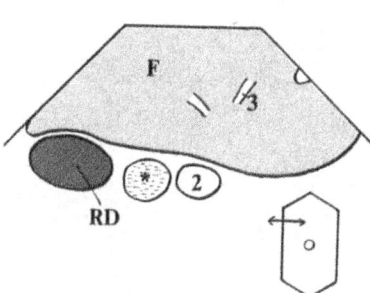

Case 81

Clinical data: A 50-year-old man presented with neurological symptoms. Computed tomography of the skull revealed multiple cerebral metastases. Investigation was aimed at detection of the primary lesion.

Description: The scan shows a homogeneous rounded hypoechogenic mass, 2.5 cm in diameter, with sharp borders, at the upper pole of the right kidney, adjoining the inferior vena cava. The investigation was otherwise unremarkable.

Diagnosis: This is easy: metastasis in the right adrenal gland.

Comments: The adrenal gland is the fourth commonest site of secondary lesions after the lung, the liver and the bones. The primary tumours may be located (with decreasing frequency) in the bronchi, breast, stomach, kidneys, pancreas or colon. Clinically latent, their incidence is increasing due to increased survival of cancer patients, but especially to improvement in the techniques of diagnosis. Microscopic involvement is actually much more important; from autopsy data, 50% of patients with carcinoma of the breast or bronchi show evidence of microscopic involvement, whereas a third of the patients have macroscopic lesions. Sonography shows a rounded or an ovalar mass that is uni- or bilateral.

82

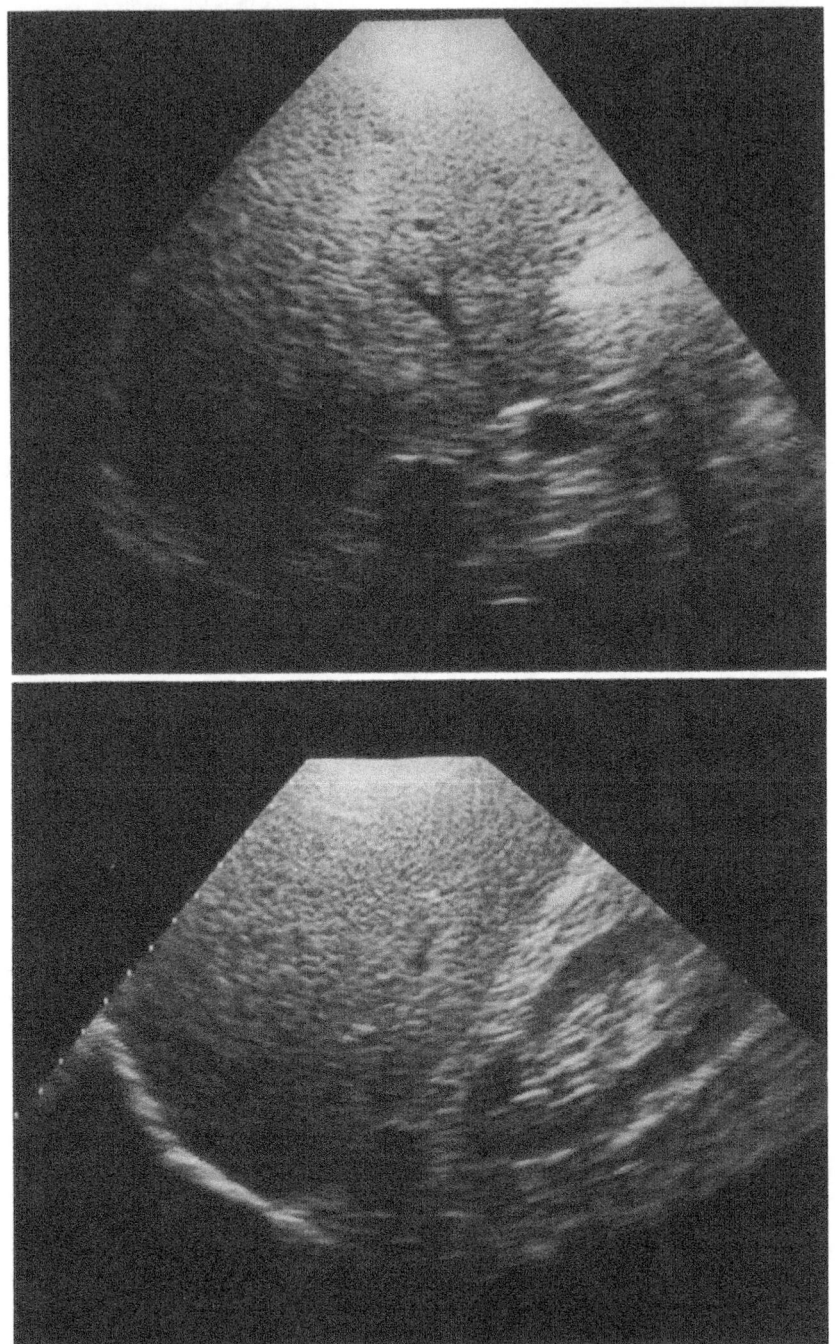

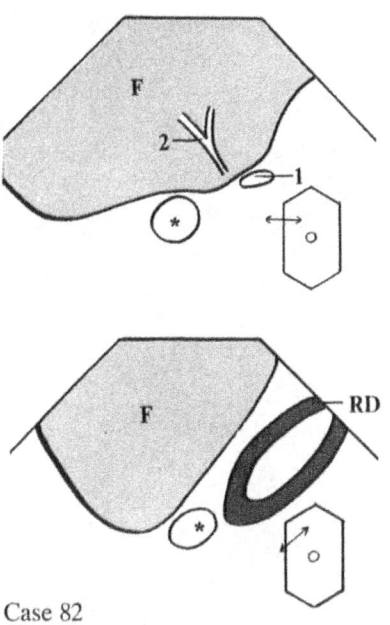

F liver
RD right kidney
1 inferior vena cava
2 right hepatic tributary
* adrenal tumour

Case 82

Clinical data: A 70-year-old woman presented with alteration of general status.

Description: A rounded mass, 1.5 cm in diameter, is seen on the medial aspect of the superior pole of the right kidney. It is hyperechogenic and homogeneous, with sharp borders but no posterior relative echo-enhancement.
It is not a primary or secondary tumoural process. Computed tomography shows this right suprarenal mass to have densities close to zero which are unchanged after contrast injection.

Diagnosis: With sonography, this is difficult. It was actually a cyst of the adrenal gland.

Comments: This appearance is atypical. An adrenal cyst is usually seen as an echo-free fluid structure with posterior relative echo-enhancement and thin walls. The presence of thin intracystic septation reflecting the echoes, or of intracystic debris, can however be responsible for the appearance described. Absence of posterior relative echo-enhancement can be due to deep location of the adrenal mass and to the low energy level transmitted by the ultrasound beam at the level.

Adrenal cysts are rare occuring in 0.6% of the total population. They are seen in all age groups but particularly in middle-aged women.

The clinical signs are inconstant or lack specificity. Vague abdominal pain is the most frequent sign.

Adrenal cysts are usually unilateral, with an equal frequency for the left and the right. Their volume varies from 1 cm^3 to several litres. They can originate from the adrenal medulla as well as the cortex. The non-involved adrenal tissue is progressively compressed and distended. Calcification is often present.

82

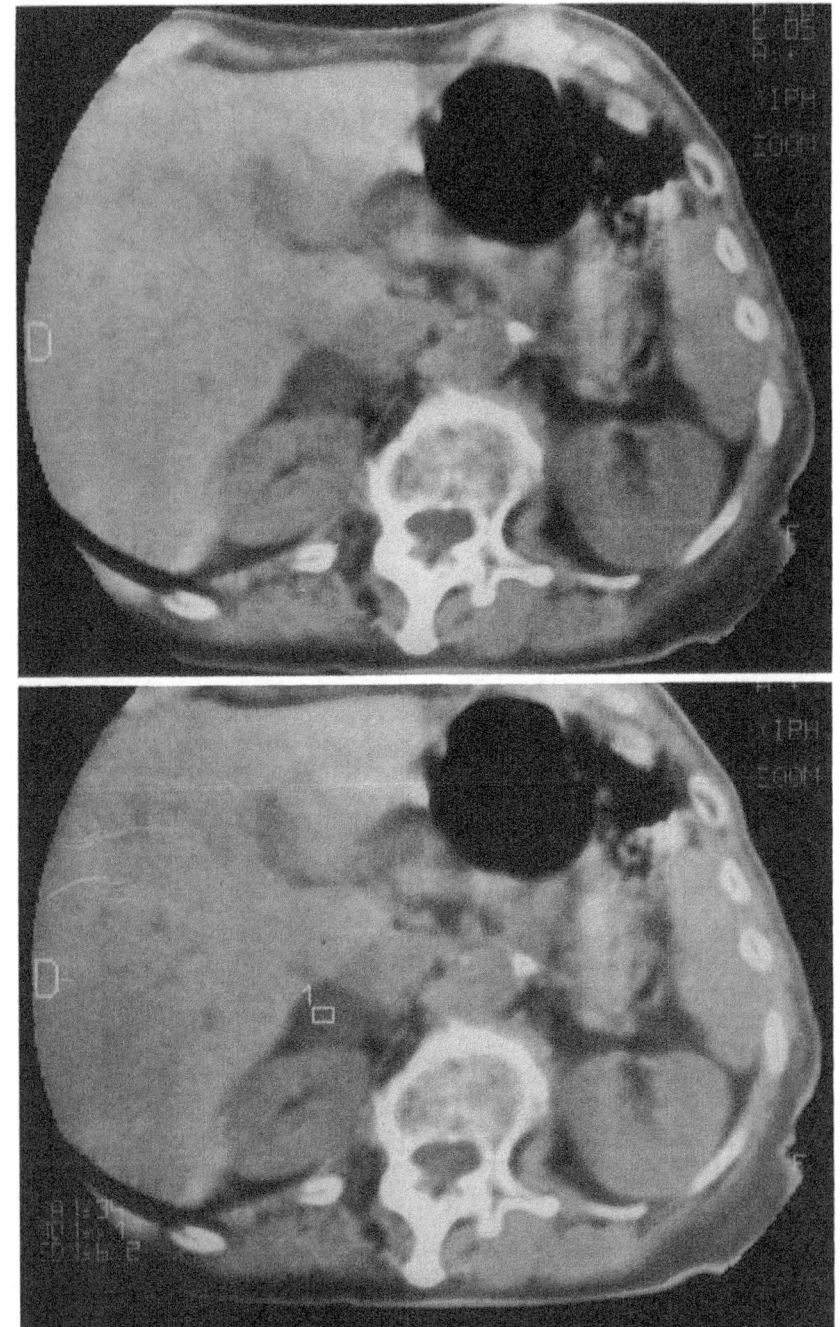

Computed tomography is the best investigation in this case. It allows one to affirm the fluid nature of the lesion.

The contents depend upon the histological type and vary from serofibrinous fluid to almost pure blood. The accepted classification distinguishes between cysts and pseudocysts. True cysts are of three types – parasitic, epithelial and endothelial cysts. The parasitic cysts are mainly echinococcal. Epithelial cysts are uncommon and include three sub-groups: true glandular cysts, which are extremely rare and are due to the distension of a pseudoacinous structure by secretory products; embryonic cysts; and finally, cystic adenomas, which are benign adenomas that have become cysts secondarily. Endothelial cysts are the most common and account for half of the cases. They are subdivided into several sub-groups: serous or lymphangiectasic cysts (closely related to cystic lymphangiomas) and angiomatous cysts. Cystic lymphangiomas are usually seen as multilocular fluid-filled liquid structures.

Finally, cysts are the commonest non-secretory tumours of the adrenals.

83

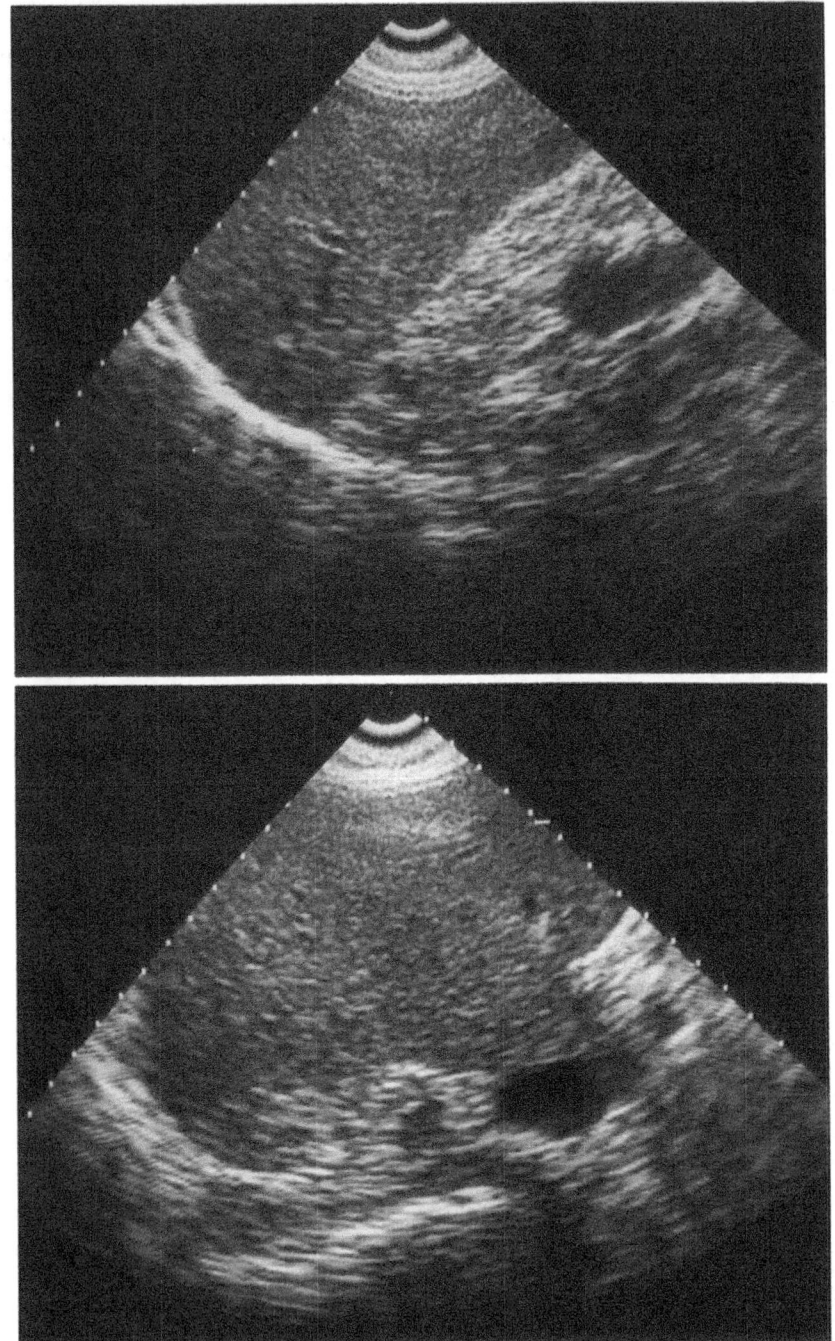

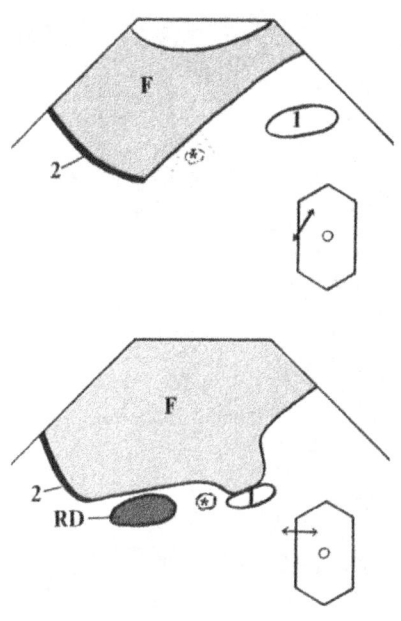

F liver
RD superior pole of the right kidney
1 inferior vena cava
2 diaphragm
* right adrenal mass

Case 83

Clinical data: This 40-year-old man has hypertension, hypokalaemia and hyperaldosteronaemia.

Description: In the right suprarenal region, there is a small, rounded hypoechogenic mass, 1 cm in diameter, without attenuation or posterior relative echo-enhancement and with smooth borders. It is situated above the superior pole of the kidney, between the liver and the inferior vena cava.

Diagnosis: There is a right adrenal mass. The definitive diagnosis was Conn's adenoma (primary hyperaldosteronism due to a secretory suprarenal adenoma).

Comments: Sonography seldom decisively detects Conn's adenoma. In 90% of cases, this consists of a small solitary lesion less than or equal to 1 cm in diameter. Sometimes the lesion is microscopic, although it is secretory. Sometimes there is also bilateral adrenal hyperplasia. This distinction is important since surgery is not recommended in the latter case. Primary hyperaldosteronism (Conn's syndrome) is, moreover, a rare cause of hypertension (1% of cases).

Computed tomography is still the best investigation here, although its accuracy is diminished because of the small size of the lesions and because they are often peripheral. Finally, the most reliable technique is adrenal phlebography combined with selective hormone assays, but it must be kept in mind that this method entails a risk of iatrogenic adrenal haematoma and is difficult to perform.

84

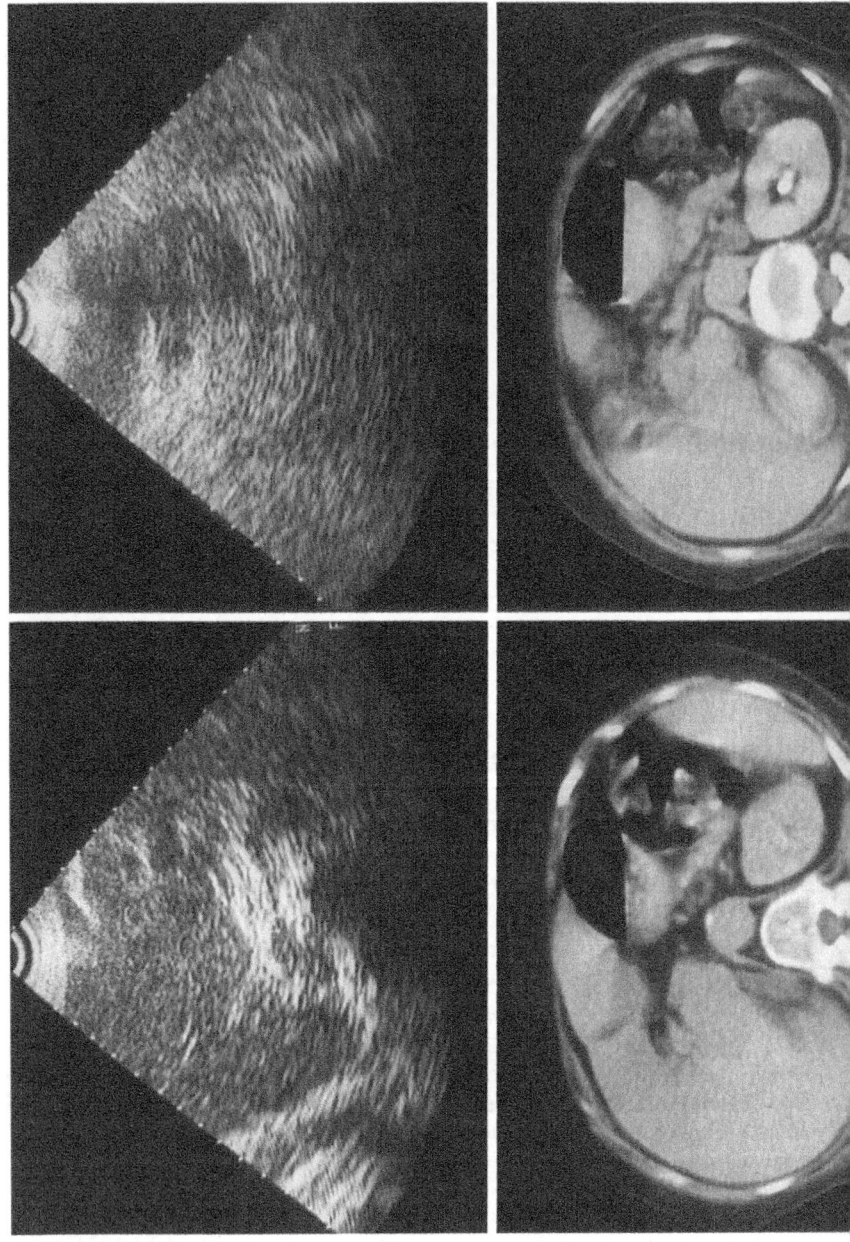

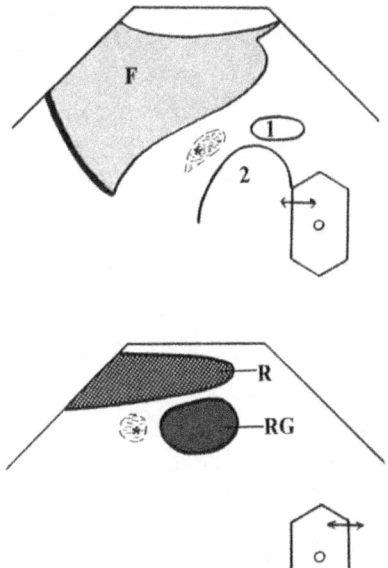

F liver **84**
R spleen
RG superior pole of the left kidney
1 aorta
2 vertebral body
* left and right adrenal

Case 84

Clinical data: A 80-year-old woman presented in poor physical condition with hypertension, pigmentation, symptoms of virilization and fever.

Description: A hypoechogenic, oblong mass, 3 cm long and 1 cm thick, is seen in the right adrenal region, in opposition to the right crus of the diaphragm. There is also a hypoechogenic, rounded mass, 1.5 cm in diameter in the superomedial portion of the left kidney.
Computed tomography confirmed hypertrophy of the right adrenal cortex, and global hypertrophy of the left.

Diagnosis: There is bilateral adrenal hyperplasia. Biochemical findings suggested a paraneoplastic syndrome. Three months later, multiple pulmonary metastases had developed. The primary tumour was not identified.

Comments: In 10% of cases, bilateral adrenal hyperplasia is due to a paraneoplastic syndrome related to abnormal adrenocorticotropic hormone (ACTH) secretion by a malignant tumour: bronchial (40% of cases), pancreatic (20%) or thymic (20%) carcinoma. It causes even, bilateral enlargement of the adrenals, which maintain a subnormal morphology, at least as concerns the concave appearance of the borders. However, a pseudotumoural appearance can also be present, similarly suggesting a paraneoplastic syndrome.

Normal sonographic findings do not exclude bilateral hyperplasia. Again, computed tomography is more useful. The degree of paraneoplastic hyperplasia allows one to exclude Cushing's disease (hyperadrenocorticism secondary to increased pituitary secretion of ACTH).

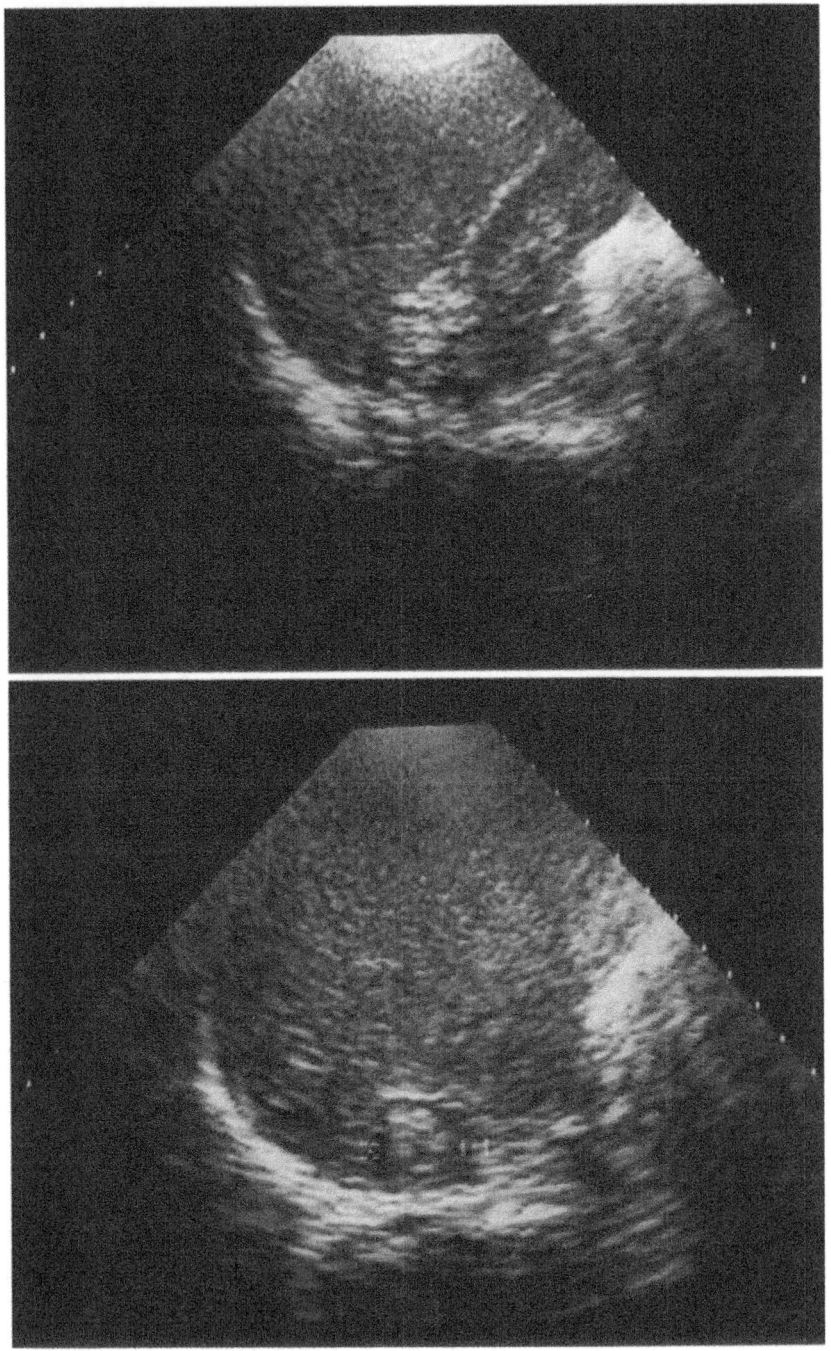

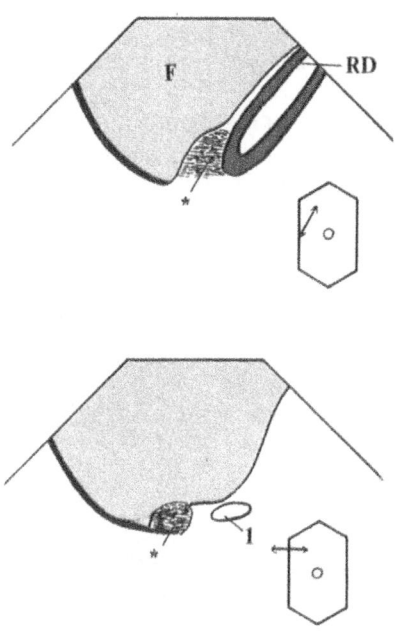

F liver
R spleen
1 inferior vena cava
* right adrenal mass

Case 85

Clinical data: A 70-year-old woman had follow-up investigations of a right adrenal mass detected 2 years previously. There were no symptoms or biochemical abnormalities.

Description: A homogeneous, hyperechogenic mass, 2.5 cm in diameter is seen at the superior pole of the right kidney. Its borders are well delineated. There is no contact with the upper pole of the kidney. The appearance is unchanged compared to previous investigations.

Diagnosis: This is difficult: myelolipoma of the right adrenal gland.

Comments: The myelolipoma is a rare tumour (1% of adrenal disorders). Its sonographic appearance is relatively specific, due to the abundant fat which produces intense echoes. There can also be calcification or heterogeneous areas subsequent to intratumoural haemorrhage. Diagnosis is made with computed tomography which shows a negative density, reflecting the presence of fat.

Among the other non-secretory tumours, besides cysts, one must mention adenomas, certain malignant corticoadrenalomas, metastases and finally some exceedingly rare tumours – haemangiomas, lymphangiomas, hamartomas, fibromas, sarcomas and schwannomas.

86

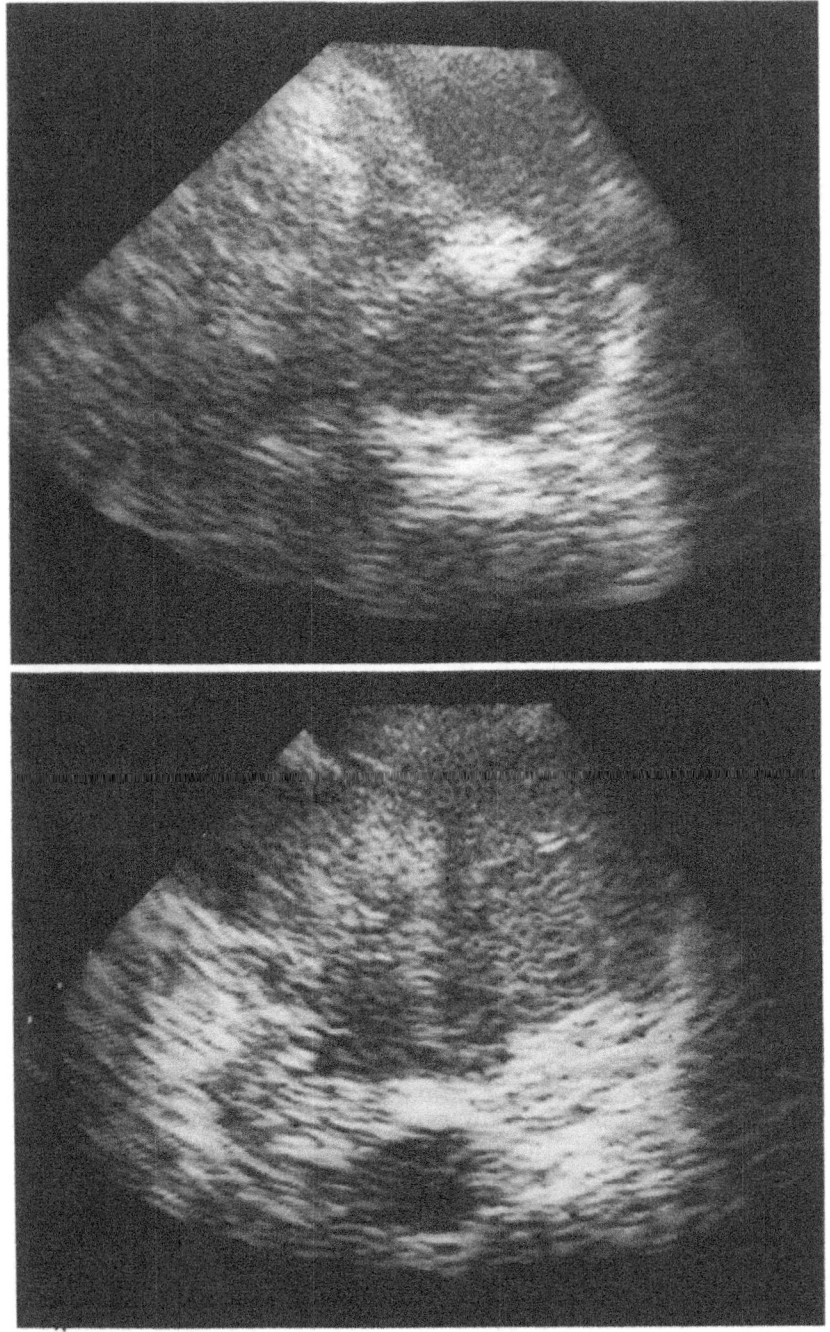

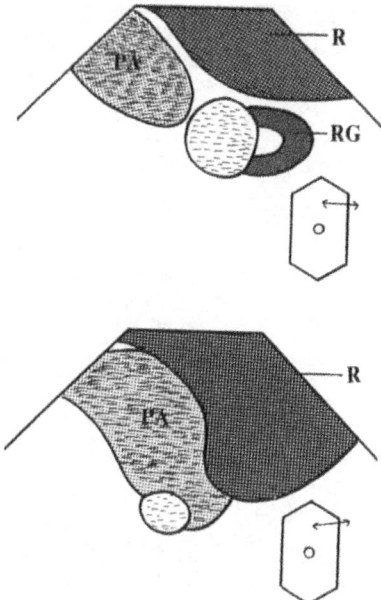

R spleen
PA tumour of pancreas
RG left kidney

Case 86

Clinical data: This 70-year-old woman has epigastric pain.

Description: A rounded, homogeneous, hypoechogenic mass with sharp limits and without posterior relative echo-enhancement, is seen at the superomedial pole of the right kidney. There is no clear demarcation between the gland and the upper pole of the kidney. The mass measures about 3 cm in diameter.
Scan B shows a voluminous mass of 5−6 cm diameter, which is echogenic and heterogeneous with poorly defined borders, located against the medial surface of the spleen.

Diagnosis: This is easy: adrenal metastasis secondary to carcinoma of the pancreatic tail. You should have noticed that this is Case 78.

Comments: The echostructure of adrenal metastases is variable. Usually they are less echogenic than the surrounding retroperitoneal fat, but they can also appear hyper- or anechogenic. Calcifications may be seen as intense echoes with or without acoustic shadow.

Usually, the upper pole of the kidney is sharply delineated from the adrenal mass. The absence of such a delineation does not exclude an adrenal lesion, and invasion of the kidney by the adrenal mass is not uncommon. Assessment of the origin is especially difficult when there is a voluminous mass. In this case too, definite diagnosis is provided by computed tomography.

Adrenal metastases occur more often in the medulla than in the cortex, and involve the left adrenal more frequently.

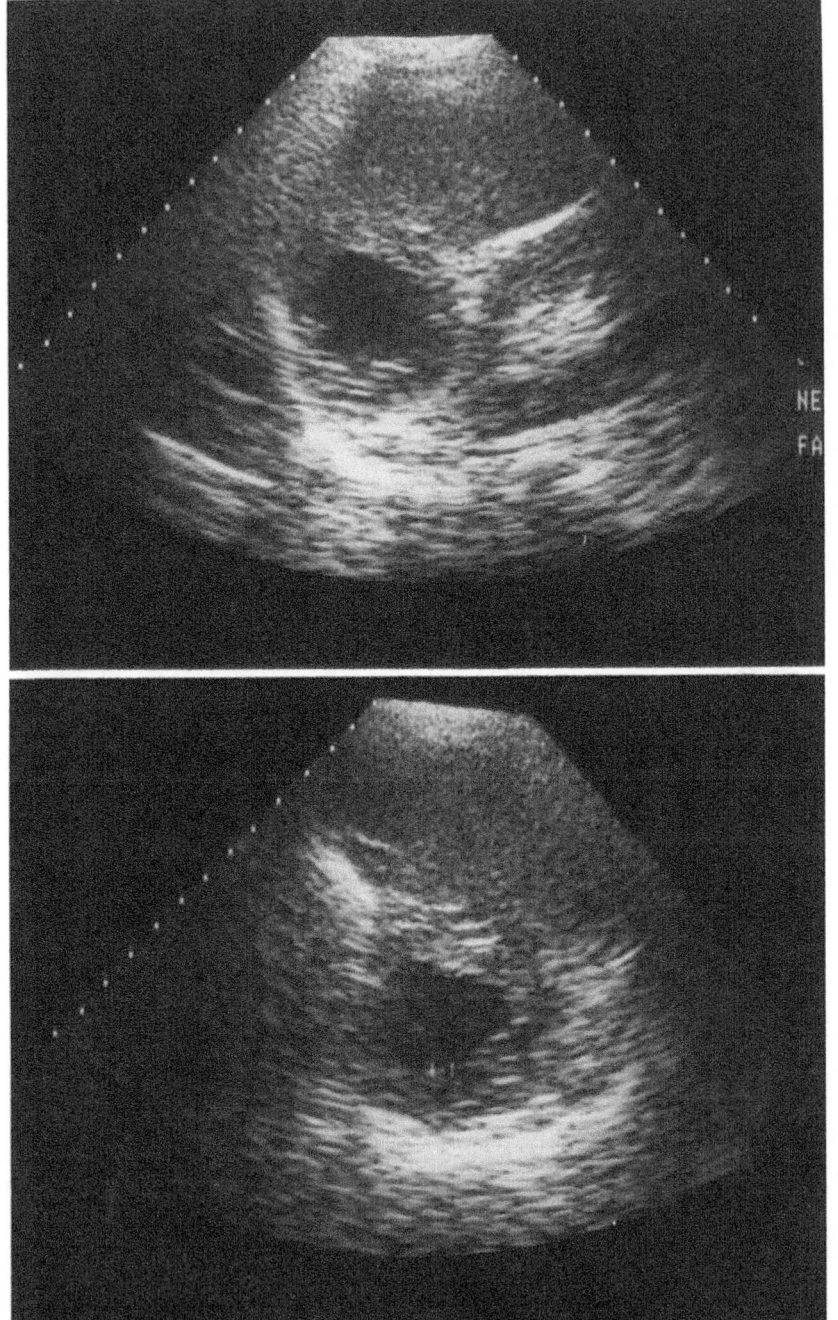

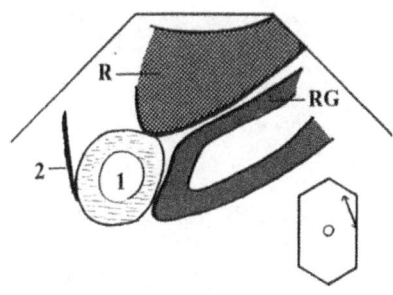

87

R spleen   **87**
RG left kidney
1 tumoural process in the left adrenal
2 diaphragm

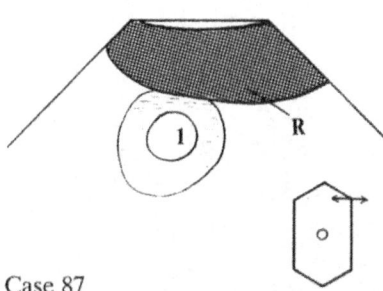

Case 87

Clinical data: A 55-year-old man has a history of surgery. The initial postoperative sonography showed a left adrenal mass. A follow-up examination was performed 6 months later.

Description: There is a rounded mass of 4 cm diameter above the superior pole of the left kidney, but clearly demarcated from the kidney. The mass consists of an echo-free centre and has a sharp medial limit. The wall has a thickness of 1 cm; its lateral limit is smooth.

Comparison with the inital examination was difficult, since the ultrasound equipment and the sonologist were no longer the same. The appearance was unchanged 1 year later.

Diagnosis: There is a cystic tumoural process of the adrenal, or pseudocyst.

Comments: We have already discussed true cysts. However, there is also another type, the "pseudocysts". These are common. They comprise 40% of all adrenal cysts. They are not lined by a cellular membrane and are usually larger than true cysts. Their origin is related to the development of an intraglandular haematoma which progressively liquifies. This haemorrhage has two types of etiology; it can result from:

– Iatrogenic or noniatrogenic trauma, infection, intoxication or embolism.
– Haemorrhage occuring within a tumour.

These structures are surrounded by a capsule, the thickness of which depends on the size of the cyst. Different studies have shown that most pseudocysts are due to haemorrhage occuring in normal glands. Tumoural pseudocysts comprise only 10%. Only histological evaluation permits the diagnosis of malignancy.

88

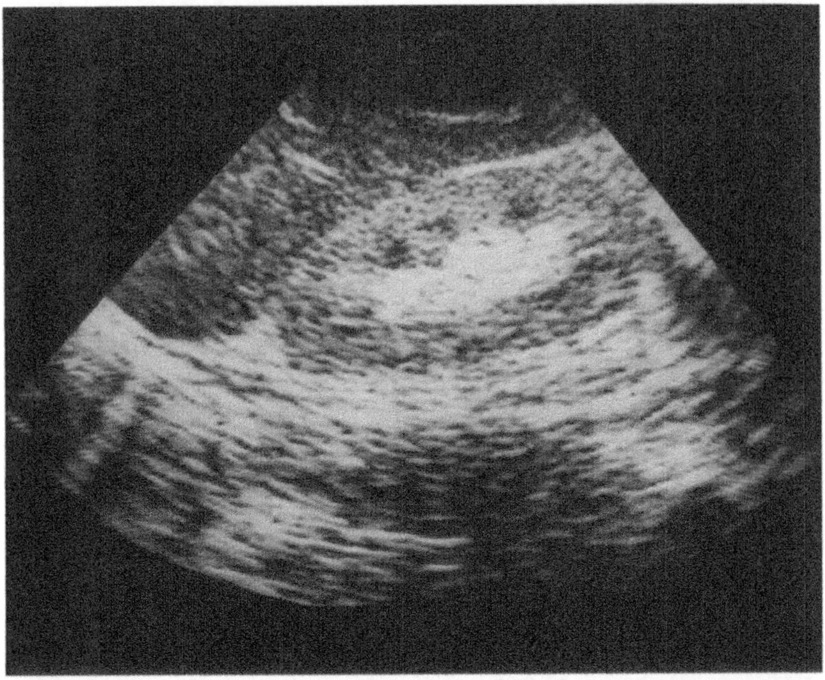

89

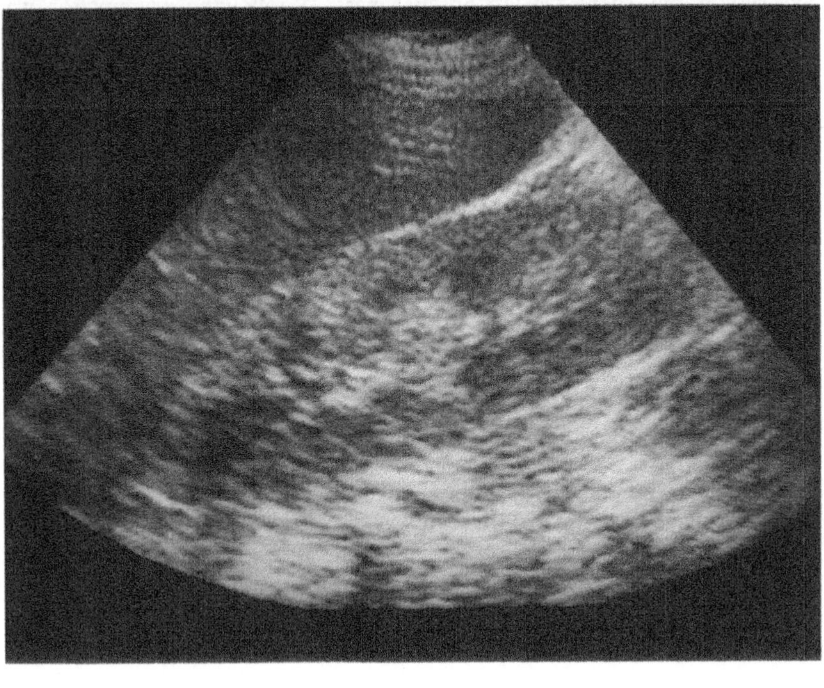

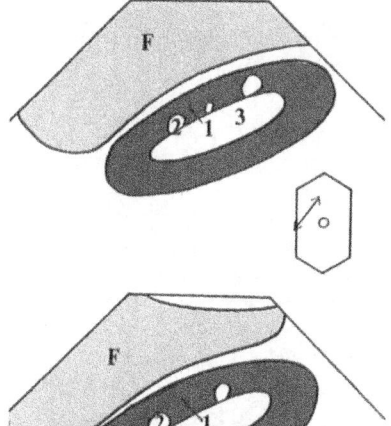

F liver
1 cortex
2 pyramids of Malpighi (enlarged)
3 hilus

Case 88 and 89

Clinical data: These two patients both have oliguria with increased serum levels or urea and creatinine.

Description: The scans are almost identical. There is enlargement of the kidney, especially its anteroposterior diameter (Scan 89). The pyramids are enlarged and show increased hypoechogenicity, reflecting oedema. The renal cortex is hyperechogenic but the corticomedullary junction is still visible. The calyces are not dilated.

Diagnosis: This is non-obstructive renal failure. In Case 88 this was due to phenacetin ingestion, which classically causes interstitial nephritis. Case 89 concerns a patient with disseminated lupus erythematosus.

Comments: Three structures are distinguishable in the normal renal parenchyma. The cortex is seen as a homogeneous, hypoechogenic band. The medulla (pyramids of Malpighi) is seen as less-echogenic triangular areas, whose bases are peripheral and whose apices are in contact with the hilar area; they are regularly distributed and separated by cortical tissue (Bertin's columns). The arcuate vessels are seen at the corticomedullary junction as fine and strongly reflective echoes. The renal cortex is always less echogenic than the liver.

Renal failure is an indication for sonography. Three possibilities must be considered: firstly chronic renal failure (with small atrophic kidneys or polycystosis); secondly, bilateral or unilateral hydronephrosis associated with contralateral atrophy; and finally, acute nephropathy. There is no correlation between the nature and the severity of the glomerular lesion and the sonographic appearance, whereas there is a relationship between the nature and the severity of interstitial changes and the echogenicity of the cortex. Localized interstitial lesions cause little modification, whereas diffuse lesions cause a very marked increase in echogenicity.

Many lesions cause hyperechogenicity of the cortex but preserve corticomedullary differentiation. These include: amyloidosis, leukaemic infiltration, acute renal thrombosis, acute tubular necrosis, chronic reflux, nephrotic syndromes, glomerulopathies, acute disseminated lupus erythematosus and nephritis.

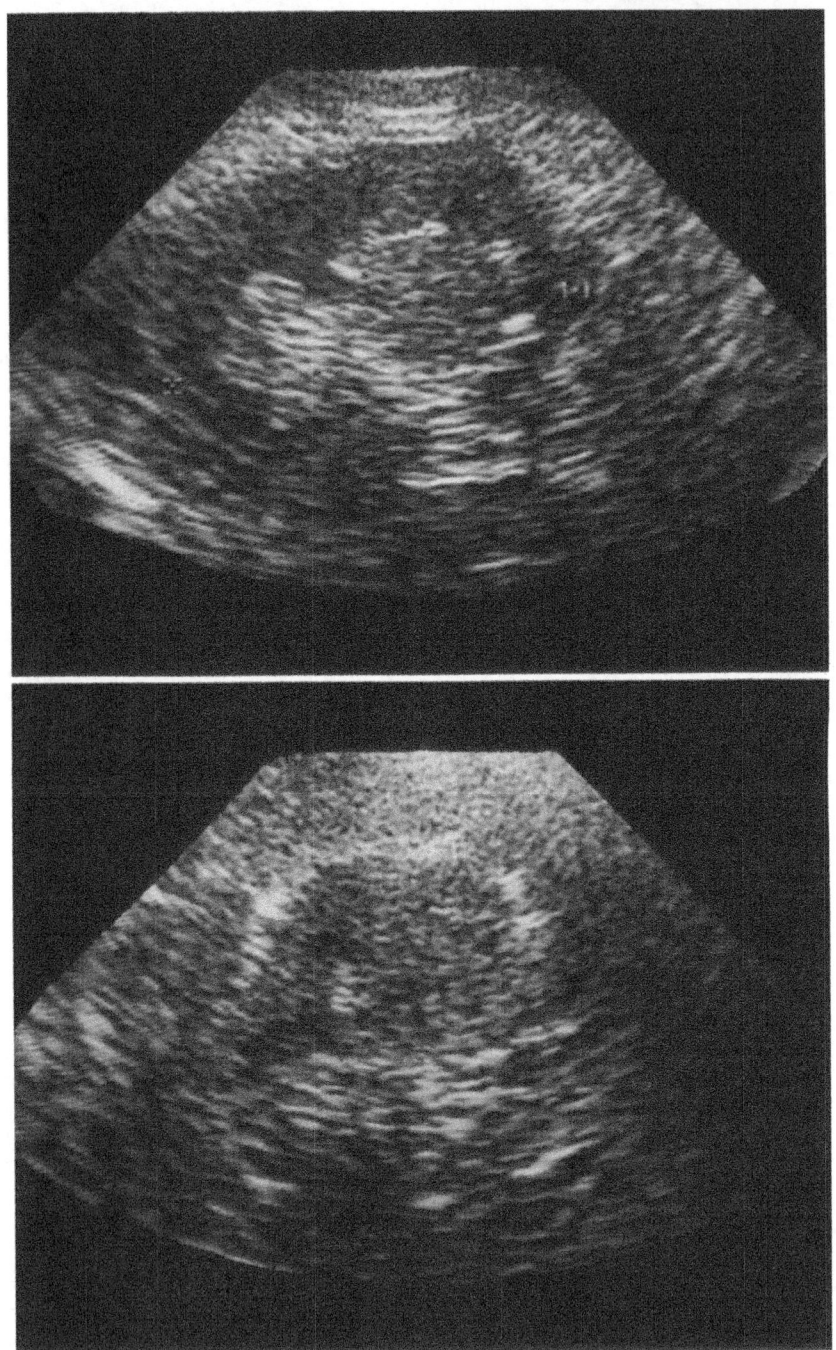

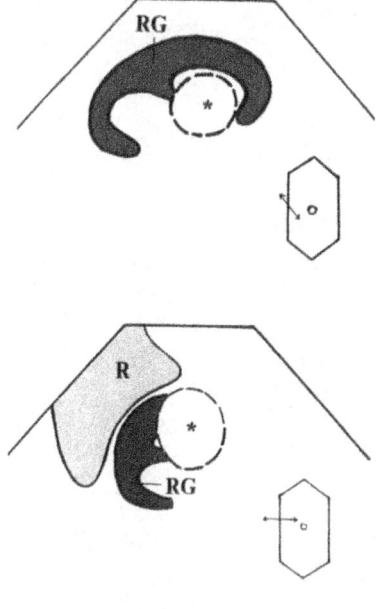

RG left kidney
R spleen
* tumoural process

Case 90

Clinical data: This 60-year-old man has had a myocardial infarct.

Description: A mass of 3.5 cm diameter is responsible for localized protrusion of the inferolateral cortex of the left kidney. The mass is homogeneous, with smooth borders, and is well delimited. It is hyperechogenic compared to the renal cortex, but hypoechogenic compared to the renal sinus.
– There is no lymph-node enlargement; the inferior vena cava and the left renal vein are unremarkable.

Diagnosis: This is the typical appearance of Grawitz's tumour in the lower pole of the left kidney.

Comments: This echo pattern is the most frequent (60% of the cases); it corresponds to type I described by Weill. Asymptomatic for a long time, renal carcinomas account for 3% of all cancers in man. The terms "clear-cell carcinoma", "nephroepithelioma", "adenocarcinoma", "tubular epithelioma", "Grawitz's tumour" and "hypernephroma" are all synonymous. It is the commonest solid primary malignant renal tumour in adults (95%). The remainder is dominated by mesenchymatous tumours (fibrosarcoma, liposarcoma, leiomyosarcoma) and embryonic tumours (nephroblastoma, often called Wilms' tumour). Most pathologists agree that renal adenocarcinomas arise from tubular cells. In 1893, Grawitz observed a certain similarity to tumours of the adrenal cortex and concluded that these tumours were due to adrenal inclusions, frequently present in the renal parenchyma, so that the terms hypernephroma and Grawitz's tumour are still commonly utilized. From a histological point of view, however, the term tubular epithelioma would be more appropriate.
These tumours are usually unilateral, but in 5% of cases they are bilateral. Let us recall the importance of early diagnosis, since the natural course results in a 1.7% 5-year-survival rate. Subcapsular forms have an 80% 5-year-survival rate. Sonography is of fundamental importance in this field. It may detect lesions which have remained undetected despite intravenous pyelography, especially lesions of the anterior and posterior surfaces. The accuracy of sonography is 95%.

91

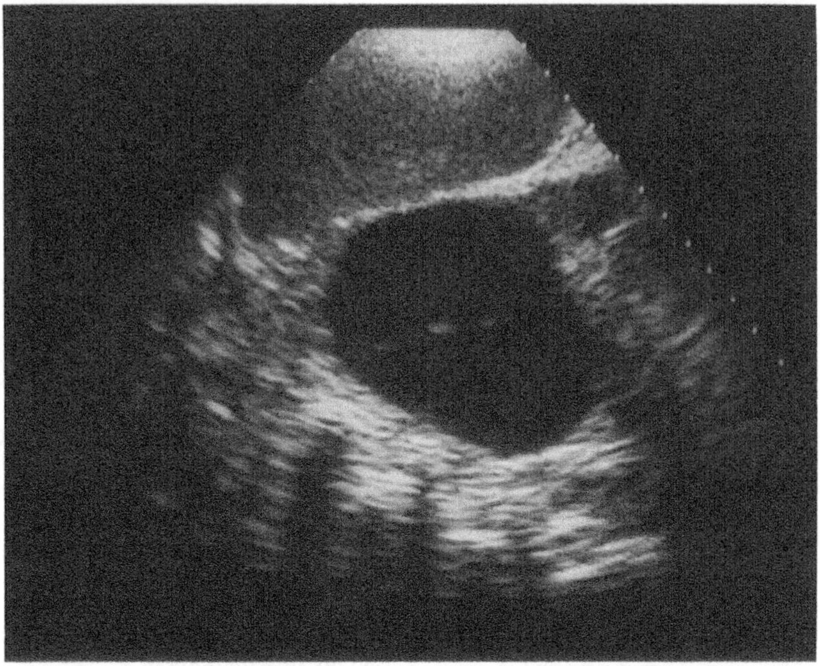

92

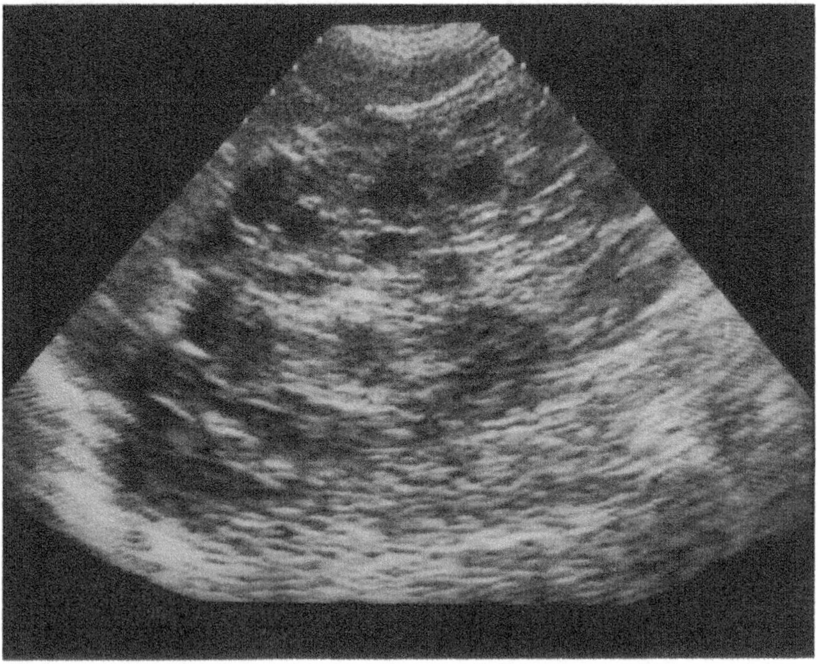

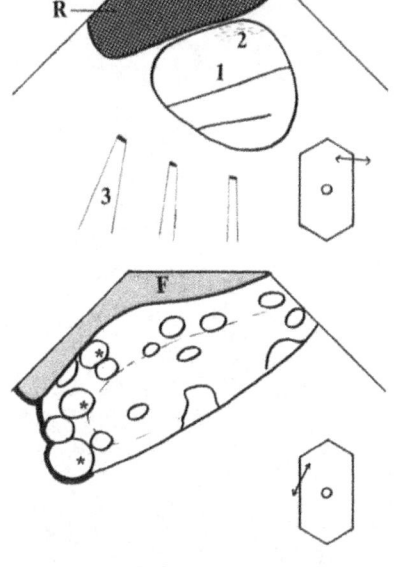

R spleen
1 intracystic septum
2 artefacts
3 costal shadows
* small cysts

Case 91

Clinical data: A 60-year-old man presented with aneurysm of the aorta abdominalis.

Description: A large echo-free oval mass, 7 cm in diameter, with thin walls and posterior relative echo-enhancement in seen at the upper pole of the left kidney. Note the presence of fine intracystic septations.

Diagnosis: This is a cyst of the superior pole of the left kidney.

Comments: Renal cysts are of variable size, from a few cubic millimetres to several litres in volume. Their incidence increases with age. They are usually oval, but a tense cyst becomes round. They can be uni- or bilateral. In 95% of cases, sonography will demonstrate the lesion.

The fine echoes behind the anterior wall are due to artefacts: they are caused by retarded echoes that originate in the tissues surrounding the cyst. When the cyst is superficial and small, these echoes may fill the structure and render the diagnosis difficult. Altering the angulation of the transducer is helpful.

Case 92

Clinical data: A 60-year-old man had recurrent pleural effusion.

Description: Multiple small cysts occupy the right kidney. The kidney is enlarged, and its structure is disorganized. The borders are uneven and poorly defined. The left kidney has the same appearance.

Diagnosis: This is easy: polycystic kidney in an adult.

Comments: Renal polycystosis in adults is usually bilateral. This is an autosomal dominant genetically transmitted condition. Sonography should assess the renal involvement but also search for hepatic and pancreatic involvement. Cerebral angiography can detect possible associated vascular malformations.

Renal polycystosis is well-tolerated for a long time; complications are mainly due to the occurrence of chronic renal failure. These complications are either lithiasis, haemorrhage or rupture of a cyst. Sonography can be used for follow-up but computed tomography is more accurate for the detection of complications.

93

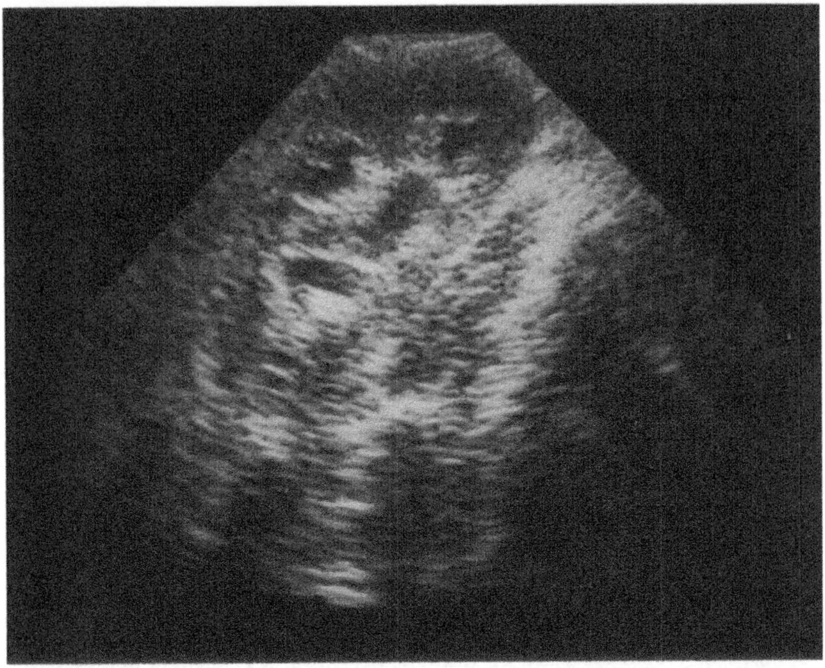

94

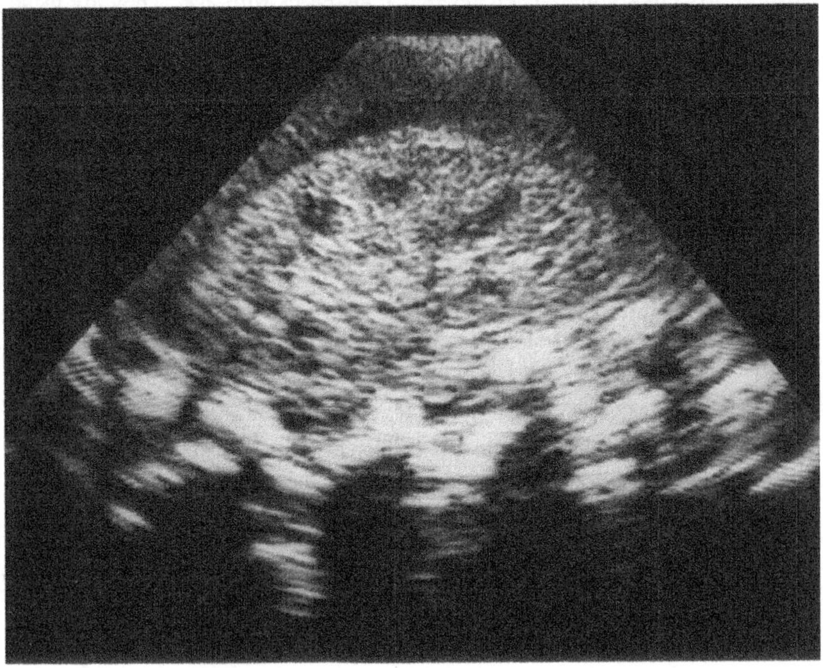

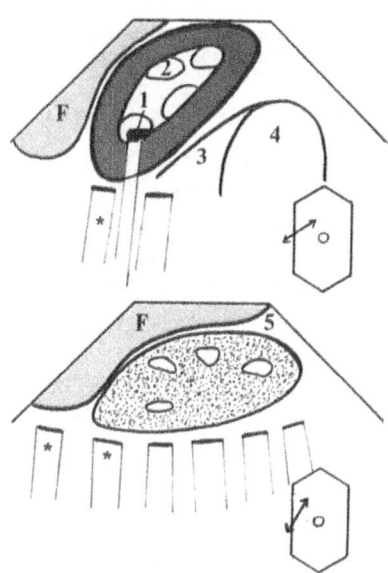

F liver   *3* psoas muscle   **93**
1 renal lithiasis   *4* vertebral body   **94**
2 calyceal dilatation   *5* ascites
            * costal shadows

Case 93

Clinical data: A 40-year-old woman complains of pain in the right hypochondrium.

Description: Several echo-free areas are seen at the corticomedullary junction. They become confluent in the renal sinus to form a larger, sharply demarcated, echo-free area, corresponding to the renal pelvis. This is the classical appearance of pyelocalyceal dilatation. Note the hyperechogenic structure with an acoustic shadow in the superior calyceal group. Also note the costal acoustic shadows (*).

Diagnosis: There is lithiasis in the superior calyceal group. Hydronephrosis is due to a lithiasic obstacle in the ureterovesical junction.

Comments: Calcification is present in 80% of renal lithiasis. The remaining 20% are composed of uric acids. Diagnosis is facilitated when there is an associated hydronephrosis. Sometimes the hyperechogenicity of the stone can be confused with the renal sinus, but the acoustic shadow remains. In fact, the important factor is the size of the stone. Stones of dimensions less than 4 mm are not sonographically detectable in the absence of hydronephrosis.

Case 94

Clinical data: This 55-year-old man has a left hilar bronchial tumour, metastatic hepatomegaly, ascites and hypercalcaemia.

Description: Note the homogeneous, diffuse and very intense hyperechogenicity of the entire renal cortex with loss of differentiation between the renal parenchyma and the renal sinus. The borders of the kidney are smooth.

Diagnosis: There is cortical nephrocalcinosis. Note the presence of ascites.

Comments: Sonographic signs of cortical nephrocalcinosis are seen earlier than the radiographic signs. Depending on their site, nephrocalcinoses are cortical, medullopapillary, diffuse or disorganized. There are various etiologies: local causes are chronic glomerulonephritis, nephritis and pyelonephritis and cortical or papillary necrosis. Among the general causes the most frequent is hypercalcaemia of diverse origins – hyperparathyroidism, bone tumours, prolonged immobilization, vitamin D toxicity, paraneoplastic syndrome. Hypercalcaemia is, however, not always associated with nephrocalcinosis. Among the other general causes, let us mention hyperchloraemic acidosis and oxalosis. Finally, there are also idiopathic nephrocalcinoses.

95

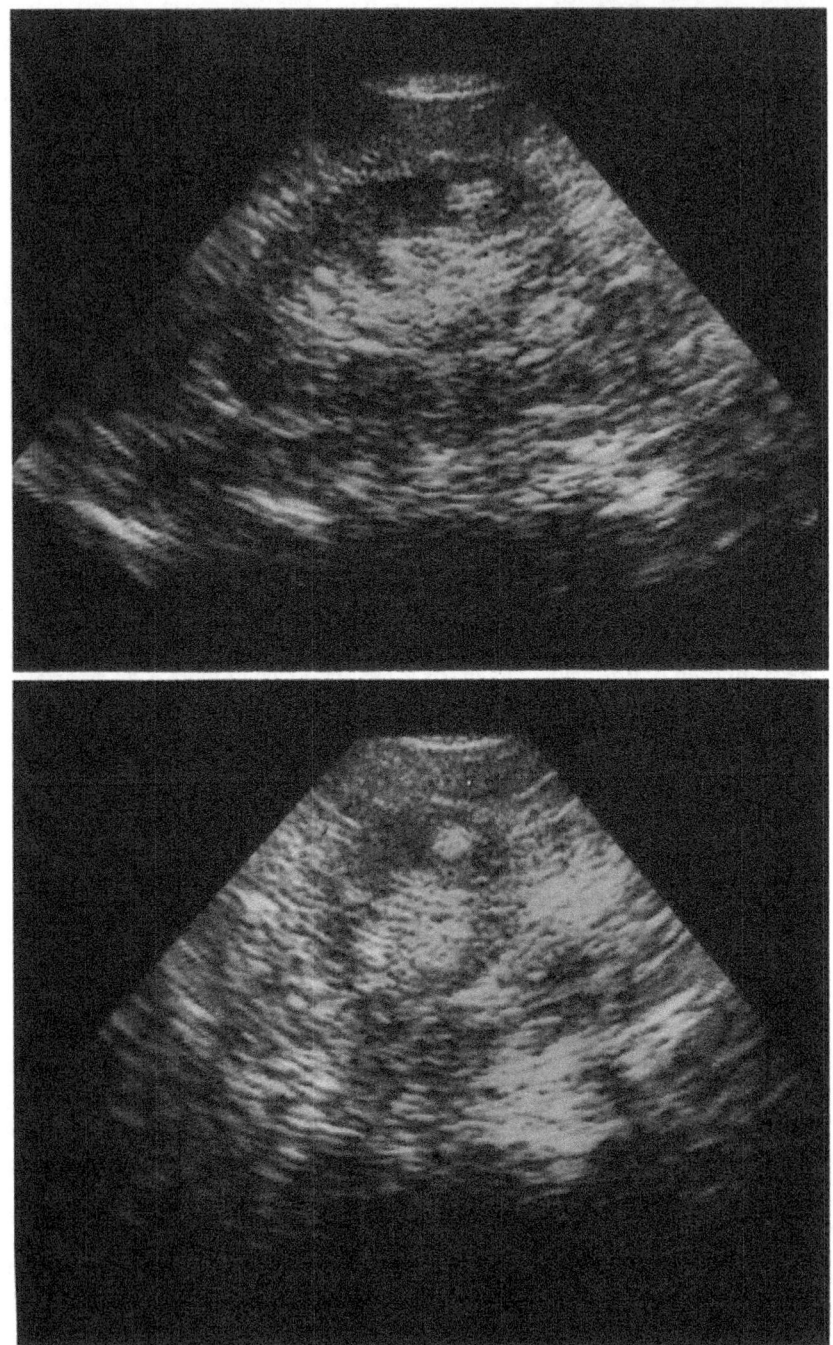

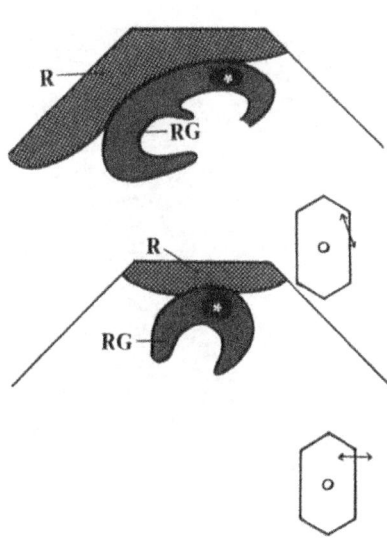

R spleen
RG left kidney
* angiomyolipoma

Case 95

Clinical data: A 60-year-old woman underwent follow-up investigation of a renal hyperechogenic structure that had been detected 3 years before.

Description: A rounded, homogeneous, hyperechogenic mass, which is sharply delimited is seen in the cortex of the inferior pole of the left kidney. There is no acoustic shadow and no deformation of the renal borders. The image is unchanged compared to the previous investigation.

Diagnosis: This is easy: small angiomyolipoma.

Comments: Angiomyolipomas are benign tumours whose reported incidence has increased with the rise of modern investigation techniques. These tumours comprise three elements in variable amounts: muscle cells, tumoural vascular structures and fat. They are usually unilateral, but can be bilateral, in which case a search for tuberous sclerosis (Bourneville's disease) is advisable. The lesions are usually asymptomatic, but can be complicated by haemorrhage.

In sonography, the angiomyolipoma appears as a hyperechogenic mass because of the presence of adipose tissue. Its intensity must be at least equal to that of echoes from the renal sinus, and the image persists with a low gain setting. Less echogenic areas corresponding to haemorrhage or to the other components can also be seen. Although it lacks specificity, the echo pattern is quite evocative. In large angiomyolipomas the detection of hyperechogenic areas is a very strong argument in favour of the diagnosis of the lesion, but it is not specific. Small angiomyolipomas introduce a new problem: being asymptomatic, they are chance findings since sonography has become a routine investigation. They are, however, discovered in 11% of autopsy examinations. The ultrasound appearance is characteristic (as in this case). It is due to the presence of adipose tissue and to the multiple interfaces of the other constituents. Computed tomography is specific because of the negative density of the adipose tissue. Arteriography remains useful in three circumstances: for diagnosis when there is little or no fat (angiomyoma); prior to limited exeresis, for locating the vascular pedicles, and in the event of intratumoural haemorrhage, when it plays both a diagnostic and a therapeutic part, in embolization.

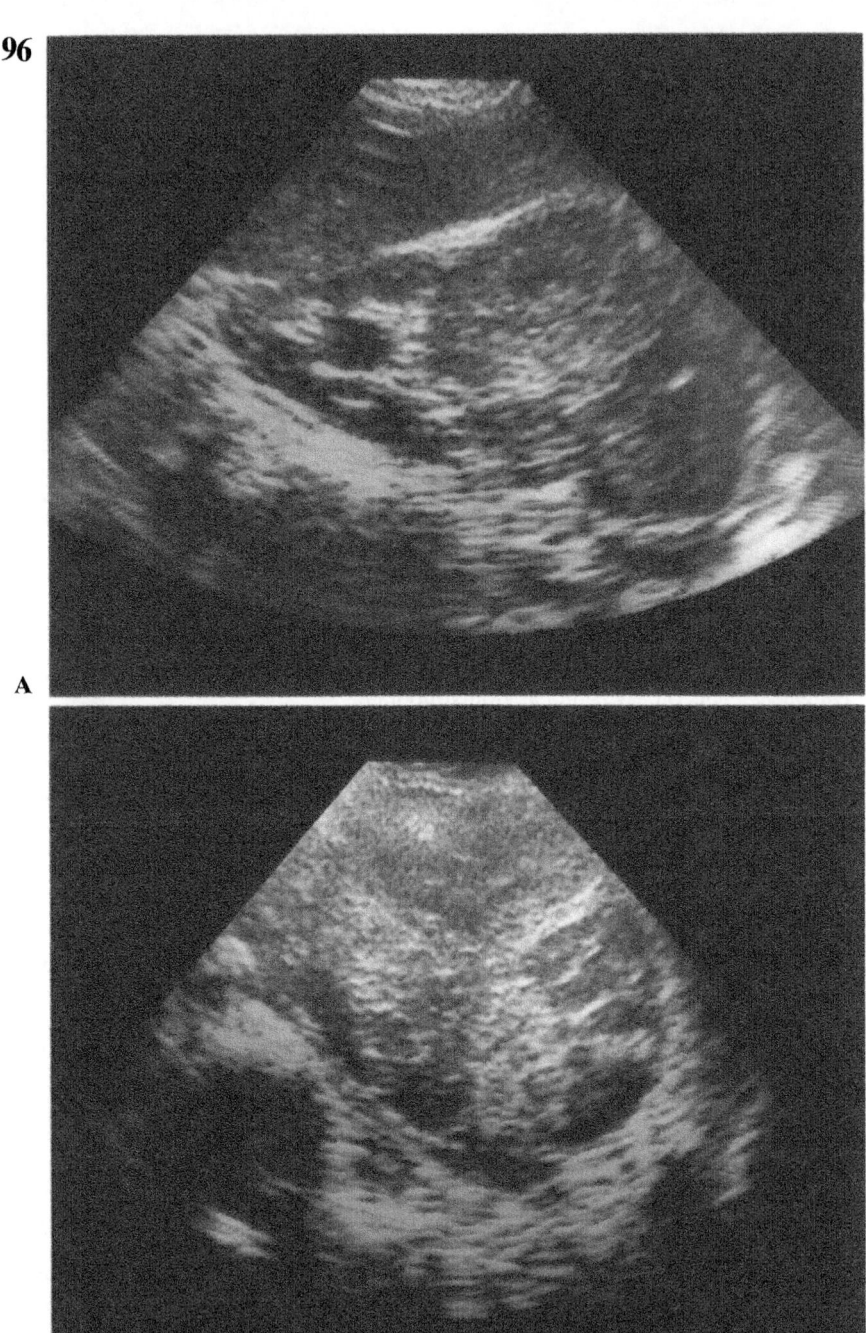

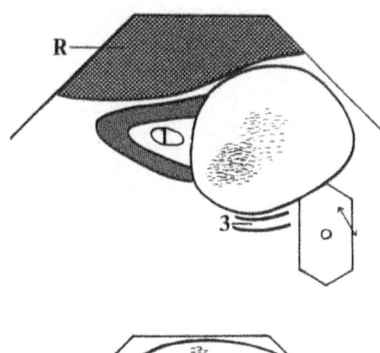

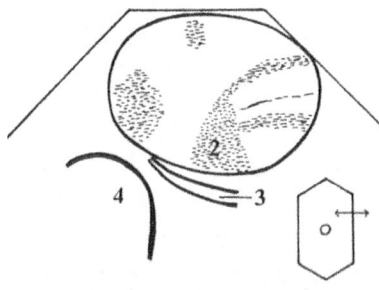

96

R spleen   **96**
1 dilatation of the superior calyceal group
2 hyperechogenic areas
3 proximal ureteral dilatation
4 vertebral body

Case 96

Clinical data: A 45-year-old Turkish woman presented with altered physical status. A mass was palpated in the left iliac fossa.

Description: The renal origin of the tumour is easily detected: a part of the renal parenchyma has disappeared; there is a voluminous mass (11.5 cm in diameter) obliterating the middle and inferior part of the left kidney. It is heterogeneous, and contains well-delimited hyperechogenic areas which are roughly triangular (Scan B). The mass is rounded with sharp borders and surrounded by a hypoechogenic line (Scan A). The echostructure of the superior pole of the kidney is normal. Note the dilatation of the superior calyceal group due to compression of the renal pelvis by the tumour.

The investigation was otherwise unremarkable: there was no lymph-node enlargement, no thrombosis of the left renal vein or of the inferior vena cava, and normal respiratory movement of the kidney.

Diagnosis: Precise diagnosis is not possible with sonography. The initial report had diagnosed a rare renal tumour and ruled out the classical hypernephroma. Histological examination of the surgical specimen revealed a Wilms' tumour in an adult.

Comments: Wilms' tumour is classically a malignant renal tumour of children. Some cases in adults have been described (2%–6% of cases, according to the authors). The histological structure shows all elements of a metanephrogenic blastema with differentiated sectors: tubular and pseudo-glomerular formations, and different tissues (bone, cartilage, fat, smooth or striated muscle and fibrous tissue).

The hyperechogenic areas correspond to adipose or fibrous tissue. Although the presence of fat is uncommon in children, it may lead to an incorrect diagnosis of angiomyolipoma. The echo-free areas correspond to haemorrhage or to intratumoural necrosis. The usually large tumour is delimited by a pseudocapsule which is seen as a hypoechogenic crown. This pseudocapsule sometimes creates an echogenic interface mimicking an extrarenal origin.

Metastases are primarily pulmonary, and then hepatic. The older the patient, the poorer the prognosis is.

97

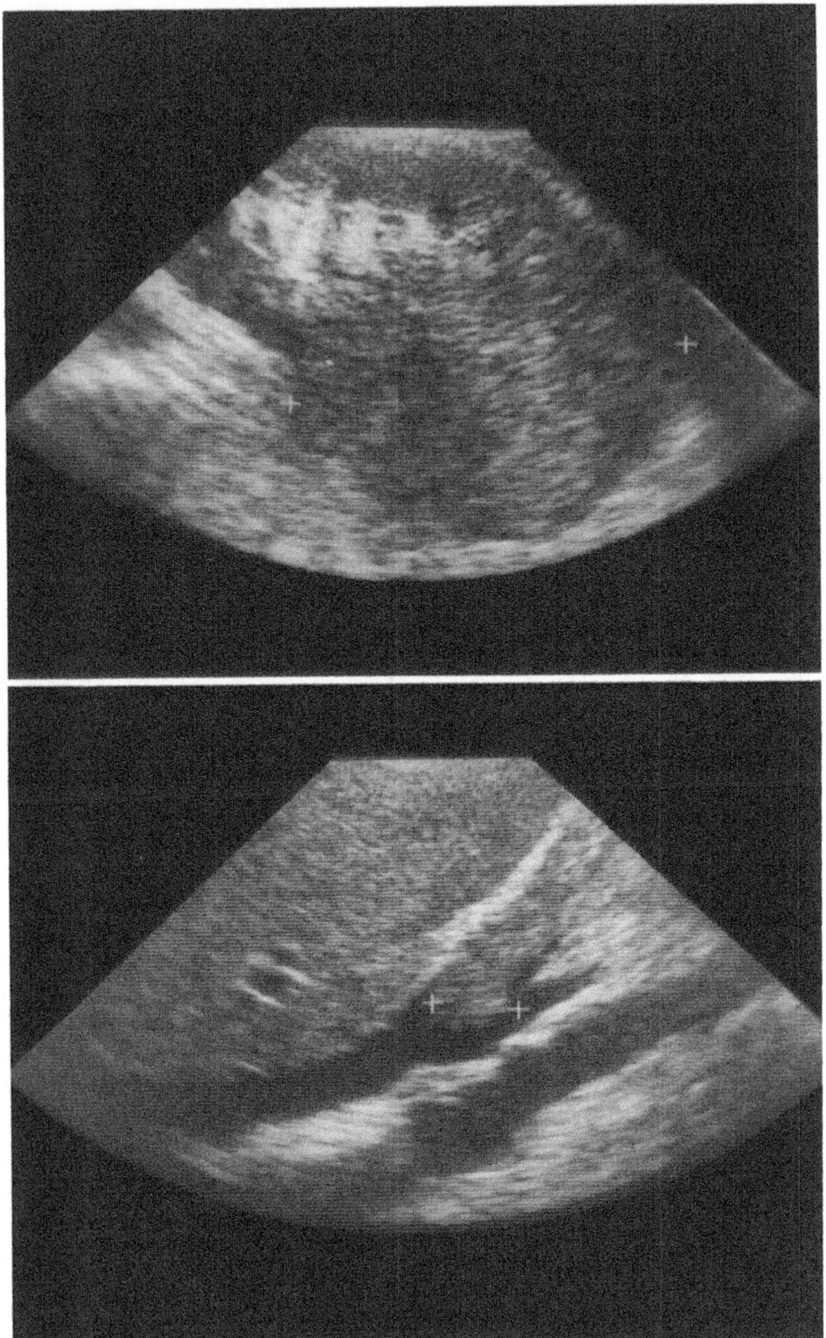

A

B

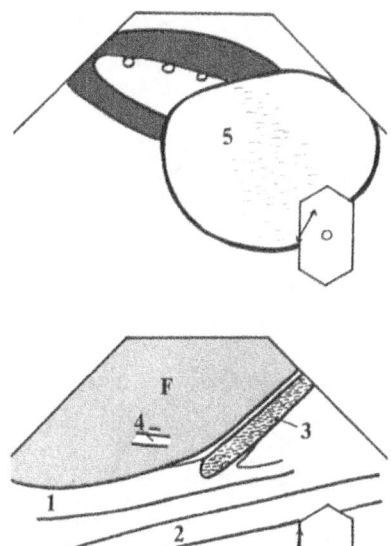

F liver
1 inferior vena cava
2 aorta
3 tumoural bud in right renal vein
4 right portal vein tributary
5 renal tumour

Case 97

Clinical data: This 50-year-old man has macroscopic haematuria.

Description: The scan shows a voluminous heterogeneous mass (13 cm in diameter) that is more echogenic than the renal cortex, located in the inferomedial part of the right kidney. The right renal vein is not detected. It is replaced by an echogenic, homogeneous tubular structure, wider than a normal renal vein, extending into the inferior vena cava, into which it protrudes (Scan B).

Diagnosis: This is easy: Grawitz's tumour of the right kidney with thrombosis of the renal vein and a "bud" in the inferior vena cava.

Comments: This echo-pattern corresponds to Weill's stage II, and accounts for 29% of cases. Venous extension, characteristic of this type of tumour, corresponds to stage IIIa of Robson's classification. Its presence changes the prognosis as well as the surgical management.

At the present time, the assessment of extension is based on sonography and computed tomography. Detection of renal vein thrombosis is more difficult on the right (due to the oblique and short vein) than on the left side. The intravenacaval tumoural bud is easily detected by sonography. Stages I and II can be detected by computed tomography. As concerns later stages, sonography and computed tomography are equally accurate. The indications for arteriography are more limited: arterial cartography before partial nephrectomy, pretherapeutic embolization and differential diagnosis.

98

B, D

A, C

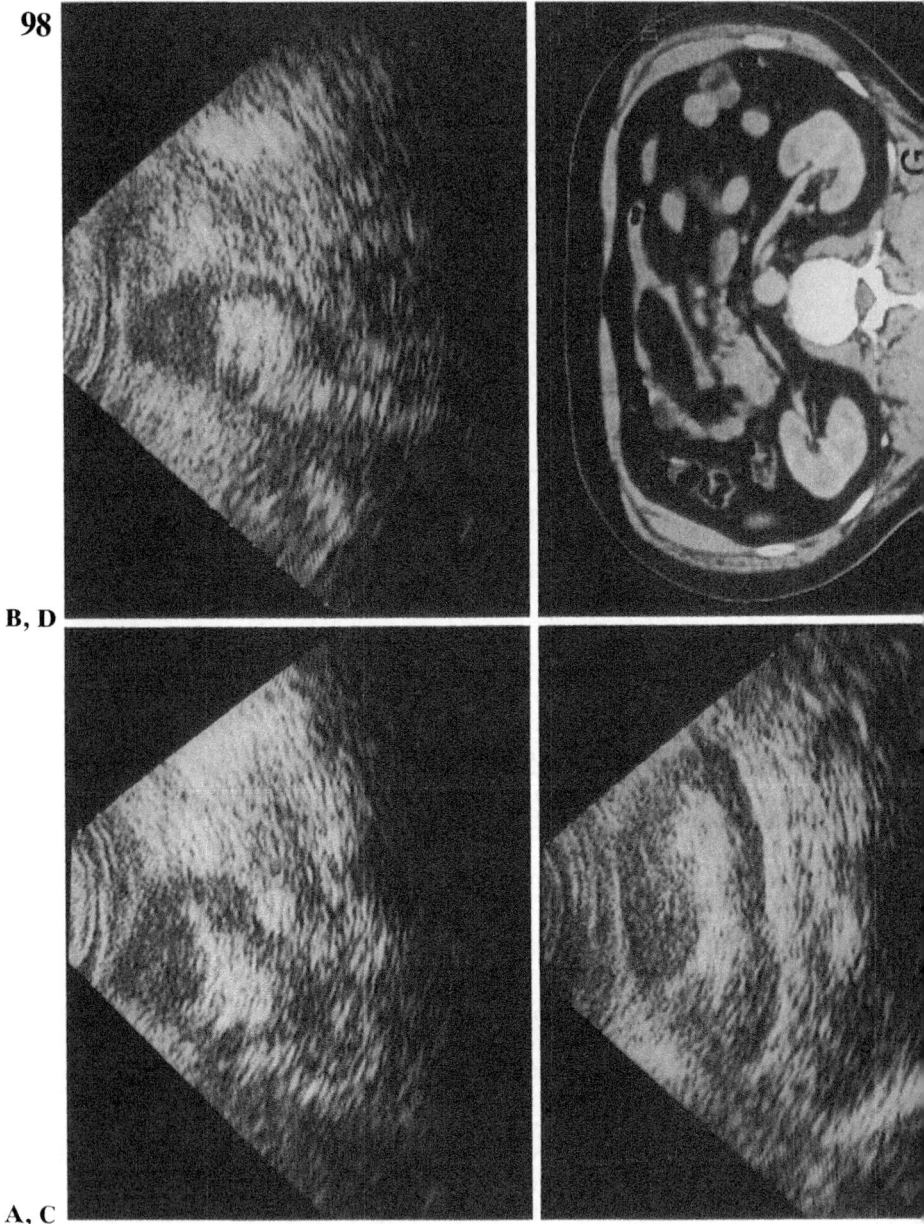

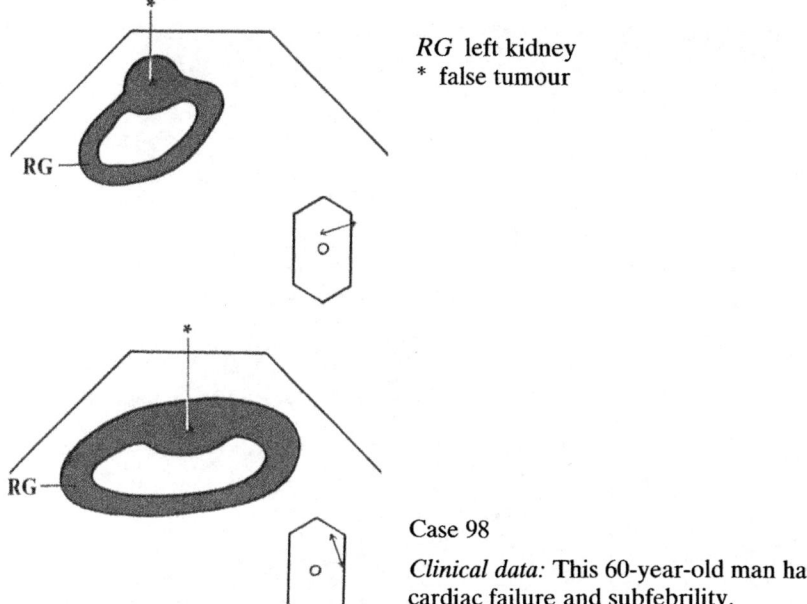

RG left kidney

* false tumour

98

Case 98

Clinical data: This 60-year-old man has cardiac failure and subfebrility.

Description: Oblique and transverse scans of the left kidney show a rounded mass, situated in the cortex, deforming the outer boundary of the kidney and protruding towards the renal sinus. It has the same echo-pattern as the renal parenchyma. It is located in the middle of the convexity. The investigation is otherwise unremarkable.

Diagnosis: This is a normal kidney. The mass corresponds to a renal pseudotumour. Computed tomography gave evidence of hypertrophy of a renal column, and foetal lobulation.

Comments: Certain anatomical variants can mimic renal tumours. The diagnosis of a hypertrophied renal column (dromadery lump) or foetal lobulation is easy with intravenous pyelography. Hypertrophy of a renal column is a single or a multiple congenital anomaly within a kidney. It is a mass of cortical tissue situated between the pyramids, protruding into the renal sinus (Scan C).

The sonographic appearance does not usually cause a problem: the echo-structure is identical to that of the renal cortex, the mass has no proper limit and the outer surface of the kidney is not deformed. In contrast, persistent foetal lobulation is responsible for an uneven boundary. When hypertrophy of a renal column and foetal lobulation are associated, sonography is more difficult, especially as the multiplicity of oblique scans creates false images (Scans A and B).

There are also aquired renal pseudotumours, which follow infections, infarcts and trauma. In such cases there is localized hypertrophy of the remaining normal parenchyma.

In some very difficult cases, computed tomography with dynamic vascular studies or renal angiography may be helpful.

99

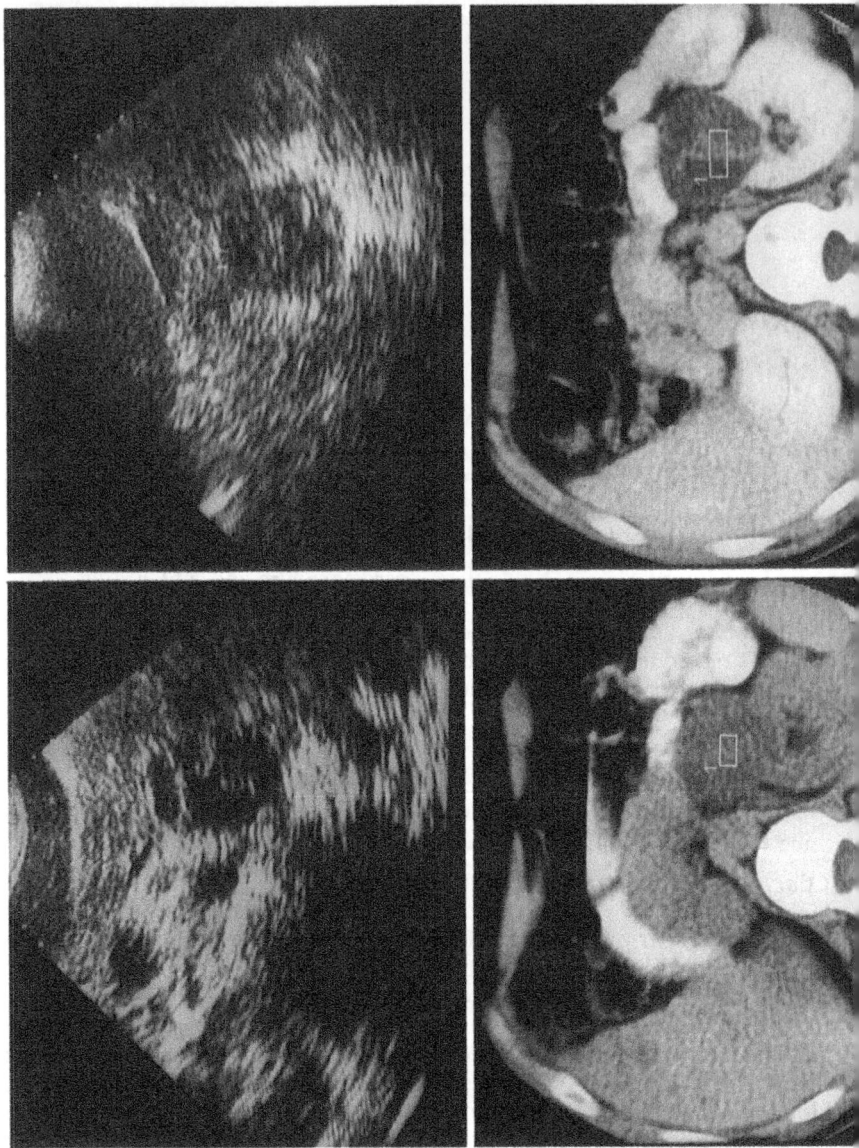

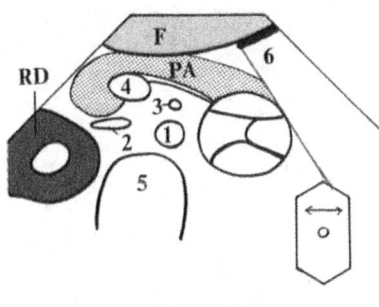

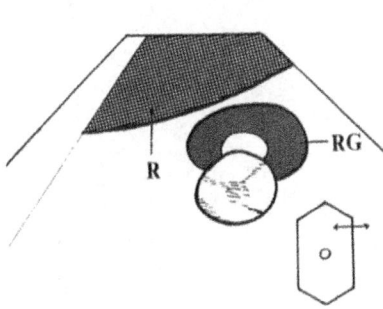

F liver
R spleen
RD right kidney
PA pancreas
RG left kidney
1 aorta
2 inferior vena cava
3 superior mesenteric artery
4 splenic vein
5 vertebral body
6 bowel gas

Case 99

Clinical data: This 30-year-old man has viral hepatitis.

Description: The scan shows a hypoechogenic mass of 4.5 cm diameter, which contains multiple septations delineating cystic structures in the superomedial pole of the left kidney. The junction angle, as well as the deformation of the superior pole of the kidney, rule out a suprarenal lesion.
Computed tomography also shows a mass with a mean density of 25 UH moderately enhanced by contrast injection: 35 UH. The structure is heterogeneous and contains purely liquid areas of 2 UH density.

Diagnosis: This is difficult: it was not a plain septated cyst, but a multilocular cyst.

Comments: The multilocular cyst, or cystic adenoma, or polycystic nephroblastoma is an uncommon benign tumour, surrounded by a capsule, containing several compartments formed by membranous septa lined with epithelium. There is no communication between the cyst and the pyelocalyceal cavities. This is a congenital lesion which is detected in children in 50% of the cases. The mass is usually avascular, but selective angiography may show thin vessels within the septa. Calcification can also be present.
    Differential diagnosis from a necrotic malignant tumour (thick and irregular walls), an intracystic tumour, or a hydatid cyst can be difficult.
    Surgical exploration is recommended since multilocular cysts may undergo degeneration.

100

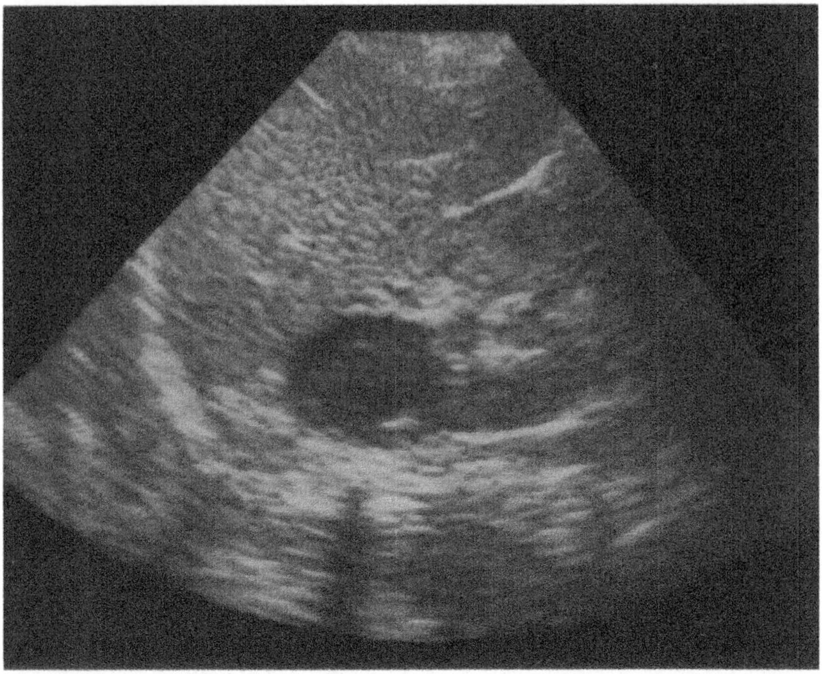

101

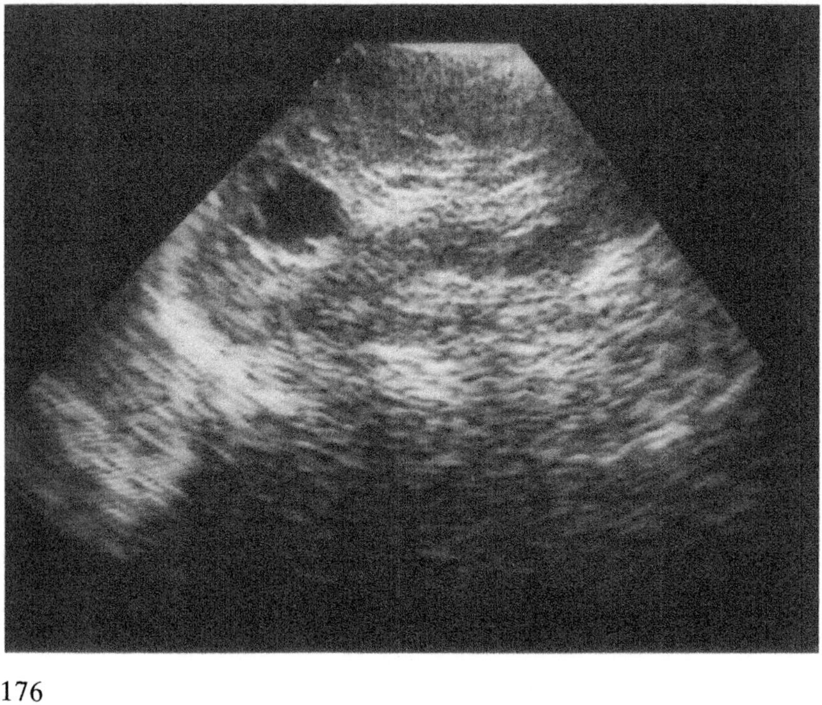

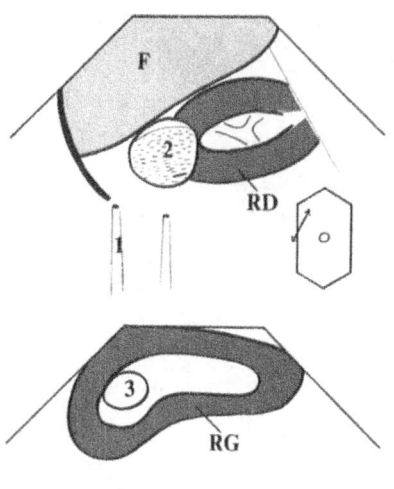

F liver
RD right kidney
RG left kidney
1 costal shadows
2 fine intracystic echoes
3 anechogenic rounded calyceal area

Case 100

Clinical data: This 20-year-old woman has acute right-sided pyelonephritis.

Description: The cyst at the upper pole of the right kidney contains fine echoes; its upper limit is convex. It is thin-walled, and a more intense echo arises from the inferior part.

Diagnosis: There is a superinfected cyst in the superior pole of the right kidney.

Comments: The multiple fine echoes in the cyst are due either to intracystic haemorrhage or to infection. It may be difficult to show the fluid level; this should be searched for in the dorsal decubitus and the erect positions. The convex upper limit seen in this case can be accounted for by recent mobilization of the patient. The diagnosis can be confirmed by computed tomography, which shows an intracystic density of about 25−35 UH, or by puncture of the cyst.

Case 101

Clinical data: This 35-year-old man was treated for peritoneal tuberculosis.

Description: There is an echo-free structure in the superior pole of the left kidney, at the corticomedullary junction. It has thin walls and smooth borders.

Diagnosis: Two hypotheses should be considered: hydronephrosis localized to the superior calyx, or parapelvic cyst. Pyelography showed the pyelocalyceal system to be normal.

Comments: Comparison with pyelography is fundamental for differentiation between localized hydronephrosis or hydronephrosis of the upper renal segment and of a parapelvic cyst. Hydronephrosis of the entire pyelocalyceal system, on the contrary, can be diagnosed using ultrasound alone. Computed tomography is never necessary.

102

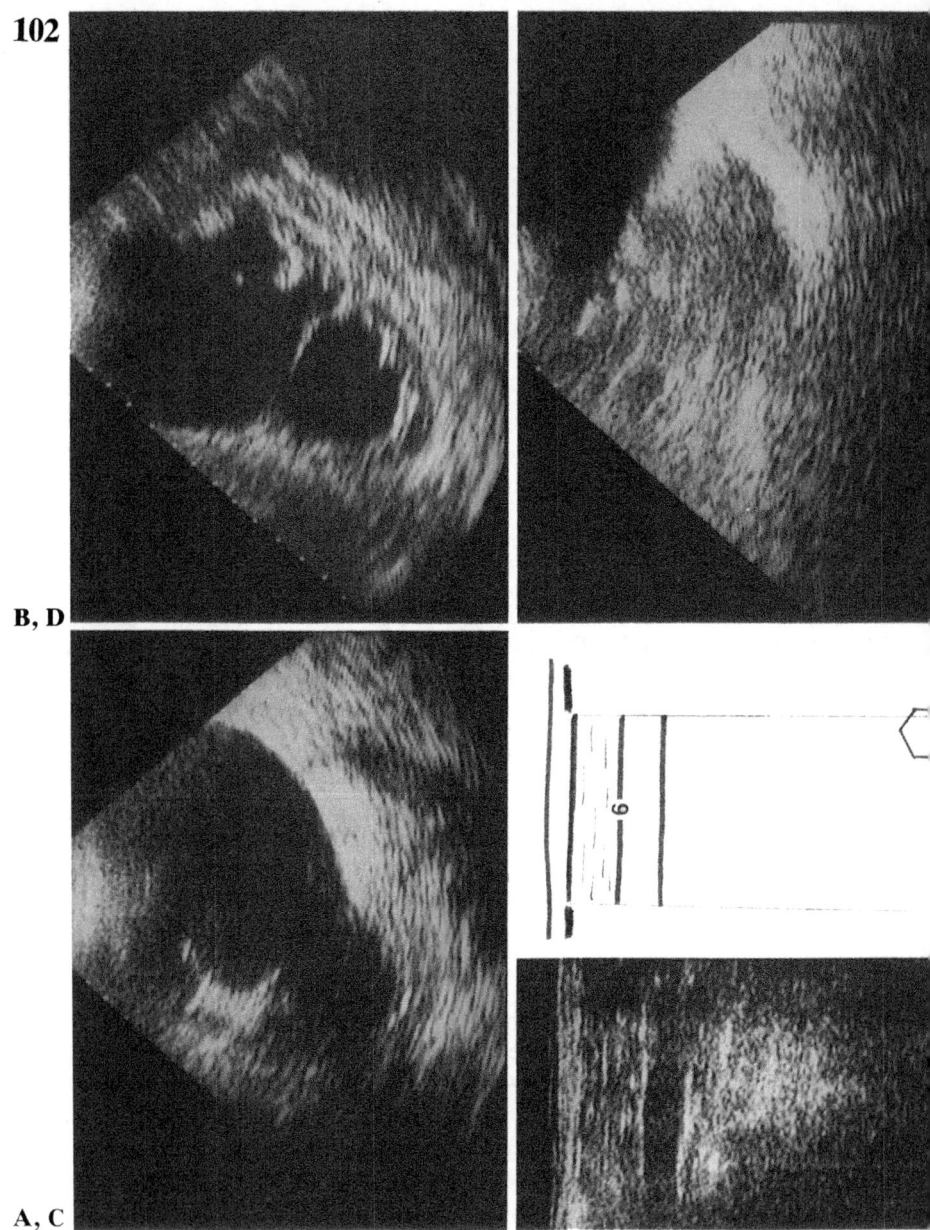

B, D

A, C

178

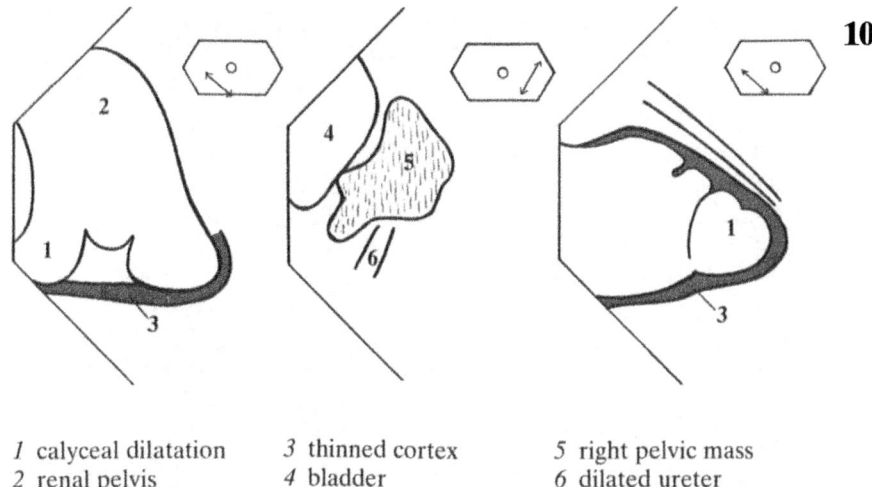

1 calyceal dilatation   3 thinned cortex   5 right pelvic mass
2 renal pelvis   4 bladder   6 dilated ureter

Case 102

Clinical data: A 70-year-old woman presented with an inflammatory syndrome. She had had hysterectomy for fibroma 15 years earlier.

Description: There is a voluminous right pyelocalyceal hydronephrosis (peripheral intraparenchymatous polycystic lesions that communicate with each other, and one large fluid mass in the right iliac fossa that corresponds to the renal pelvis). Thinning of the cortex indicates that the lesion is longstanding. The ureter is visible up to the renal pelvis, where a voluminous, homogeneous hypoechogenic mass, 6 cm in diameter, is seen to extend to the right laterovesical region (Scan D).

Diagnosis: There is right uretero-hydronephrosis in a tumour of the residual uterine stump.

Comments: Differential diagnosis from polycystosis is usually easy because of the dilatation of the renal pelvis and the rounded, communicating pyelocalyceal cavities. Bilateral pyelocalyceal dilatation is significant only when the bladder is empty. Exploration of the pelvic should always be combined with exploration of both kidneys, and vice versa. Thinning of the cortex is related to the duration of hydronephrosis. Visualization of the dilated abdominal and pelvic parts of the ureter is sometimes difficult. Is some cases it may therefore be impossible to exclude obstruction of the pelviureteric junction, or the proximal ureter as the underlying lesion.

With minor hydronephroses differential diagnosis from lipomatosis of the renal sinus can be difficult. Also, with major hydronephroses, renal-pelvis dilatation can be confused with other types of large multilocular "pouch" (a septate cyst, cystic lymphangioma or mesenteric cyst).

103

B, D

A, C

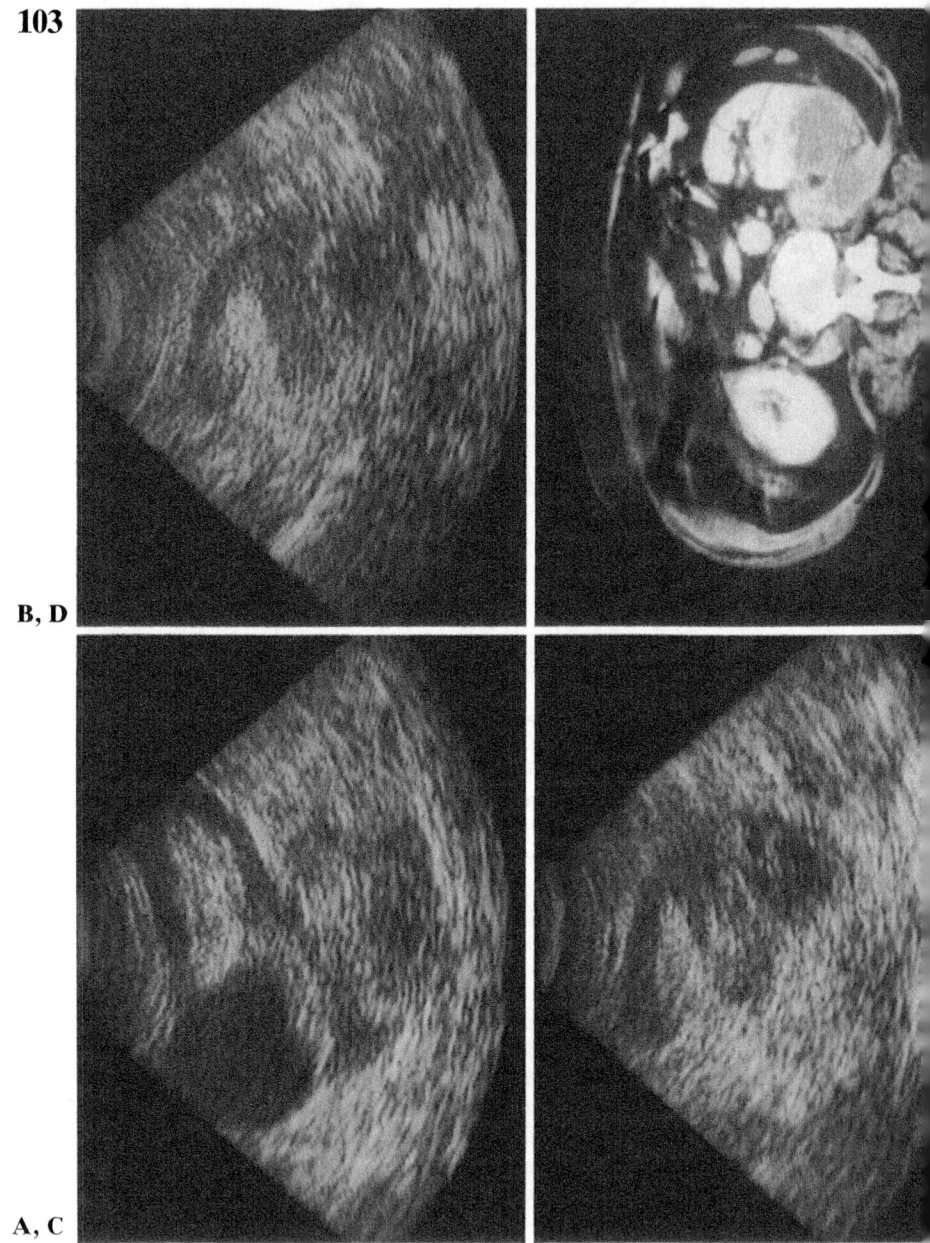

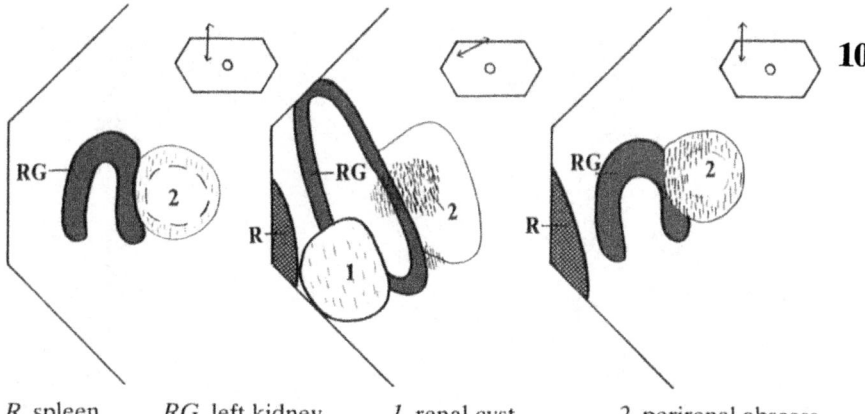

R spleen   *RG* left kidney   *1* renal cyst   *2* perirenal abscess

Case 103

Clinical data: A 70-year-old woman with longstanding fever has a history of recent urinary tract infection.

Description: There is a large cyst in the superior pole of the right kidney, with some fine central echoes (Scan A). A heterogeneous, oval mass, with a hypoechogenic centre and a poorly demarcated, thick echogenic wall, is seen on the posterior and medial part of the kidney (Scan B). It displaces the cortex, which has an altered echostructure and contains hyperechogenic, linear structures. Note also that the kidney is displaced anteriorly (Scan C) and that it remains fixed during respiratory movements.

Diagnosis: This is a perinephric abscess, situated on the posterior aspect of the kidney, confirmed by computed tomography, from a superinfected cyst in the right kidney.

Comments: A perinephric abscess is an uncommon and severe complication of primary or secondary pyelonephritis or ascending nephritis. It requires drainage, which can be carried out after sonographically-guided puncture and insertion of a catheter. The causative organism is usually *Staphylococcus,* but gram-negative organisms can be found. In the present case, it was a colibacillus.

The collection is usually seen in the posterior perirenal space and it usually remains confined to the perirenal area. In the case shown, there was extension to the posterior pararenal space. Rupture can occur through the inferior part of the perirenal space with extension to the true pelvic cavity.

Although sonography remains a sensitive investigation (with a visualization limit of 1.5–2 cm) it lacks of specificity. When the clinical data are not pathognomonic, the question of perirenal haematoma or a tumoural process arises. Computed tomography is actually the most accurate investigation, affirming the presence of an abscess when there is a mass whose density is greater than that of a cystic structure, and which is surrounded by a variably thick capsule, whose density in enhanced by contrast injection. Computed tomography permits one, moreover, to assess the involvement of the perirenal fasciae and the retroperitoneum as a whole.

104

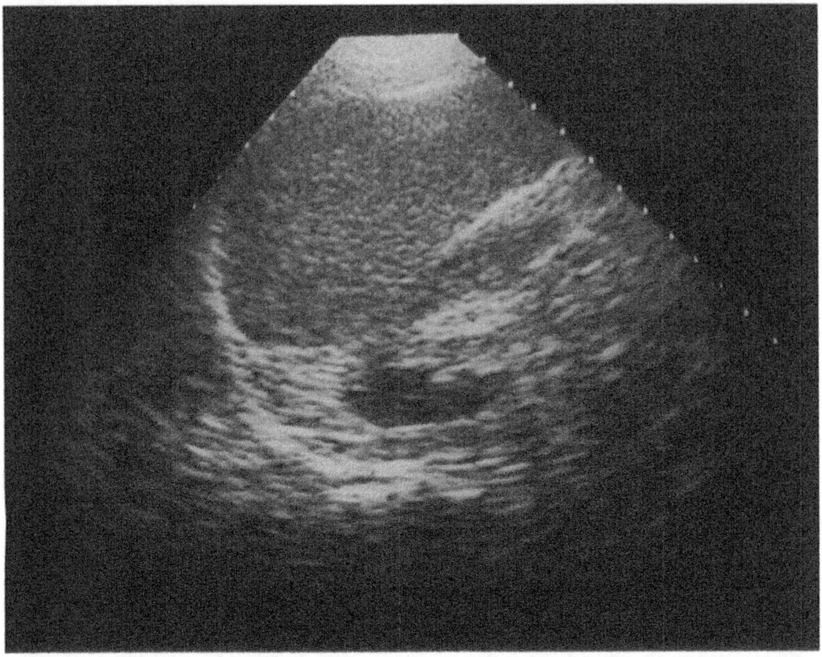

105

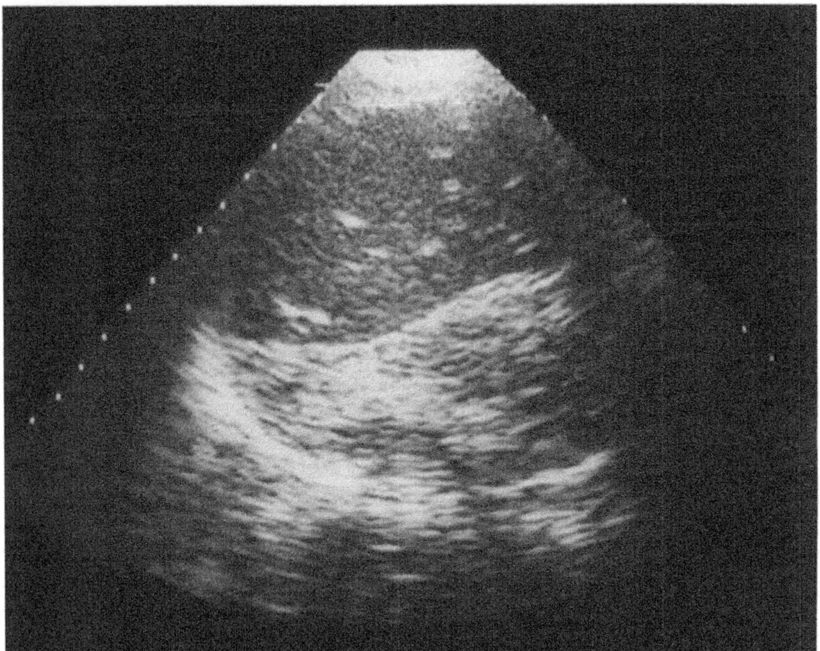

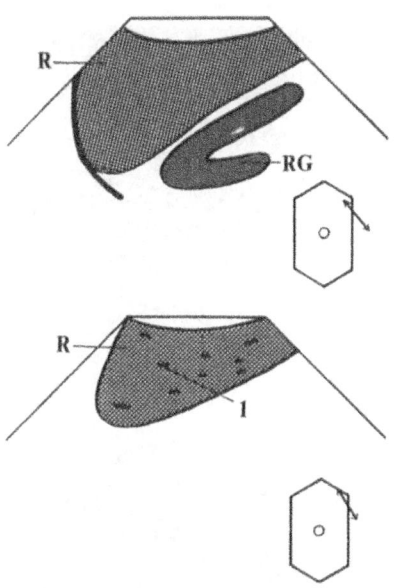

R spleen
RG left kidney
1 splenic calcification

Case 104

Sonographic investigation of the spleen does not require preparation. Transverse and longitudinal scans are performed via the left posterolateral intercostal, or left recurrent subcostal approach. Two morphological types are distinguished: "compact" and "spread" spleens. The normal spleen shows considerable variations in size between individuals, and even in the same person, depending on age and nutrition. The mean dimensions are: 12 cm, craniocaudal; 7 cm, anteroposterior; and 3–4 cm, transverse diameter. Whereas the lateral surface is convex and smooth, the medial, visceral surface is variable and can have important lobulations between the pancreas and the kidney, forming true pseudotumours. Its echostructure is homogeneous and less echogenic than the liver. Splenomegaly is only considered to exist when at least two dimensions are increased.

Case 105

Clinical data: A 50-year-old Indian man complains of pain in the abdomen.

Description: The spleen has a normal volume and contains numerous small hyperechogenic areas, 0.3–0.5 cm long, without posterior relative echo-attenuation.

Diagnosis: There is calcification of the spleen.

Comments: The absence of an acoustic shadow is due to the small size of the calcifications. When they are multiple and small they suggest two possibilities: phleboliths and tuberculosis. More rarely, the lesion is a splenic infarct, parasitosis or brucellosis.

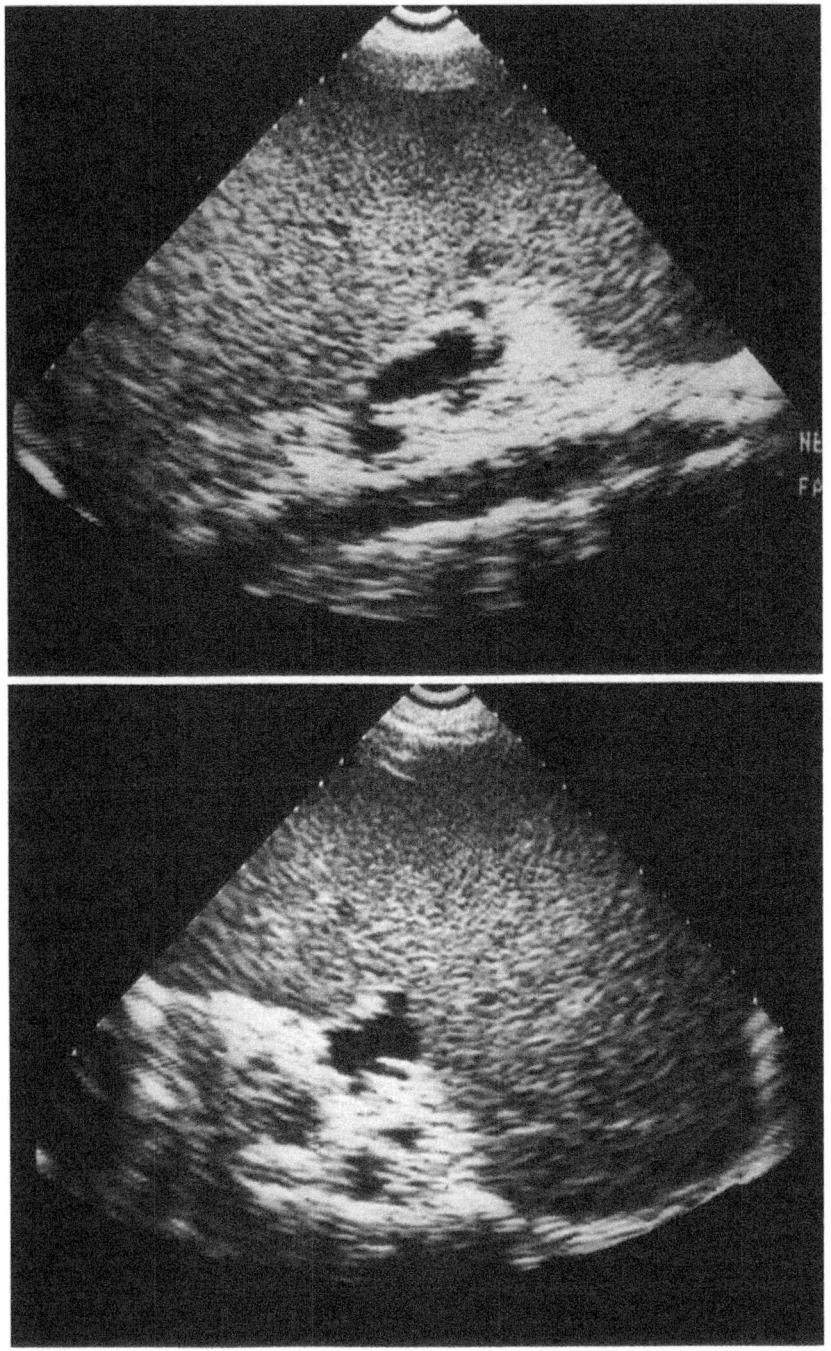

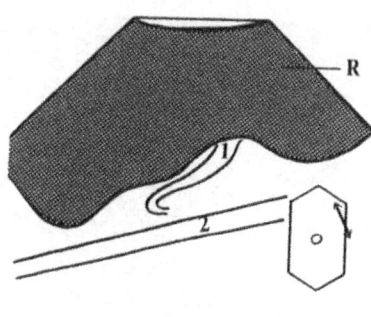

R spleen
1 dilated splenic pedicle
2 abdominal aorta

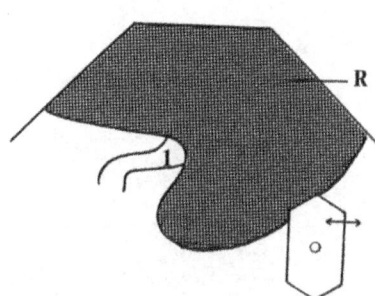

Case 106

Clinical data: This 50-year-old man has pyelonephritis.

Description: There is obvious splenomegaly: the craniocaudal diameter is 20 cm. The echostructure is homogeneous. Note the large size of the splenic pedicle.

Diagnosis: This is easy: polycythaemia rubra vera (Vaquez' disease). The splenomegaly is so significant that myeloid metaplasia of the spleen is to be suspected.

Comments: The sonographic diagnosis of splenomegaly is easy. There are numerous etiologies: portal hypertension, haematological diseases, infection and parasitic diseases. Neoplastic conditions of the spleen itself are much more rare.

Lymphomatous spleens have various appearances; diffuse infiltration with a homogeneous echostructure, well-defined hyperechogenic nodules, hyperechogenic areas or a combination of both patterns may be seen. Increased echogenicity in splenomegaly due to malignant infiltration is not specific, since this feature is also present in chronic inflammatory conditions and in benign conditions. The etiology of this hyperechogenicity is poorly understood; it is said to be proportional to the degree of diffuse infiltration of the spleen rather than to the nature of the disease.

On the other hand, the absence of splenomegaly does not rule out lymphomatous infiltration.

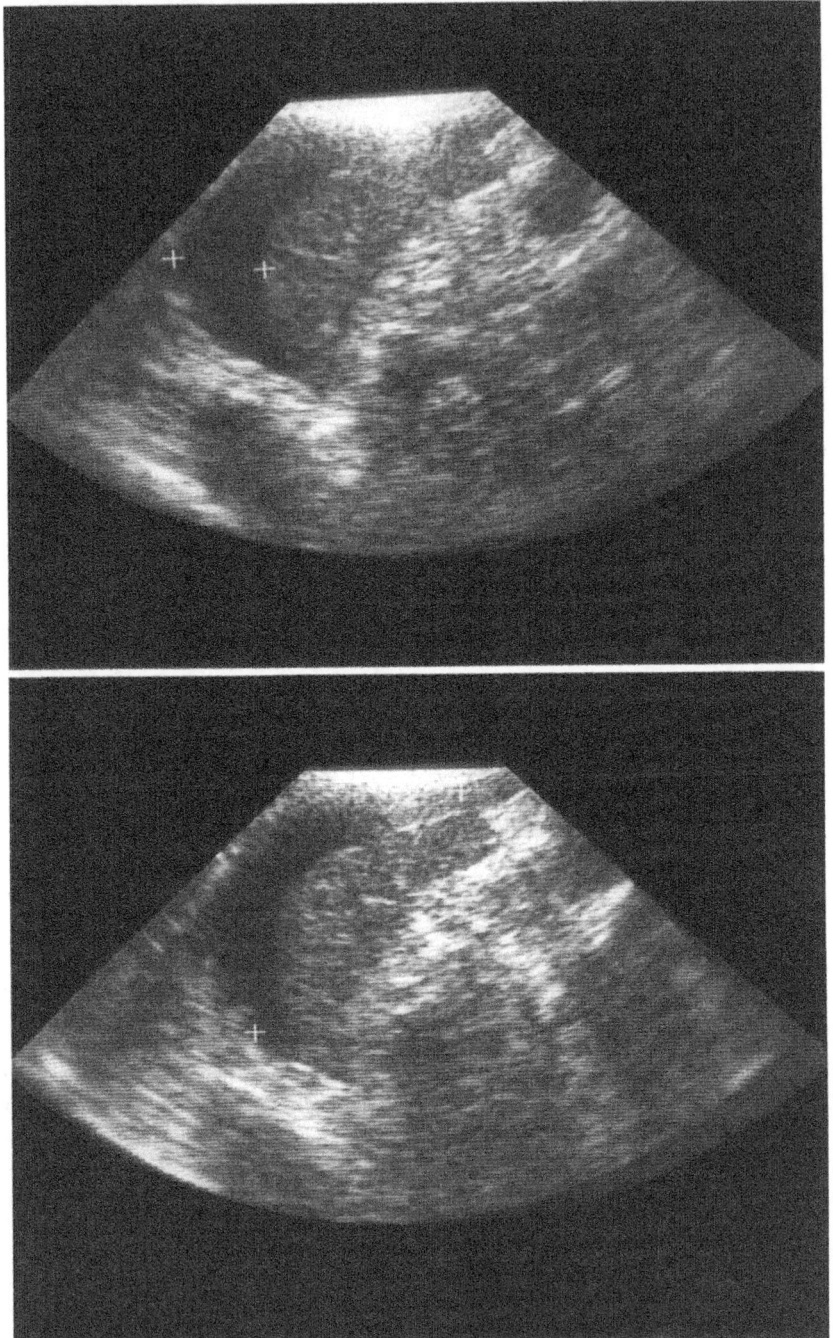

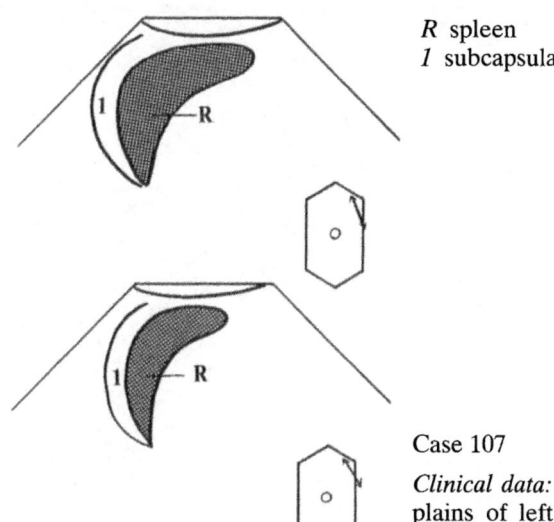

R spleen
1 subcapsular haematoma

Case 107

Clinical data: A 25-year-old man complains of left hypochondrial pain following a motor vehicle accident.

Description: An echo-free band is seen between the left cupola of the diaphragm and the superior splenic surface. The band obviously indicates a fluid structure. Otherwise the spleen has a normal volume and a homogeneous echostructure.

Diagnosis: This is easy: post-traumatic subcapsular haematoma of the spleen.

Comments: Subcapsular splenic haematomas can be either post-traumatic, or spontaneous (in patients taking anticoagulative drugs or with an abnormal spleen). When the haematoma is small and located in the space between the spleen and the kidney, its origin may be difficult to determine.

Splenic lesions are variable and changeable. Four main types are to be distinguished:
a) A large heterogeneous spleen with hyperechogenic images
b) Anechogenic areas corresponding to more-or-less-discrete intrasplenic haematomas
c) Non-mobile peripheral "arcuate" images, corresponding to a subcapsular haematoma (Case 107)
d) Rectilinear anechogenic bands corresponding to tears

Sonography helps detect intraperitoneal effusion in the most inferiorly located areas when the patient is in the dorsal decubitus position, i.e. fluid in the hepatorenal space, the pouch of Douglas and the paracolic recess. Although sonography is very accurate in detecting fluid in the peritoneal cavity, it is less trustworthy in detecting the intrasplenic lesion itself. Let us also recall the notion of biphasic rupture, and the significant proportion of spleens which are not well visualized, in emergency investigations or in difficult patients. It should also be kept in mind that ultrasound scanning must be performed prior to puncture-lavage of the peritoneum.

108

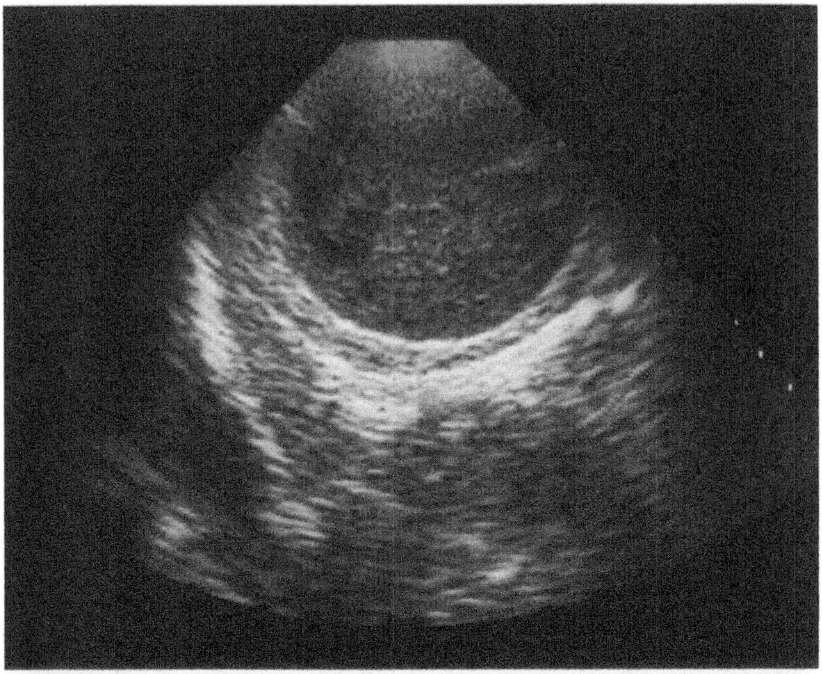

A

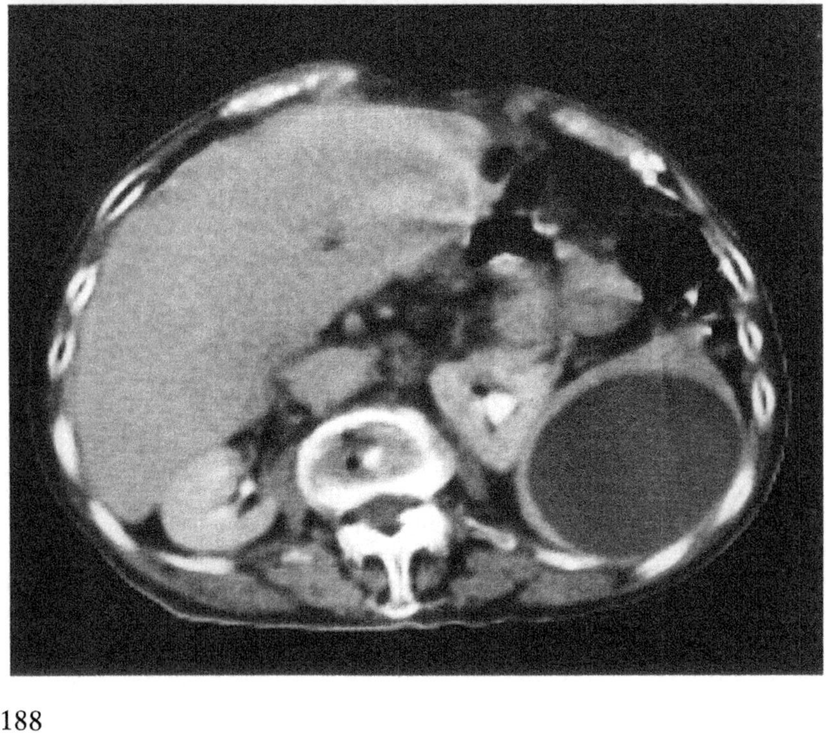

B

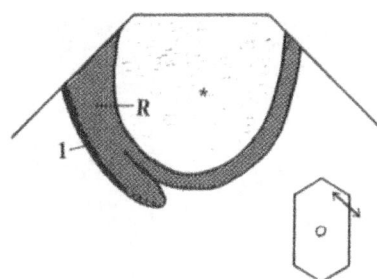

Case 108

Clinical data: A 75-year-old woman complained of episodic diarrhoea.

Description: A rounded mass, 8 cm in diameter, with sharp borders, is seen in the splenic parenchyma, which is displaced and reduced to a thin strip. The left kidney is displaced anteriorly (Scan B). The mass is hypoechogenic and heterogeneous; there is no posterior relative echo-enhancement.

Computed tomography confirms the presence of an intrasplenic mass of 15 UH density, unchanged after contrast injection. There is no calcification.

Diagnosis: This is easy: splenic epithelial cyst.

Comments: Different acquired or congenital cystic structures may be seen in the spleen, as follows:
- False cysts can result from undiagnosed traumatic of spontaneous haematomas, or from an attack of pancreatitis. The false cyst is the commonest intrasplenic mass. Very often the spleen is not enlarged. Compression of the splenic parenchyma may result in true ischaemic splenic atrophy. Parietal calcification can also occur. Sonography will show only a plain cyst.
- Parasitic cysts, especially the echinococcal type, are common.
- Some vascular tumours can take on a cystic appearance e. g. haemangiomas and cystic lymphangiomas; this type is less frequent.
- True cysts with cellular peripheries include two groups:
  · Epithelial cysts, which are mainly epidermoid can be complicated by painful intracystic haemorrhage, intraperitoneal rupture and superinfection. Sonography shows a sonolucent mass with peripheral trabeculation. When central echoes are present, these are due to intracystic clots or to desquamated keratin (this case).
  · Endothelial cysts are congenital. They are plain serous cysts that are seen as a sonolucent mass. They should also be searched for in the liver and in the kidneys.

Splenic cysts are most often asymptomatic. They can also be responsible for pain in the left hypochondrium.

109

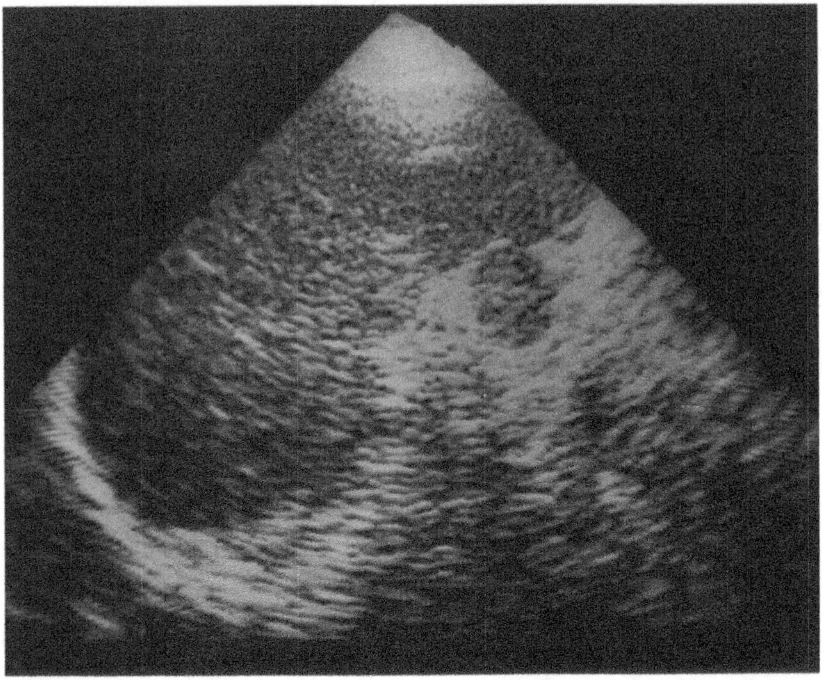

110

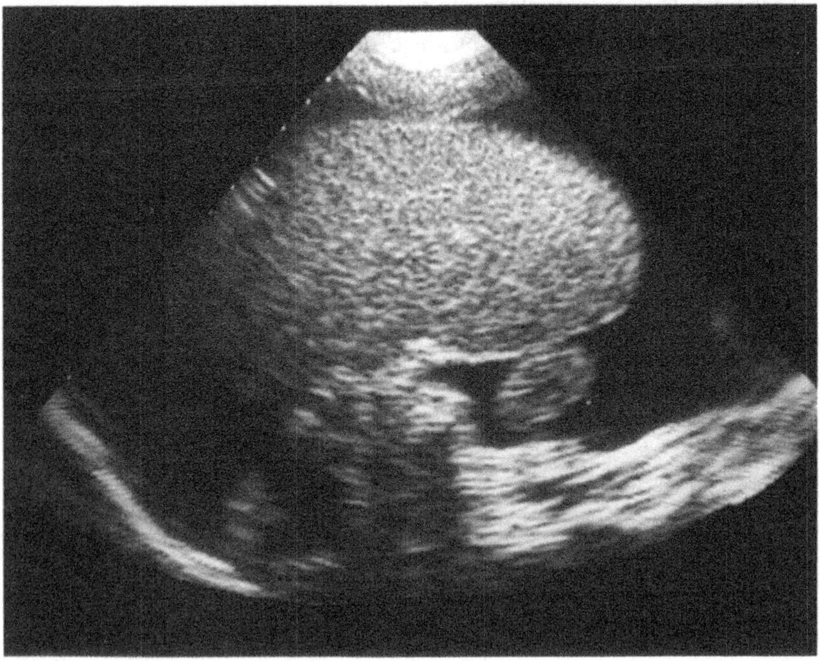

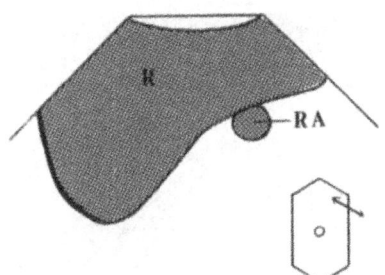

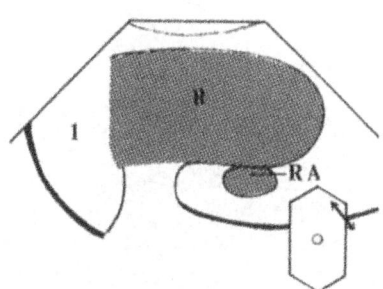

Cases 109 and 110

Clinical data: These two patients both have a history of alcoholism. Investigations were aimed at detecting decompensation.

Description: There is clear evidence of splenomegaly (case 109, and ascitic decompensation (case 110). In both cases, you must have noted the presence of a small rounded structure, about 2 cm in diameter, with smooth borders and a homogeneous echostructure, appended to the splenic parenchyma.

Diagnosis: This is easy: accessory spleen.

Comments: This is a normal variant. Accessory spleens are found in 10% of randomly selected autopsies. They are small nodules of splenic tissue, which are most often located near the hilum. There are no diagnostic problems with this simple form. Sometimes diagnosis is less easy, for instance when the accessory spleen is completely isolated from the spleen and is seen in the vicinity of the pancreatic tail, the lesser omentum, the mesentery or the retroperitoneal space, or also when it is connected by a thin band of tissue. It may also be larger and mimic a tumoural process. In case of doubt, the diagnosis can be confirmed by scintigraphy.

There may be multiple accessory spleens. They are more easily detected when the spleen is enlarged. When they persist after splenectomy they can become very large and be a cause of recurrence especially of haematological diseases. They can also be the site of intrinsic splenic pathology, infarct or trauma.

111

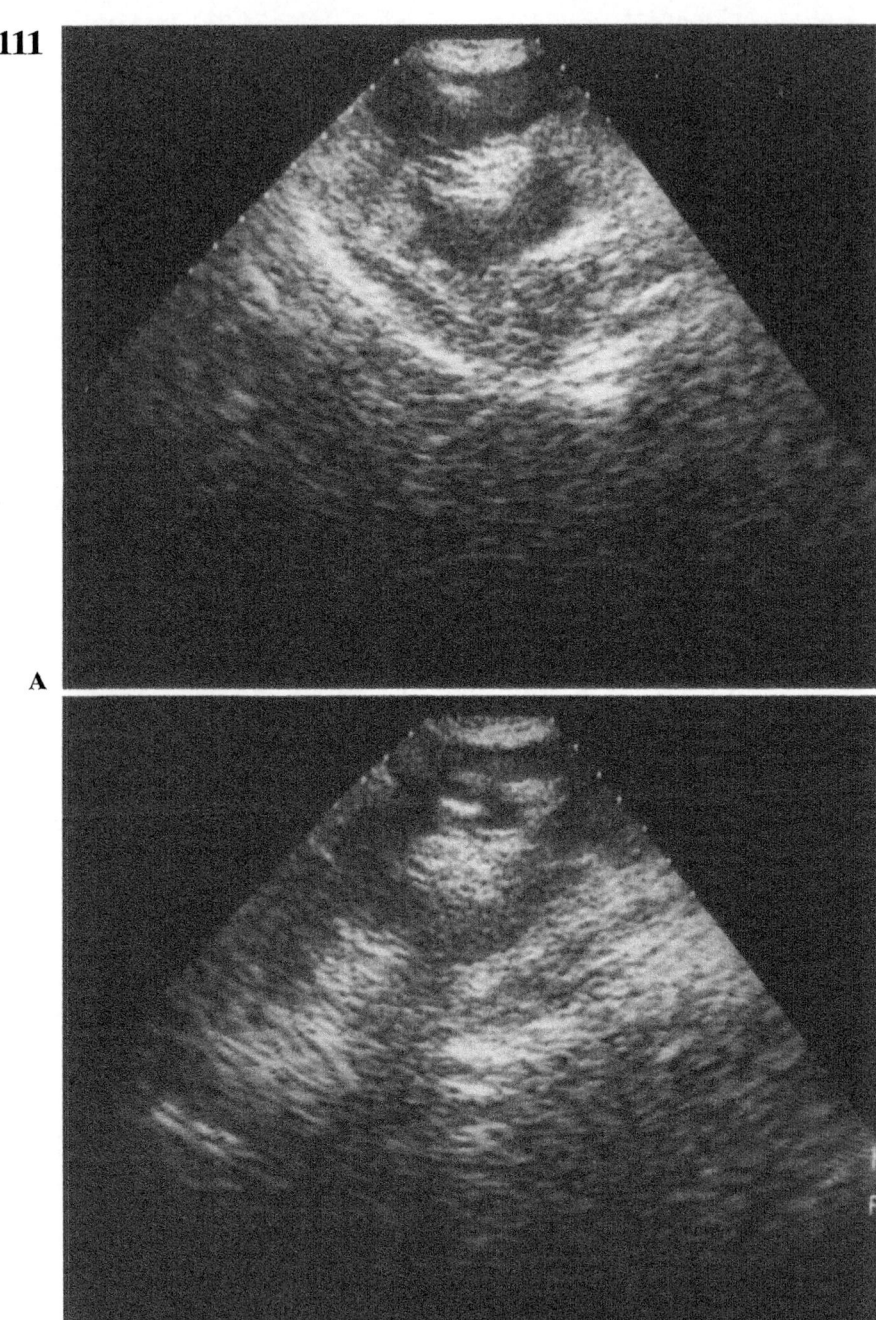

A

B

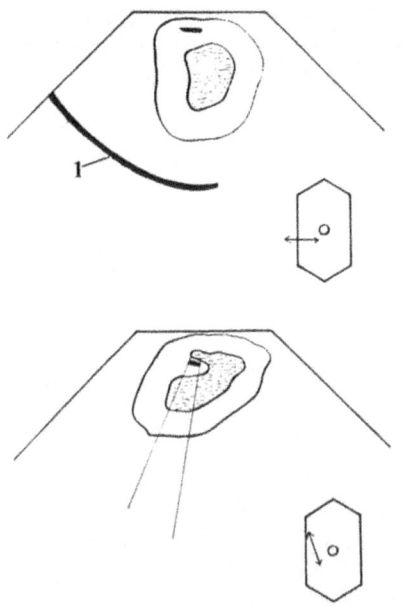

Case 111

Clinical data: This 65-year-old woman has severe anaemia.

Description: Scanning shows a mass in the right iliac fossa, which measures 6 x 4 cm and is composed of a hyperechogenic centre, surrounded by a 2 cm-thick hypoechogenic area, with irregular outer borders. Note its subcutaneous location and its relationship to the upper part of the ilium.

Diagnosis: This is easy: cancer of the caecum

Comments: This typical image is called "pseudo-kidney". It differs from the kidney, however, by the absence of the normal internal structures, namely the pyramids, arcuate vessels and calyces. The hyperechogenic centre corresponds to mucus and air confined within the tumour (you should have noted the acoustic shadow in Scan B). It may be central or eccentric. The surrounding hypoechogenic area corresponds to the pathological colonic wall. The absence of brownian movements and the persistance of the mass should be assessed by two successive investigations.

This image is pathognomonic of a gastrointestinal lesion, but it does not imply malignancy or colonic location. It can also be seen in inflammatory processes and in involvement of the small intestine or stomach. The precise diagnosis can be made with appropriate studies after barium ingestion.

One should not consider as pathological the cocardiform (rosette-shaped) image, with a thin wall (under 5 mm), that is frequently seen in the gastric wall (Case 54 C). Localized hypertrophy of the intestinal wall suggests adenocarcinoma rather than lymphomatous infiltration.

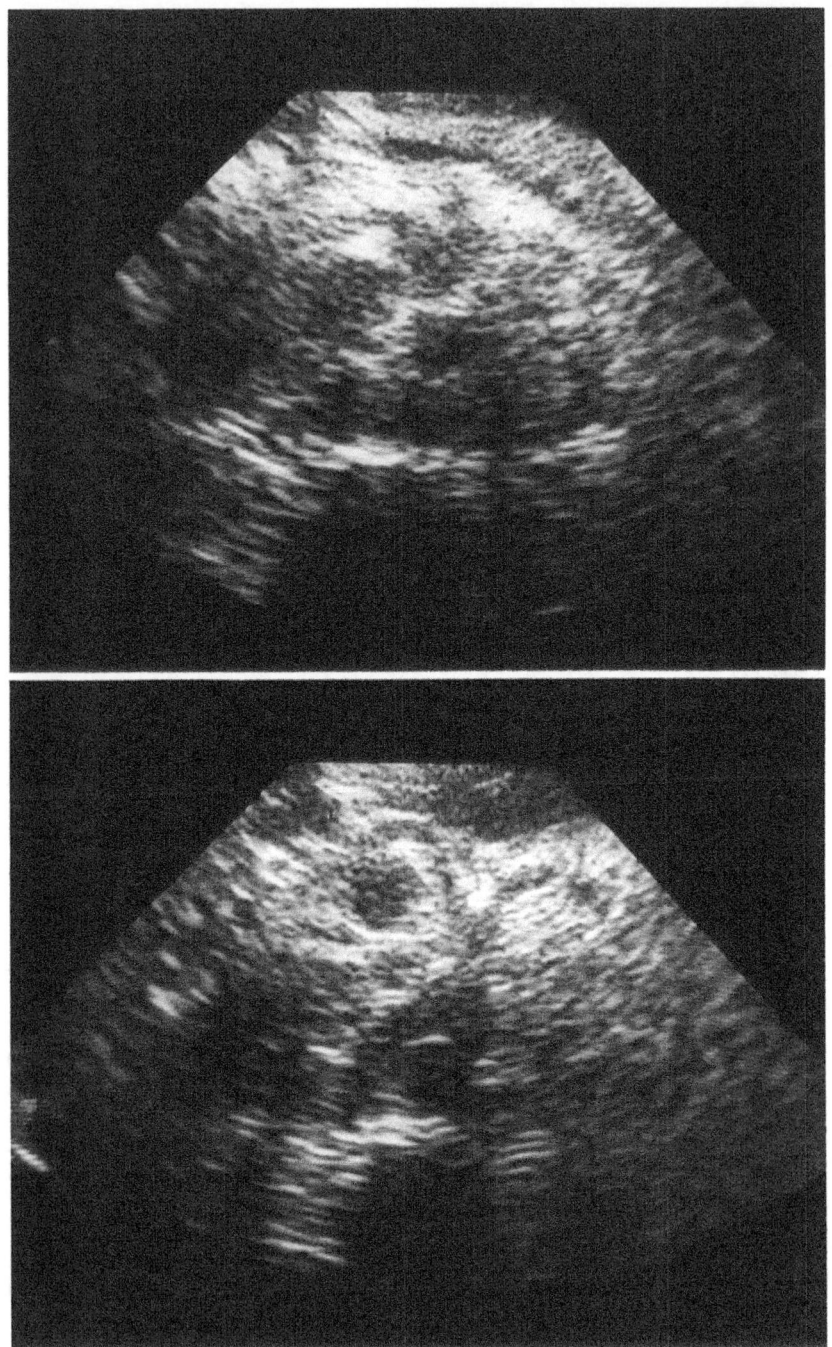

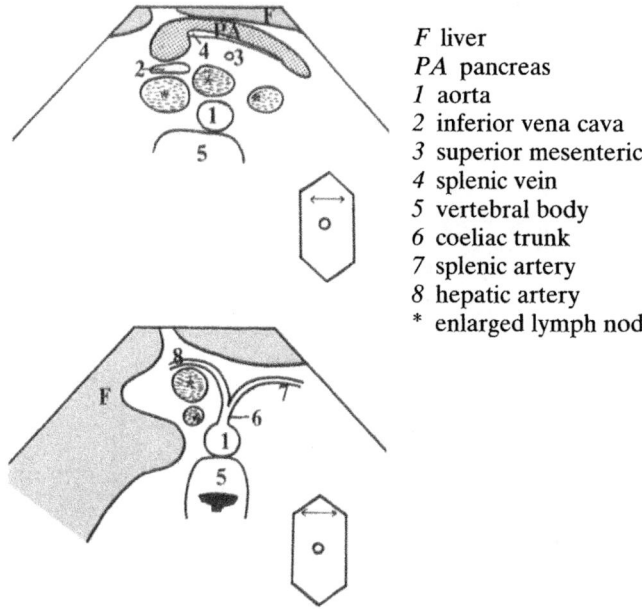

F liver
PA pancreas
1 aorta
2 inferior vena cava
3 superior mesenteric artery
4 splenic vein
5 vertebral body
6 coeliac trunk
7 splenic artery
8 hepatic artery
* enlarged lymph nodes

112

Case 112

Clinical data: A 28-year-old man has a palpable mass in the left hypochondrium.

Description: Anomalies are seen in the retropancreatic and lumbo-aortic retroperitoneal regions. We will first describe the pancreatic region. This shows multiple nodular hypoechogenic structures, 1.5−2 cm in diameter, which are homogeneous, have distinct borders and lack posterior relative echo-enhancement. They correspond to lymph-node enlargement. The more craniel scan shows three lymph-node aggregates which have caused anterior displacement of the superior mesenteric artery, the inferior vena cava, the splenic vein and the body of the pancreas. The caudal scan shows a lymph-node aggregate that has displaced the hepatic artery superiorly.

Comments: Normal lymph nodes are not visualized, because they are too small and their echostructure resembles that of the adjacent tissues. When affected by disease, they become enlarged and their echostructure changes. They are detectable by sonography when they are larger than 1 cm.

In the upper retroperitoneal (coeliac and pancreatic) region, and in the right renal hilum, lymph nodes are usually easily visible, whereas in the lower regions they are often obscured by overlying bowel.

Sonography has an accuracy of about 80% in the detection of upper retroperitoneal lymph nodes. Computed tomography has better accuracy for the aorticorenal and pelvic nodes.

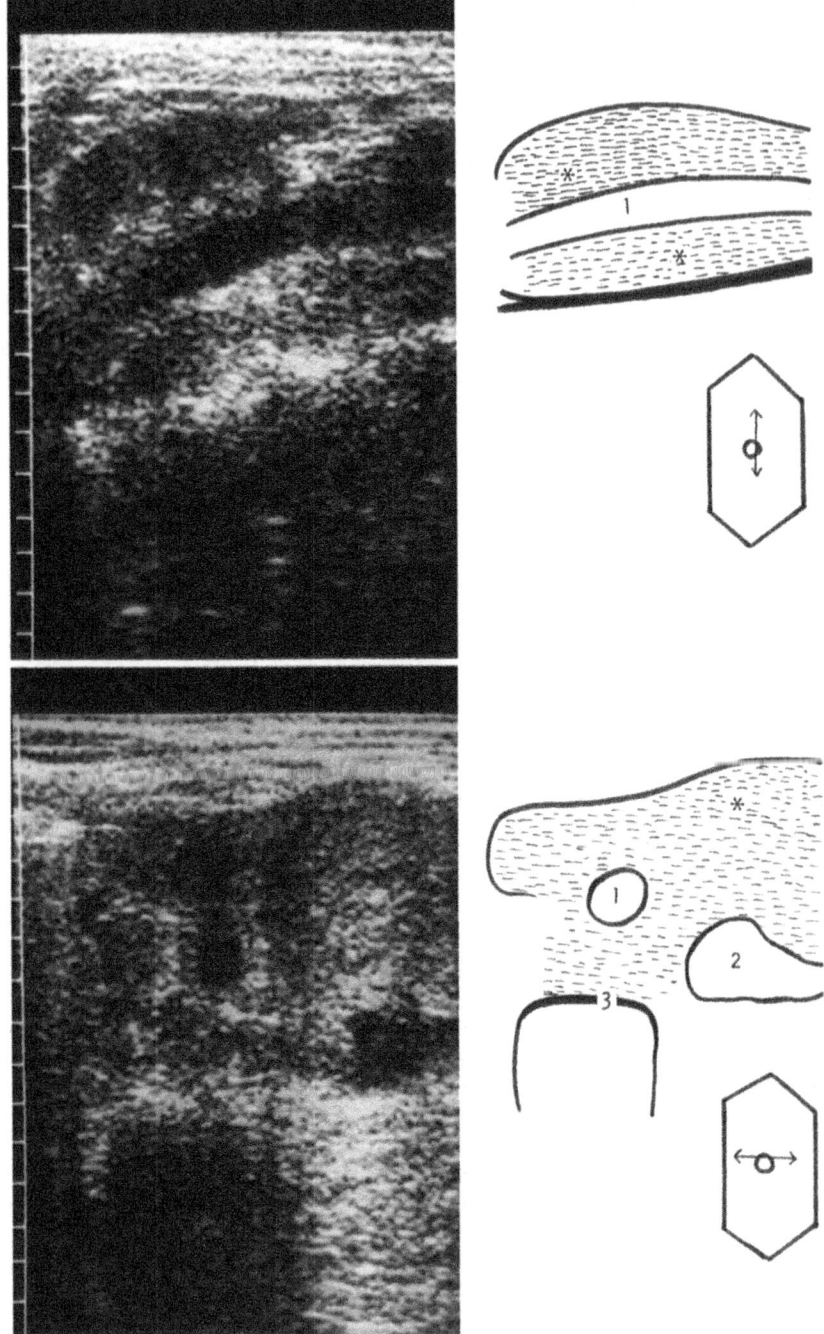

1 aorta
2 intratumoural necrosis
3 vertebral body
* retroperitoneal masses

Case 112 (continue)

Description: This patient also had lymph-node enlargement in the lower retroperitoneal area. Utilization of a linear scanner permits better appreciation of a large mass, insofar it avoids compressing the echoes of superficial structures and deformation of the linear, deeper structures. The scan shows a huge mass encasing the aorta und the inferior vena cava. It is about 7 cm thick and invades the entire lumbo-aortic region; it also extends into the left iliac fossa. Its borders are smooth and its echostructure is heterogeneous. The inferior vena cava is displaced superiorly. In the inferior part of the mass, a poorly demarcated hypoechogenic area reflects intratumoural necrosis.

Diagnosis: There are enlarged retroperitoneal lymph nodes secondary to seminoma. The nature of the lesion could not be determined from the abdominal sonogram.

Comments: The testicular lymphatics accompany the blood vessels and end in the lateral aortic and pre-aortic lymph nodes. Seminomas metastize to the para-aortic lymph nodes, which are then markedly enlarged. They are often not opacified with lymphangiography.

Classically, the lymph nodes are homogeneous and hypoechogenic, with distinct borders. Nodes with metastatic infiltration are more echogenic than those of lymphoma, in which it is much more difficult to visualize the aorta. There is no correlation between histology and echogenicity. Histological assessment cannot be made on the basis of sonography. The same is true for computed tomography.

When the lymph nodes are very large and confluent, the differentiation of lymph-node enlargement from a retroperitoneal tumour may be difficult.

113

B, D

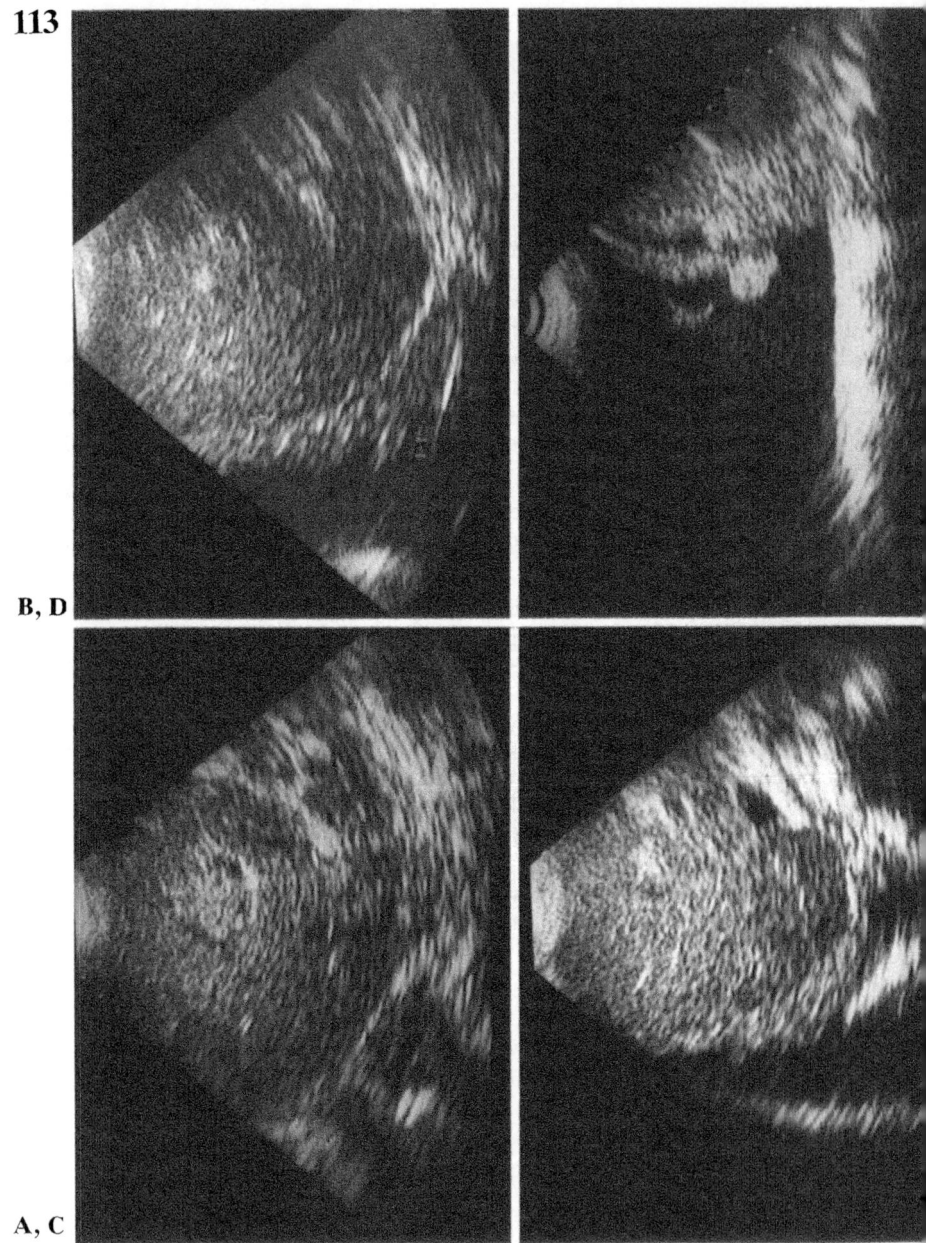

A, C

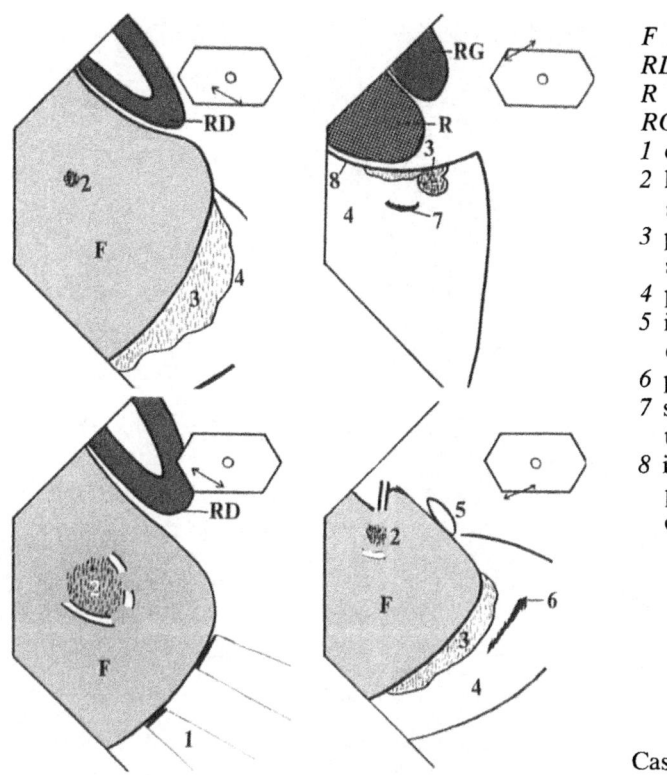

F liver
RD right kidney
R spleen
RG left kidney
1 costal shadows
2 hepatic metastases
3 pleural metastases
4 pleural effusion
5 inferior vena cava
6 pulmonary air
7 strip of atelectasis
8 intersplenodiaphragmatic ascites

Case 113

Clinical data: This 60-year-old man with a carcinoma of the colon was operated 2 years ago.

Description: You should have noted three types of anomaly.
– Hyperechogenic areas in the hepatic parenchyma are causing displacement of the venous structures (Scan A).
– There is a layer of ascites between the spleen and diaphragma (Scan D).
– A bilateral pleural effusion permits visualization of a thick, supradiaphragmatic mass of tissue, with an irregular superior border, on the right side (Scans B and C). On the left there is a hyperechogenic nodular structure above the diaphragm (Scan D).

Diagnosis: This is easy: These are, of course, hepatic metastases. However, there are also supradiaphragmatic metastases.

Comments: Pleural effusion facilitates the visualization of metastatic pleural nodules. The cupola of the diaphragm should always be examined during hepatic sonography; detection of minor pleural effusion by sonography is often easier than with poor-quality radiographs of the lungs.

Sonography of the thoracic wall is moreover useful in two circumstances: after unsuccessful pleural puncture, and for visualization and possible puncture of a parietal mass.

114

B, D

A, C

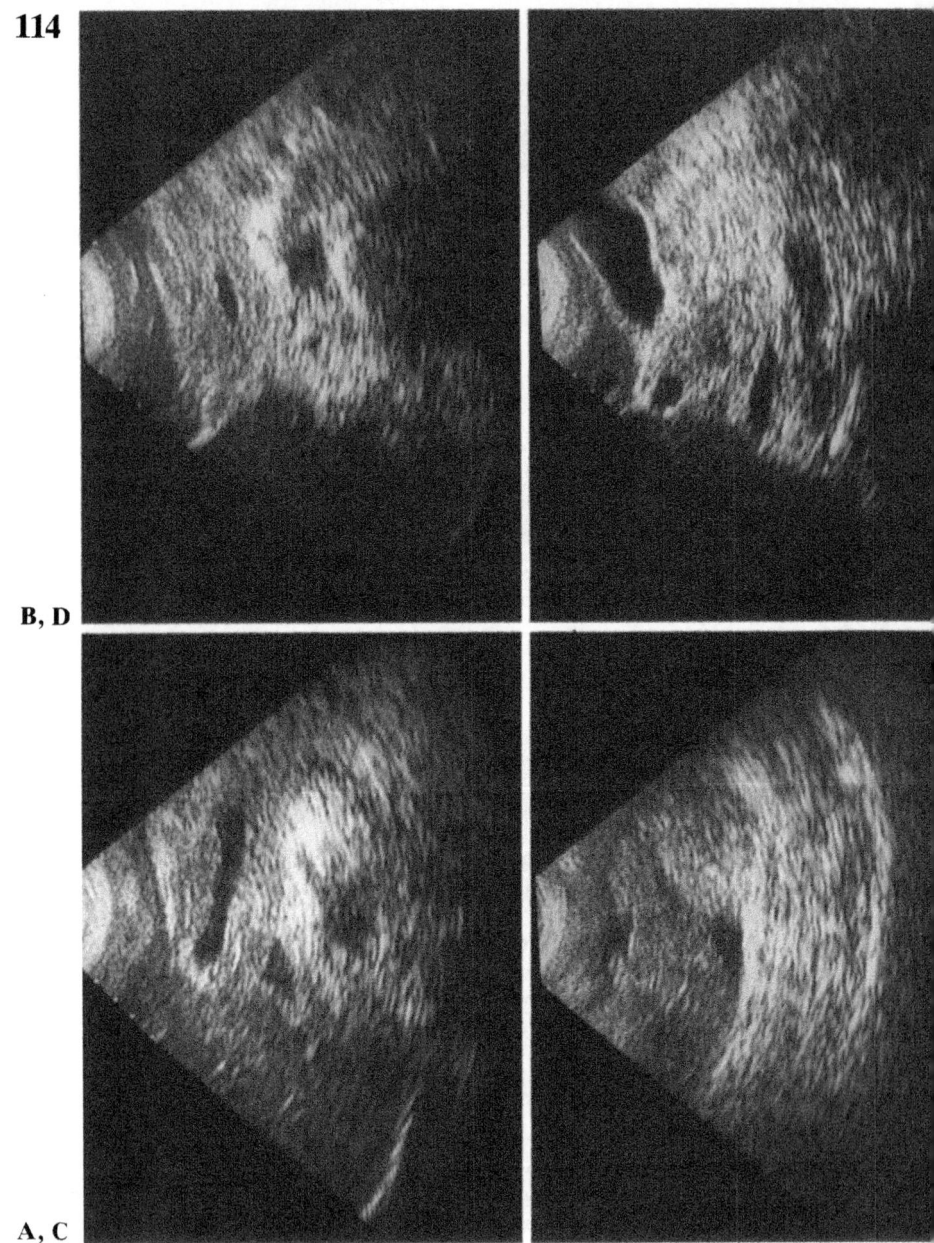

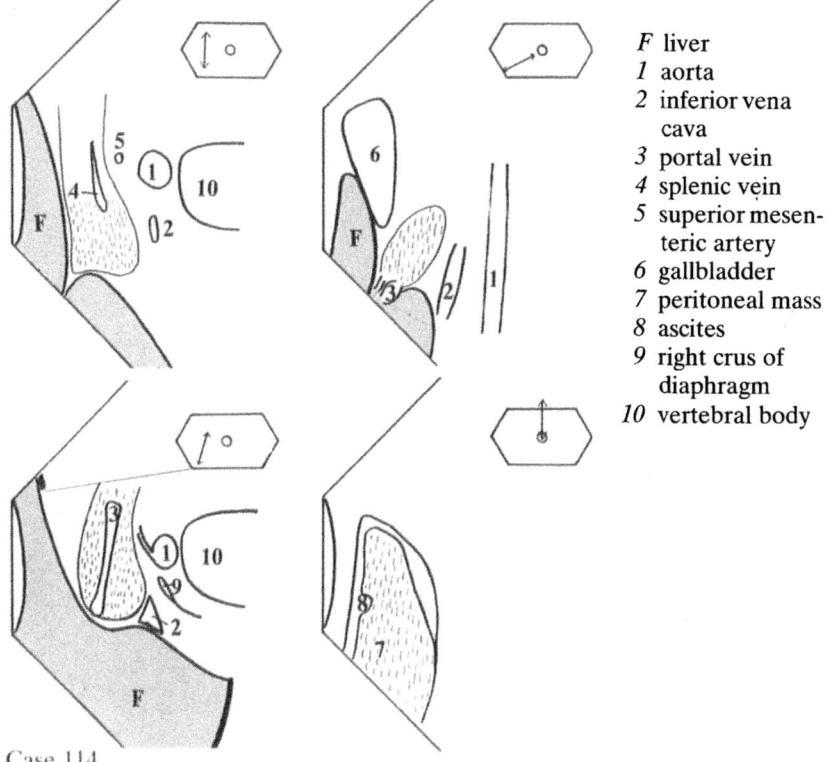

F liver
1 aorta
2 inferior vena cava
3 portal vein
4 splenic vein
5 superior mesenteric artery
6 gallbladder
7 peritoneal mass
8 ascites
9 right crus of diaphragm
10 vertebral body

Case 114

Clinical data: This 60-year-old woman has diffuse abdominal pain and abdominal distension.

Description: You must have noted the following points:
a) There is a cuff, less echogenic than adipose tissue, encasing the portal vein and compressing the inferior vena cava (Scans A and D).
b) The body and tail of the pancreas are enlarged and there is tissular infiltration between the superior mesenteric artery and the splenic vein with moderate compression of the latter (Scan B). The biliary system is not distended.
c) In the left paraumbilical region the scan shows a large hypoechogenic and homogeneous mass, which is delimited by a small amount of ascites and clearly differentiated from the bowel loops. It measures approximately 4 cm x 2 cm; its borders are irregular (Scan C).

Diagnosis: This is difficult: the lesion proved to be a peritoneal mesothelioma.

Comments: Peritoneal tumours are common, and generally malignant. Most of them are secondary deposits (ovary, stomach, and more rarely, breast). Peritoneal mesothelioma is a very rare tumour. Small masses (2–3 cm) are only visible when there is ascites. The sonographic appearance is that of irregular masses or of infiltration. The nodular form is not seen in mesotheliomas, since it corresponds to a very early stage and mesothelioma develops very rapidly.

Subject Index